# ADULT REHABILITATION:
## A Team Approach for Therapists

# ADULT REHABILITATION:
## *A Team Approach for Therapists*

*Edited by*

Martha K. Logigian, M.S., O.T.R.
Assistant Professor of Occupational Therapy,
University of New Hampshire, Durham;
Instructor, Tufts University,
Boston School of Occupational Therapy

Little, Brown and Company   Boston

Library of Congress Catalog Card No. 81-83249

ISBN 0-316-53083-2

Printed in the United States of America

HAL

*Cover Design by Weymouth Design*

*To Rick, with love*

# CONTENTS

*vii*

# PREFACE

This text presents an overview of rehabilitation programs developed to meet the needs of patients with a variety of physical disabilities. It is designed for students and health professionals, particularly entry level clinicians in the disciplines of occupational therapy, physical therapy, speech-language pathology, and recreational therapy. Emphasis is placed throughout on the function of the interdisciplinary rehabilitation team.

The book is organized into chapters covering: normal aging, oncologic rehabilitation, orthopedics, rheumatic diseases, burn rehabilitation, cardiac and pulmonary rehabilitation, stroke and speech-language rehabilitation, brain trauma, and spinal cord injury. Each chapter describes specific disease processes in general medical terms, associated rehabilitation problems, and evaluation of suggested treatments for the resulting physical and emotional dysfunction. Wherever possible, we have consolidated multiple sources of rehabilitation and educational materials to provide practical information for therapists and their patients. Every effort has been made to present current and comprehensive therapy programs, recognizing that the role of team members and the therapeutic regimen may vary among institutions.

Increasing demands are being placed on rehabilitation professionals to have greater knowledge of anatomy, physiology, psychology, and medicine, as well as an understanding of the therapeutic programs provided by the interdisciplinary team. To meet these needs, we have tried to provide the basic clinical information required by each discipline. In addition, in recent years rehabilitation programs have expanded to include treatment of the cardiac patient and cancer patient. Moreover, given the age group often seen in rehabilitation facilities, therapists are increasingly called upon to meet the needs of the elderly. Thus, we have devoted sections of the text to these issues.

Although this is a basic text on rehabilitation, it is our intention to provide a foundation for more effective therapy programs. Ultimately we hope that the body of scientific knowledge in this volume stimulates further research, adding to our understanding of rehabilitation and patient care.

Special thanks to Rita Hammond for the illustrations, Charlene Arthur for her contribution to the oncology chapter, Dave Boisvert for his contribution to the cardiac rehabilitation chapter, Barbara Ward (Allied Health Editor) for her continual encouragement, Martin Samuels for his inspiration, and my husband Rick for his patience and support.

M. K. L.

# CONTRIBUTING
# AUTHORS

*Susan Koch Clark, O.T.R.*
Staff Occupational Therapist, Hunterdon Medical
Center, Flemington, New Jersey

*Beth Edelstein, O.T.R.*
Assistant Director, Occupational Therapy,
Massachusetts Rehabilitation Hospital, Boston

*Judith Falconer, M.P.H., O.T.R.*
Senior Occupational Therapist, The London
Hospital, London, England

*Judith G. Helman, O.T.R.*
Staff Therapist, Department of Rehabilitation
Services, Brigham and Women's Hospital, Boston

*Laura-Lee Hollander, M.P.H., O.T.R.*
Community Health Education Coordinator,
Faulkner Hospital, Jamaica Plain, Massachusetts

*Marilyn Lee Holzer, O.T.R.*
Staff Occupational Therapist, Stroke Unit,
Massachusetts Rehabilitation Hospital, Boston

*Bess Kathrins, R.P.T.*
Director of Rehabilitation Services, Greenery
Nursing Home, Brighton, Massachusetts

*Richard J. Kathrins, R.P.T.*
Director of Physical Therapy, Central
Massachusetts Rehabilitation Hospital, Worcester

*Elaine LaCroix, M.H.S.M., O.T.R.*
Clinical Director of Occupational Therapy,
Department of Rehabilitation Services, Brigham
and Women's Hospital, Boston

*Nancy G. Lefkowitz, M.S.*
Director, Speech-Language Pathology,
Massachusetts Rehabilitation Hospital, Boston

*Alice Crow Seidel, M.P.H., O.T.R.*
Assistant Professor of Occupational Therapy,
University of New Hampshire, Durham

*Frances Senner-Hurley, M.S.*
Clinical Supervisor, Speech-Language Pathology
Unit, Massachusetts General Hospital, Boston

*Ellen Herz Silverman, O.T.R.*
Staff Therapist and Consultant, Pennsylvania
Home Health Services, Broomall

*Janice Giuggio Simari, O.T.R.*
Lecturer, Boston University, Sargent College and
Tufts University, Boston School of Occupational
Therapy

*Denise A. Stiassny, O.T.R.*
Research Assistant, Psychology Service,
Boston Veterans Administration Medical Center

*Nancy H. Wall, M.Ed., O.T.R.*
Clinical Module Coordinator, Tufts University,
Boston School of Occupational Therapy

ADULT REHABILITATION:
*A Team Approach for Therapists*

# 1 NORMAL AGING

*Laura-Lee Hollander*

## What Do We Mean By Aging?

Aging is a complex process that occurs on several levels: cellular, biological, psychological, and social. It is the accumulation of many universally experienced events that affect the life span of every individual.

To understand and study the natural effects of aging, one must define senescence: *senescence* is the increasing vulnerability of an organism progressing through life. Therefore, in describing the changes that occur in older people, distinction must be made between natural aging and diseases that affect the organism. This is particularly important with a disease such as arteriosclerosis, which affects so many elderly persons. It is well acknowledged that aging is not synonymous with disease, nor are there diseases exclusively characteristic of old age. In this chapter, the normal process in the absence of disease is discussed.

Aging can be defined as changes in a living system that occur over a period of time. *Primary aging* is time-relative, sequential, and results in functional decline essentially as the result of heredity. *Secondary aging* is a process of changes manifested when environmental stress is superimposed on the basal state. Generally, this process includes: biological aging—changes in physiology that occur with time; chronological aging—indicating the number of years a person has lived according to a birth date; psychological aging—occurring at different phases throughout life, and includ-

The discussion of visual loss was written by Beth Edelstein.

ing changes in sensory, cognitive, and personality components; and sociological aging—occurring as roles, status, and functions of an individual change within society.

As insights are gained about aging, society will need to explore ways to support them, as possible control brings with it a moral responsibility to respond to the simultaneous social consequences that may occur. If human beings can look forward to prolonged healthier life, a readjustment in cultural perspectives concerning work, marriage, leisure time, and the exploration of all potential resources will be necessary. We will be challenged to a general restructuring of our attitudes and priorities.

## Cultural Attitudes

In our society there is no exact point at which adulthood begins. It gradually evolves from adolescence, and at some time full adulthood is attained. There are, of course, many biological and social indicators that are used to imply transition from one level to the next. Age status systems such as the one that typifies American society define expectations and roles using chronological age. Although people differ in the rate and manner in which they age, our culture distributes privileges, obligations, and rewards to groups based on the number of years they have lived. This phenomenon, known as *age-grading*, refers to a social organization of the life span into stages or time periods in which individuals are socially categorized. These arbitrary definitions subsequently create expectations for specific behavior and participation in certain activities. Rites of passage signify progress from one age-graded phase to the next. These were originally celebrated by tribal groups to signify adult status, and indicated the appropriate behavior for an age norm. Modern society indicates this transition through formal means such as weddings or less formal events such as going to college, beginning a career, or buying a house. Although less ceremonial, these activities are theoretically symbolic of a status shift to further maturity and responsibility. Each developmental task prepares an individual for the milestones to follow, and continuity is thereby assured as passages through the stages are ordered without major disjunctions [47, 52].

What are the events that socially define an older person? This passage is gradual and the rites are unceremonious, commonly acknowledged when a sixty-fifth birthday is reached or mandatory retirement occurs. Preparation for retirement frequently is the impetus to redefining social roles that are forced on an older person. Unlike all previous transitions, aging clearly signifies the final one in the life cycle. In essence, old age tends to imply restricting opportunities rather than expanding alternatives, the latter having been the pervasive theme for previous stages.

Chronological age influences social definitions. It may reflect accumulated experience and biological and social changes that have occurred; however, it is questionable if chronological age is a valuable index of stages of adulthood. In other cultures, capacity for work and valued social roles are maintained as long as biological and psychological faculties last. In American culture, old age begins at age 65 . . . ready or not.

Age-grading has perpetuated the greatest myth about aging. We are led to believe that older people are a homogeneous group. Gerontology, the study of aging, has attempted to dispel this myth, as professionals in a variety of disciplines examine the tremendous variability that exists among older people. The multitude of problems, potentials, and differ-

ences that they offer challenge us to seek increasing options in life-styles for this diverse population. Frequently, the notion of homogeneity is reinforced by the media as they portray negative stereotypes. Appearing before the House Select Committee on Aging, Maggie Kuhn, founder of the Gray Panthers, testified [24]:

Television still reinforces society's pervasive age bias. What do we see? When old people are portrayed, we are usually stereotyped. In appearance our faces are blank and expressionless, our bodies are bent over, and the 'senior shuffle' is just a step away from the embalming room. Our clothing also reflects low self-esteem. Old men are shown wearing baggy, unpressed suits. Old women's clothing is frumpy and ill-fitting. Our voices are high-pitched and querulous. The personalities of old people are likewise stereotyped. We are shown as stubborn, rigid, inflexible, forgetful and confused. By comparison to other age groups, old people are depicted as dependent, powerless, wrinkled babies, unable to contribute to society. The strength of old age—the vitality and wisdom of those who have survived—is seldom portrayed.

In addition, generalizations about specific age groups are influenced by the ideals of our culture. Old age is accorded little prestige in a society that idolizes youth and the acquisition of material goods.

Myths that portray the old as unproductive, generally ill, inflexible, senile, uninvolved, asexual, isolated, and passive only add to the existing distaste our society has about growing old. Why has this prejudice become a commonly accepted attitude? Many sociologists believe that our cultural emphasis on productivity and technological expertise encourages the extinction and devaluing of those unable to contribute. Others feel that prejudice against the old is merely a poorly masked fear of our own aging and ultimate death.

Obviously, some of these characteristics may be true for some individuals over 65, but they can be found in all other age groups as well

[34]. Aging as a reality does not parallel the stereotypes; however, despite increased public education, the myths persist. Even people who may be aging with few problems see themselves as atypical in an otherwise depressing scenario. The most insidious effect of these misconceptions and age biases is the limited use of a great resource.

Gerontology confronts our society's social policies, traditions, priorities, and health care, and identifies impediments to significant life. It affirms aging as a process of growth and development from birth to death. Gerontologists do not view this as a singular experience; rather they emphasize the interrelationship of biological, psychological, and social elements occurring over a period of time.

To say that old age is not without difficulty would be misleading. What we need to learn is that later life can be a time of growth. It is important to assess our personal attitudes about aging and our own mortality, as these feelings largely determine our effectiveness with older people. Robert Butler coined the word *ageism* to describe an innate prejudice against the elderly he feels exists to some extent within all of us [7]: "Ageism can be seen as a process of systematic stereotyping of and discrimination against people because they are old, just as racism and sexism accomplish this with skin color and gender. Old people are categorized as senile, rigid in thought and manner, old-fashioned in morality and skills.... Ageism allows the younger generation to see older people as different from themselves; thus they subtly cease to identify with their elders as human beings."

In any helping relationship a sense of satisfaction is felt if there exists a potential for helping the person seeking assistance; effectiveness and professional worth are reinforced if positive changes occur. Unfortunately, because much of society considers older people incapable of change, the desire to work with them professionally is minimal. Interestingly, those who have worked with them no matter the setting or the therapy have found that with

intervention, the elderly are capable of positive physical and psychological changes. Thus the theory of the unchangeable aged can be exploded providing both the older person and the therapist believe it possible. Obviously, older people have fewer years to live; therefore a sense of satisfaction must and will come from enabling them to enjoy those remaining years more fully.

## Demography

Demographic data are used in gaining an understanding of where older people are situated in a modern industrialized society. They also help detect and interpret trends that serve as a base for relevant program planning. The dramatic increase in the number of older persons in the United States has had a great impact on social, political, and economic levels.

Most available statistical data in the United States use the age boundary of 65 years and over when categorizing older persons. It is interesting to note, however, that dramatic improvements in life expectancy in Western industrialized countries have occurred in the twentieth century. In 1900, the average life expectancy was 47.3 years, compared to over 71 years today in the United States. This gain has been attributed to improved health care, a higher standard of living, medical advances, and more extensive public health programs. At present, however, life expectancy has appeared to stabilize, and predictions for the future indicate an unchanged rate.

Since 1900, the number of elderly in the United States has increased dramatically, and for each succeeding decade a larger proportion of the total population is represented by this age group. In 1900, approximately 3 million persons were age 65 and over; in 1940 it grew to 9 million, and in 1979 the elderly population was estimated at 24.4 million, or 11 percent of the total. Three factors have influenced this rapid expansion, the most important of which is probably the high birth rate of the late nineteenth and early twentieth centuries. The second factor is the decline in mortality as a result of medical progress and technology. These advancements were especially advantageous in reducing the death rate among infants and youths, allowing a larger portion of the population to survive to age 65. Today, approximately 72 percent of all newborns are expected to live to this age. The third factor is the high rate of immigration prior to World War I. The Bureau of the Census [51] has projected that by 1990 there will be 27.7 million elderly, 28.8 million by 2000, and 40.2 million by the year 2020.

There is a significantly uneven distribution by sex for the population 65 years and older, as throughout the industrialized world men have shorter life expectancies than women. In 1977, between the ages of 65 and 74, there were 130 women per 100 men; after age 74 there were 176. Among those age 85 and over there were 217 women to 100 men. This distribution has a significant impact on marital status and living arrangements. Generally, in the United States twice as many older men (70 percent) are married, while 2 to 3 times as many women are widowed (54 percent in 1971). These statistics help us to understand the much higher proportion of older women living alone. It is important to note further that only 15 percent of older women and 7 percent of older men are living with their children or relatives. The value of independence, prevalent in the American culture, continues to play a significant role in the lives of older persons. Many feel that they become more dependent and often suffer a role reversal that is considered degrading if they live with their children. Living alone may result in isolation and loneliness, but it is the preferred option for the majority of the elderly.

## Economic Statistics

Social security was never intended as the sole source of support for the elderly, however, it remains the most prevalent source of income for retired persons. Income from wages is next in importance, assets in real estate and investments are third, and some form of public assistance is fourth. What is most sobering about these statistics is that for many people, social security as the sole support offers an income that is below federally established poverty levels. These guidelines distinguish 1 out of every 5 older persons to be impoverished. There is also a sharp contrast in adequate income for elderly couples compared to single persons.

The economic situation of older people remains a serious problem despite attempts to increase benefits through Medicare, social security, and supplementary programs. A relatively fixed income cannot withstand the pressures of inflation, and the reality of financial insecurity can cause this period of life to be stressful, frustrating, and desperate for many.

## Physical and Biological Changes

As one of many changes of aging [29], the respiratory system demonstrates loss of efficiency. Specifically, this can be seen in a reduction of total lung capacity and vital capacity, decrease in the resiliency of the lungs, an increase in residual volume, and thickening of support membranes between the alveoli and the capillaries.

Typical skeletal changes such as stooped posture, stiffened joints, and porous bones often result in decreased mobility and efficiency. Reduction of height and poor posture may result from progressive calcification and eventual ossification of vertebral ligaments. This mineralization usually involves the elastic fibers, erosion and ossification of cartilaginous joint surfaces, and degenerative changes of the synovium that can lead to stiffening of the joints. The fibrocartilaginous discs undergo atrophic changes, and are responsible for increased curvature of the spine. Degenerative changes in rib cartilage, ligaments, and joints contribute to respiratory impairment. Changes in the temporomandibular joint and loss of teeth may cause difficulty in speech and eating. Finally, with age the bones become porous, lighter, and less elastic, resulting in osteoporosis.

Many changes in the brain have been identified associated with aging. Included are progressive atrophy of the gyri and widening and deepening of the sulci, loss of bulk, dilatation of the ventricles, loss of neurons, and an increase of corpora amylacea (small, sandlike substances). Within the nervous system, atrophy of the medullary olives, decrease in Purkinje cells in the cerebellum, trunk instability, and loss of some proprioceptive, kinesthetic, vestibular, and visual mechanisms all can occur.

The muscular system demonstrates decline with muscle atrophy, hypotonia, and weakness. As a result of muscle deterioration, respiratory efficiency and excretory function can be affected.

There is a decline in cardiac output at rest, and the heart loses some of its capacity for responding to extra work. There is an increase in both peripheral resistance to blood flow and systolic blood pressure.

The glomerular filtration rate of the kidney in an 80-year-old is approximately 50 percent of that of one in the 20s. Renal blood flow is also about 50 percent. Polyuria is common. Intrinsic aging of the gastrointestinal system produces a decline in gastric volume, loss of digestive acid, reduction of digestive enzymes, diminished peristalsis, and atrophy of the mucosal lining. It should be noted that constipation is a common complaint in the elderly, with multifactorial etiology related to changes in motility of the bowel, and decrease of dietary bulk, fluid intake and exercise.

Wrinkling of the skin is often attributed to decreased blood supply and changes in collagen and elastic fiber that result in loss of elasticity and resiliency. When the skin of an older person is stretched, the folds become more delineated as they return to place. In addition, skin undergoes an atrophic process, with many pigmentary discolorations (brown or yellow). Red blotches are usually caused by changes in the blood vessels beneath the skin. Small wartlike growths (senile keratoses) may be noticed, and fissures may appear about the mouth because of atrophy of the epidermal layer. Atrophy of nail tissues

causes the nails to become more brittle and grow more slowly. There is loss of hair pigmentation that results in graying or whitening, probably caused by a decrease in enzyme activity. The tongue and gums become reddened, and gum shrinkage may cause eating and teeth-cleaning problems. Atrophy of subcutaneous tissue, decrease in size and number of sweat and oil glands, and changes in the autonomic nervous system make the body's temperature regulation inefficient. Because of this, older persons lose their ability to sweat, and consequently the skin becomes dry.

## Sensory Loss

Sensory changes do occur with age and can influence an individual's ability to function. Sensory loss can affect relationships with other people and interaction with the physical environment. It can lead to misrepresentation of the impaired person by incorrect labeling as demented, obstinate, or maladjusted, when in actuality there is a loss of hearing or vision. Diminution of the sensory systems is gradual, thus making adaptations possible that enable the person to cope with activities of daily living. Therapists must be aware of these changes so that adequate spatial, visual, and acoustical changes can be made in settings that consider the special needs of the elderly. If sensory changes are not identified, unnecessary social isolation, paranoia, frustration, and accidents may result. Keen observation and sensitivity are necessary on the part of the therapist to help identify age-related sensory changes before they develop into more extreme functional and behavioral problems. It is imperative to detect these special needs and create suitable environments for persons adapting to sensory change, so that with adequate information and encouragement they can function at maximum capacity.

### GUSTATORY AND OLFACTORY LOSS
Taste and smell show age-related changes that functionally appear as inability to distinguish

among various foods or smells. As nutrition is closely linked to these senses, the implications are vitally important to consider. Many people rely on the appearance, smell, and taste of food for the inspiration to eat. If these sensations are diminished, the appeal of and interest in food may be lessened. In addition, diet restrictions, of salt, for example, can contribute to the unpalatability of food.

It is important to create a pleasant mealtime atmosphere. A social setting that is enjoyable can make people feel more like eating. Talking about the food, its flavor and smell, may make it appear to taste better. Preparing food that has distinctive textures and temperatures and the use of condiments can be important for maintaining a person's interest in eating. One potential hazard for the older person who lives alone and has a poor sense of smell and taste is the difficulty recognizing spoiled foods. Individuals should be encouraged to keep track of the age of foods in the refrigerator. People with impaired sense of smell might also be unaware of the presence of leaking gas, and should check the pilot lights of gas stoves regularly. These precautions can be easily taught and incorporated into home visits so that family and friends also learn to check these areas.

## HEARING LOSS

Hearing impairment is considered to be one of the most detrimental of the sensory losses, as it may significantly interfere with communication. Depending on the severity and extent of loss, impaired hearing frequently inhibits social interaction and might deter older persons from participating in situations in which oral communication is important.

This sensory change is estimated to be 10 times greater in the older age group than in the younger population. It is also known that hearing loss is found more frequently in men than women at all ages. A report by the National Center for Health Statistics, Health Resources Administration indicated that the incidence of auditory problems among residents of nursing homes is about 5 times higher than that found among the rest of the United States population [38]. It is felt that statistics assessing hearing impairment among aging individuals are conservative. Practicing audiologists estimate that approximately 50 percent of the 22.4 million people over 65 possess some degree of hearing loss. Nevertheless, the majority of older persons have little difficulty conversing. More frequently, those with sensory-neural hearing loss will complain of their inability to detect sounds of high frequency, especially in noisy surroundings. Usually, both ears are affected with unusual symmetry, and this may be accompanied with a high-pitched noise called *tinnitus.*

*Presbycusis* is a condition associated with advancing age. There are 4 major types, primarily involving high frequencies.

### SENSORY PRESBYCUSIS

In the inner ear, vibrations are transformed into nerve impulses by the cochlea. Inside this spiral cavity is the organ of Corti, which is covered with tiny hair cells that set off electric potentials and receive messages from the auditory nerve. The auditory nerve then carries the sensations to the brain, where they are perceived as sound. It is thought that the most predominant cause of sensory presbycusis is atrophy of the organ of Corti, and degeneration of hair cells at the basal end of the cochlea and moving toward the apex. The condition is manifested by abrupt loss of high tones in middle age and progresses slowly. It does not impede the understanding of speech, because speech frequencies are not affected. It is believed that its etiology is deteriorating function as the years accumulate. It is the least common of the 4 types of presbycusis.

### NEURAL PRESBYCUSIS

This generally occurs late in life, although it can begin at any age. It results from the loss of neurons in the auditory pathways and cochlea. It usually becomes apparent when 30 to 40 percent of the neurons are lost or damaged, and results in loss of speech discrimination. Speech patterns may be altered as the condition worsens because of the inability to perceive higher frequencies, such as those in the consonant sounds. Therefore differences of tone may continue to be heard, but words will not be made out.

It is important to realize that amplification does not benefit these individuals. Delivery of higher-frequency sounds is not facilitated by increasing volume, which only results in amplifying unintelligible sounds. Lowering the voice while still conversing distinctly and clearly can improve communication because of diminished tones of speech sounds.

STRIAL PRESBYCUSIS
This may often affect several members of a family. It has a slowly progressive onset seen mainly in the third to sixth decades of life. The striae vascularis, blood vessels in the wall of the cochlea, show pathological changes that cause a flat hearing loss while maintaining good speech discrimination. Atrophy may result in this area caused by arteriosclerotic changes in the cochlea. Older people afflicted with strial presbycusis may benefit greatly from hearing aids, as the residual effect is mainly flat hearing loss.

INNER EAR CONDUCTIVE PRESBYCUSIS
This condition is not, evidently, caused by histological changes. It is believed that there is an increase in stiffness of the supporting structures of the cochlear duct that may cause a mechanical type of conductive loss. The greatest impairment is produced at the basal end of the basilar membrane.

It should be mentioned that no single reason for presbycusis can be distinguished. Researchers agree that the destruction and loss of sensory and neural components regardless of age are caused by environmental noise and ototoxic drugs [23]. The detrimental effects of accrued environmental factors have been demonstrated in studies that assessed the hearing of older industrial workers. In addition, Ro-

sen, et al. [46] showed that aged populations in nonurban, less noisy areas tend to have better hearing than urban dwellers. Genetic factors have also been shown to play a role in hearing loss in older people. The combination of these 3—environmental noise, ototoxic drugs, and heredity—is the most prominent cause of the destruction of neural and sensory elements in the cochlea.

Decreased efficiency in hearing can have significant and complex effects on interpersonal relationships as well as interactions in the environment. It can serve to shut off the individual, increasing feelings of isolation, rejection, distrust, and withdrawal. Speaking with one who suffers from hearing loss requires extra energy, and may stress family and friends and contribute to closing off the person from activities and decision making. Oyer and Oyer [42] reported that husbands of women with severe loss of hearing scored high on a test for marital tension.

To understand the emotional component of its loss, it is necessary to discuss the 3 psychological levels of hearing: symbolic, signal or warning, and auditory background. Communicating by the use of words is the symbolic level. The warning, or signal, level is the use of sounds such as sirens, screams, or bells to warn of impending danger. In regard to isolation and withdrawal, the auditory background level is most significant. It is known to function at the most subconscious level of hearing. Examples are birds chirping, traffic noises, trees rustling, people talking in the background, and a ticking clock. Usually, we are unaware of these sounds, as they are automatically screened out so that we can focus on more immediate demands. In addition, such sounds tend to be faint and are the first ones lost when hearing impairment occurs. As this loss in older people progresses slowly, this level of hearing fades over many years. An individual may be unaware that this is occurring and may merely feel that the world is less active and stimulating. Although the effect is subtle, the repercussions are serious, as sensory stimulation is essential to alert, adequate psychological and physical activity.

When an individual constantly needs to listen more attentively, an element of strain develops that may not be alleviated in social situations. Listening becomes a conscious, voluntary activity that requires attention and concentration. It is not surprising that frustration and tension might provoke a person to become socially reclusive.

Acquired hearing loss may lead to an inevitable deterioration in the individual's security and self-esteem. Those with impaired hearing live with uncertainty as they cannot benefit from the warnings provided by sounds. In addition, hearing provides a means of monitoring thoughts and feelings useful in maintaining emotional stability, as it enables comparison of these concepts with others. When impairment is present, monitoring feelings, attitudes, and ideas becomes more difficult.

Therapists must use keen observation skills to ascertain signs indicating hearing loss. The following behavior in an otherwise alert and functional person may be strong indicators of impaired hearing, and should be impetus for obtaining more extensive information:

Lack of attention during informal conversations

Frequent requests to repeat what has been said

Limited initiative to be involved in social activities

Confusion as to what has been said

Constant visual scanning of the speaker's face

REHABILITATION

The primary goal in any rehabilitation program is to increase effective communication. Auditory training and speech-reading refer to a wide variety of techniques used in such a program. This training helps an individual use the full potential of residual hearing. It includes hearing aid orientation, the dynamics and control of conversational situations, and mastery of speech-reading (also known as lip-reading). The last involves visual awareness of lip, facial, gestural, and environmental clues.

The therapeutic approach to aural communication is multifaceted, and includes amplification, knowledge of language, and awareness of situational limitations, lip movements, facial expressions, and gestures. The first step in rehabilitation is to determine the usefulness of a hearing aid. In cases of neural presbycusis, it may not be effective, as it primarily amplifies sound and does not assist one to distinguish speech components. If amplification is indicated, an audiologist can provide important services in choosing the proper hearing aid, and in assisting the user during adjustment to it. Audiologists are trained to determine whether or not a person can benefit from an aid, what type should be used, the ear or ears that should be fitted, and the specific characteristics an aid should have. When orienting the person, emphasis is placed on the proper way to wear the aid, how to operate it particularly when using the telephone, its care, and how to correct common problems that occur.

Education and counseling help the individual understand the nature of the hearing loss and gain insight into coping strategies. The person is encouraged to list by priority those communicative environments in which improved function is desired, and to become more assertive in changing them. In addition, factors of language necessary for comprehension of spoken messages are practiced. Instinctive aspects of language often become repressed as an individual becomes more isolated from communication.

Counseling should include discussion of an individual's specific problems and suggestions for coping with them, the normal hearing process, and difficulties in communication. It is important that whenever possible a spouse or significant other participates in the counseling. Simulating hearing loss for this person is a useful technique in helping to create empathy with the impaired relative or friend.

The following are suggestions to facilitate

8

communication with a hearing-impaired person:

1. Gain the person's attention before speaking by touching the person. He or she will hear better while watching the speaker.
2. Be aware if there is a better ear, and position yourself so you speak toward that side.
3. Talk at a moderate rate; speak clearly and use supportive gestures.
4. Avoid shouting, as it only increases unintelligible sounds; it is more important to lower the pitch of your voice. Also, telephone bells, doorbells, and emergency alarms need to be low-toned.
5. If a person relies on lip-reading, remember that good lighting on the face of the speaker is necessary.
6. If it appears you are not being understood, rephrase your thought, using longer phrases that involve lip and facial movements that are more easily interpreted.
7. Be sensitive to the fact that the hearing-impaired person may not follow a topic shift. Try to indicate a change in a thoughtful way.
8. Be aware that background noise such as other conversations or traffic can interfere with hearing.
9. Reassure the individual that this problem may be normal to aging, and that is is possible to help by educating others in how best to communicate.
10. Exercise patience.

Communication is essential for rewarding and successful interaction in our daily living, thus hearing loss is considered particularly devastating. A therapist's sensitivity and knowledge of this impairment as an age-related change can help improve the quality of life for a large segment of the older population. Some communication devices include:

A special alarm clock that shakes the bed or produces a flashing light

Doorbell attachments that activate a flashing light or air fan

Variety of telephone and television amplifiers

Teletypewriter terminals (TTY) that allow a caller to communicate with other TTY users through the regular telephone system

Sound lamp that will go off in response to any number of auditory signs including the doorbell, baby crying, or telephone

Closed-circuit captions that can be seen on television sets equipped with a special decoding device

A vibrating alarm timer

KINESTHETIC LOSS

Kinesthesia, the ability to perceive changes in body position, decreases in advancing age with neuromuscular decline. It may precipitate postural and gait changes, such as a posture of greater flexion with the feet everted for a wider base of support, and shorter steps taken with the feet not lifted as high. Thus the foot spends more time in the support phase than in the swing phase of walking, and longer contact with the ground is maintained. In addition, balance may be affected, increasing the risk of falling. Body sway, the natural motion of the body when standing, also increases after age 50, adding to existing instability.

Therapists should educate their older clients about increased vulnerability in movement, and attention should be given to ensuring safety. Recommendations such as grab bars for the tub or shower, tub seats, nonskid treads placed in the tub, and detachable shower heads to permit sitting when showering can be useful. Removing or securing scatter rugs and simplifying the home environment by eliminating unnecessary clutter and furniture can be helpful.

VISUAL LOSS

PHYSIOLOGICAL CHANGES

Loss of skin elasticity produces wrinkling and drooping eyelids [28]. Within the outer fibrous layer of the eye, senile plaques and degenerative infiltrates are sometimes found in the conjunctiva. The cornea may develop arcus senilis, a circular infiltration of degenerative material within the limbus. Flattening of the curvature of the cornea can produce distorted vision [53].

Within the vascular layer, degenerative changes in the choroid occur. The pupil aperture becomes smaller, allowing less light to enter the eye [18]. Changes in the refractive media affect the vitreous as it exhibits an increase in "floaters" (small dark particles), detachment, and liquefaction. The growth rate of the lens decreases in senescence and the lens loses its elasticity, changing from a consistency of soft plastic to one almost glasslike in character [53]. In addition, it has increasing difficulty changing shape with accommodation, and may have a yellow appearance that is believed to interfere with color discrimination [8, 56]. Degenerative changes of the retina and choroid may result from arteriosclerosis of the vessels in these structures [53].

FUNCTIONAL CHANGES

Visual acuity, peripheral vision, and accommodation decline during aging [3, 18]. With lessened accommodation, the older person may find that material must be held at greater distances to be seen clearly, and glasses are often required for reading. Functions associated with light sensitivity such as dark adaptation, glare recovery, illumination, and contrast requirements are adversely affected. Moreover, decline in visual memory, visual perception, and color discrimination have been reported [1, 16, 54]. The ability to discriminate colors is thought primarily to affect colors in the blue, green, and violet range of the spectrum [16].

As a result of these changes, the elderly can experience difficulty adapting to the environment and performing daily tasks. The degree of difficulty will depend on the extent of the loss, adaptation to aging, level of motivation, mental acuity, status of other sensory systems, family support, general health, and environ-

TABLE 1-1. *Guide Based on Visual Acuity*

| Visual Acuity | Function |
|---|---|
| 20/20 | Adequate for all activities |
| 20/40 | Generally adequate for driving |
| 20/70 | Generally adequate for most daily activities (personal care, homemaking, mobility); reading may be difficult |
| 20/200 | Will probably have difficulty reading; mobility will generally be preserved in familiar surroundings |

Source: A. Sloane. *So You Have Cataracts, What You and Your Family Should Know.* Springfield, Ill.: Thomas, 1970.

TABLE 1-2. *Guide Based on Visual Acuity and Visual Field*

| Visual Acuity | Visual Field | Function |
|---|---|---|
| 3/200 or better | 50 degrees or greater | Adequate for mobility |
| Less than 3/200 | Less than 50 degrees | Difficulty will probably be encountered in mobility tasks |

Source: G. Fonda. *Management of the Patient With Subnormal Vision.* St. Louis: Mosby, 1970.

mental factors. A key issue is the individual's reaction to visual loss. Difficulty in adjusting could cause withdrawal, loss of self-esteem, and extreme dependency. To determine the relationship between the amount of visual loss and functional abilities, several guides have been established (Tables 1-1 and 1-2).

EVALUATION

A comprehensive evaluation is required to determine a person's skills, attitude, and learning capacity. Assessment of functional tasks in a variety of environmental settings will aid in evaluating deficit areas, and serve as a guide for establishing a program to meet the needs of the individual. An ophthalmological assessment is critical, and should include a comprehensive examination and history to determine the need for standard glasses, low-vision devices, surgical correction, and medication.

REHABILITATION

There are several methods that therapists can employ to help the elderly with visual impairment to accomplish daily tasks: education, environmental modification, vision techniques, optical and nonoptical devices, and blind techniques. In addition to the discussion of these, the reader is referred to the suggested reading at the end of this chapter for futher information.

EDUCATION

Education should be directed toward the patient, family, health professionals, the elderly, and local businesspeople. It can be provided on a group or individual basis. Topics might include normal vision, age-related changes, pathological eye conditions and their prevention, medication and its side effects related to vision, coping mechanisms, and availability of community resources for the visually impaired older person. Various media could be used for instructional purposes (Table 1-3).

ENVIRONMENTAL MODIFICATION TECHNIQUES

This is a term given to a number of methods of adapting the environment to aid in the safe and independent accomplishment of daily tasks. The majority of techniques involve control of lighting, glare, and contrast as means of aiding acuity, perception, and other visual functions. Although many are simple adaptations, their value should not be underestimated. They can produce dramatic improvement in functional skills, and should be considered when adapting an elderly person's home or rehabilitation facility, or when consulting with architects on the design of housing for the elderly.

Visual acuity is highly dependent on proper illumination. Because less light reaches the retina of the older person, increased illumination is required (Table 1-4). In addition to proper wattage, lighting should be evenly distributed, constant, and uniform. Bulbs should be kept clean, as dust may diminish illumination. Adequate lighting must be provided outside and inside the home, including outdoor walkways, stairs, and surrounding grounds, indoor hallways, closets, staircases, and work areas. Large windows and a southern exposure will generally add to lighting [10]. Electric lamps with flexible or gooseneck arms are excellent sources of supplementary lighting, as they allow precise directing of the light. Lamps should be placed on the nondominant side for reading and writing [32], and within 1 foot of work material [31, 32] (Figure 1-1). Other useful sources of supplementary lighting include night lights, small pocket flashlights, and standard flashlights. Devices such as mirrors are available with built-in light and can be useful.

Techniques of controlling glare include adjusting curtains and blinds, using shaded lamps with frosted bulbs, avoiding surfaces and objects that produce glare, or positioning them in relation to the lighting source. Table 1-5 indicates common sources of glare and suggests alternatives.

Improvements in contrast will enhance visual acuity, depth perception, and color discrimination. Multicolored objects should be avoided. Hanging or protruding objects and clutter should be eliminated. Bright colors will stand out, but colors in the blue-green-violet spectrum should not be used in close proximity, as discriminating among them can be difficult.

These basic concepts can be incorporated into daily life in a number of practical ways. The edges of steps, the first and last step, and the edges of shelves can be painted in a bright color to aid depth perception. Brightly colored cabinet knobs, elevator buttons, clothing buttons, drawstring pulls, light switches, and wall outlets will help the elderly person in locating them. Tablecloths or trays that provide contrast with the tableware can be useful. Measuring spoons and cups and oven dials with large, brightly colored digits can be obtained. Dark colored rugs should be used that contrast with

TABLE 1-3. *Source Listing*

| Name of Supplier | Large-Print Books, Newspapers, Magazines | Talking Books/ Cassettes and Machines | Other Accessory Aids | Optical Aids | Absorptive Aids | Educational Materials |
|---|---|---|---|---|---|---|
| American Foundation for the Blind 15 W. 16th St. New York, NY 10011 | | | x | x | | x |
| American Optical Corp., Inc. Optical Products Division Southbridge, MA 01550 | | | | x | | |
| American Printing House for the Blind 1830-1839 Frankfort Ave. Louisville, KY 40206 | x | | x | | | |
| APOLLO Lasers, Inc. 6357 Arizona Circle Los Angeles, CA 90045 | | | | CCTV | | |
| Bausch & Lomb, Inc. 635 St. Paul St. Rochester, NY 10146 | | | | x | | |
| Designs for Vision, Inc. 120 E. 23rd St. New York, NY 10010 | | | | x | | |
| G. K. Hall & Co. 70 Lincoln St. Boston, MA 02111 | x Book club | | | | | |
| Howe Press Perkins School for the Blind 174 N. Beacon St. Watertown, MA 02172 | x | x | x | | | |
| Keeler Optical Products, Inc. 456 Parkway Broomall, PA 19008 | | | | x | | |
| Library of Congress Division of the Blind and Physically Handicapped Washington, DC 20542 | x | x | | | | |

TABLE 1-3. *(Continued)*

| Name of Supplier | Large-Print Books, Newspapers, Magazines | Talking Books/ Cassettes and Machines | Other Accessory Aids | Optical Aids | Absorptive Aids | Educational Materials |
|---|---|---|---|---|---|---|
| Lighthouse N.Y. Assn. for the Blind 111 E. 59th St. New York, NY 10022 | | | x | x | x | x |
| Luxo Lamp Corp. Monument Park Port Chester, NY 10573 | | | Lamps | | | |
| Nat'l Assn. for the Visually Handicapped 305 E. 24th St. New York, NY 10010 | x | | | | | x |
| Nat'l Soc. for the Prevention of Blindness 16 E. 40th St. New York, NY 10016 | | | | | | x |
| New York Times 220 W. 43rd St. New York, NY 10036 | x | | | | | |
| Pelco Sales 351 E. Alondra Blvd. Gardena, CA 90248 | | | | CCTV | | |
| Readers Digest Pleasantville, NY 10570 | x | | | | | |
| Recreational Innovations, Inc. P.O. Box 203 Saline, MI 48176 | | | | | x | |
| Selsi, Inc. 40 Veterans Blvd. Carlstadt, NJ 07072 | | | | x | | |
| Visualtek 1610 26th St. Santa Monica, CA 90404 | | | | CCTV | | |
| Volunteer Services for the Blind 919 Walnut St. Philadelphia, PA 19107 | x | | | | | |

CCTV   = closed-circuit television

TABLE 1-4. *Illumination Requirements According to Age*

| Age (Years) | Illumination Recommended for Close Tasks (Watts) |
|---|---|
| 30 | 120 |
| 40 | 145 |
| 50 | 180 |
| 60 | 230 |
| 70 | 300 |
| 80 | 415 |

Source: From C. Verner and C. Davidson. *Physiological Factors in Adult Learning and Instruction.* Tallahassee, Fla.: Research Information Processing Center, 1971.

FIGURE 1-1. *The speech language pathologist can enhance communication skills in the elderly individual with use of a writing guide and adequate lighting. (Courtesy Massachusetts Rehabilitation Hospital, 125 Nashua Street, Boston.)*

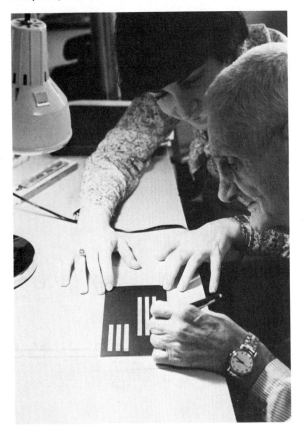

TABLE 1-5. *Glare Sources and Methods of Control*

| Glare Source | Alternative |
|---|---|
| White and cream color paints | Medium-toned colors |
| High-gloss paints | Flat paints |
| Shiny plastic placemats and tablecloths | Fiber-woven or dull plastic materials |
| Shiny metal kitchen and bathroom fixtures | Dull plastic or wood accessories |
| Highly polished floor surfaces | Carpet, dull-finished tiles, unpolished floors |
| Shiny metal pots, pans, and utensils | Dull metal, plastic, ceramic, or wood materials |
| Pictures framed with glass | Nonglare glass |
| Bright sunlight | Avoid travel in sunniest part of day and plan travel that is in a direction away from the sun |

Source: From M. C. Cristarella. Visual functions in the elderly. *Am. J. Occup. Ther.* 31:432, 1977.

furnishings. A syringe can be held over a dark surface to draw insulin. Medication labels can be rewritten using white matte paper and dark, thick print. When reading and writing, a dark blotter should be placed on the work surface. It is important to remember that the quality and color of paper, spacing, margins, sentence length, and the color ink will affect contrast and readability. The darker the ink and the lighter the paper the easier the material is to read. Stationery in the blue-green-violet color spectrum should be avoided. Mimeographed materials are difficult, as they typically have poor contrast. Dark lines can be drawn on checks or letters to assist in signing one's name. Telephone numbers can be underlined with a black fiber-tip pen to enhance readability. When involved in leisure craft activities, dark colored wools and multiple colors in the blue-green-violet spectrum should be avoided.

VISION TECHNIQUES

To enhance the field of vision that may be re-

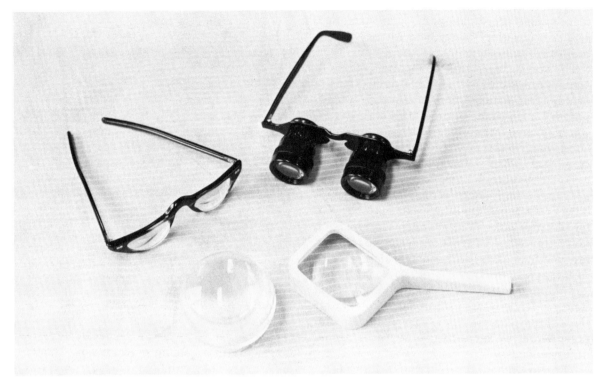

FIGURE 1-2. *Optical low-vision devices, starting at the upper left and proceeding clockwise: spectacle, telescopic, hand-held and stand magnifiers. (Courtesy Massachusetts Rehabilitation Hospital, 125 Nashua Street, Boston.)*

stricted, scanning techniques may be useful. This involves turning the head from side to side to permit taking in the total visual field. Many will do this automatically.

### DEVICES

There are many devices available for the visually impaired to assist them with daily functioning. These include optical low-vision aids, and accessory and absorptive aids.

Most optical low-vision aids are magnifying devices that enlarge the object of view. They are available in various forms to meet specific needs: hand-held, stand, spectacle, telescopic, and closed-circuit television (CCTV) (Figure 1-2). They are designed for monocular or binocular use. Frequently, the individual is instructed to use the eye that is better for the

type of task being attempted. Because the devices are task-specific, an individual may require several aids to accomplish the variety of daily activities.

Hand magnifiers are a familiar monocular aid. They are versatile and can be used for a variety of short-term, near, and intermediate distance tasks such as reading a recipe, a telephone number, or a menu. In addition to the standard model, they are available with built-in illumination, in pocket and folding styles, and in models that can be worn around the neck or clipped to a lamp so that hands can remain free for an activity.

Stand magnifiers are useful for short-term reading or hobbies such as stamp collecting. It may be the device of choice for an individual with tremors, arthritis, or other difficulty affecting hand coordination. They are manufactured in a variety of styles with or without built-in illumination.

The spectacle aid may be monocular or binocular, and is the most suitable device for the avid reader, particularly one who enjoys reading for long periods of time. The elderly person may have difficulty adjusting to the shortened reading distance, the restricted field of view, and the appearance.

The telescopic aid is perhaps the most versatile. It can be monocular or binocular, handheld or spectacle-mounted, and may be used for distance tasks such as watching television or reading signs. In addition, it can be used for intermediate tasks, and can be adapted with caps for close work. Focusing may be difficult, and the telescope produces a restricted visual field, which may be a significant problem for the elderly who may have visual field limitations. Their appearance and cost are additional disadvantages.

The closed-circuit television (CCTV) is an electronic magnification aid that uses a zoom lens to project an enlarged image on a screen. The enlargement is manifold, which makes this a useful device for the individual with severe decline in visual acuity or visual field, and for one who has difficulty adjusting to other devices. It can be used for reading and writing. Its disadvantages are cost and fixed location.

Proper lighting is crucial when using optical devices, as many of them, because of close working distance, obstruct lighting. The elderly may experience fatigue and difficulty adjusting to the devices because of different reading method, speed, and distance, and restricted visual field. They may prefer the hand and stand models, as they are generally easier to use. Most of these devices are available in a wide range of strengths. In general, as the power of the magnifier increases the visual field, focal distance, and size of the magnifier decrease. These devices should be prescribed by an ophthalmologist following a comprehensive evaluation to rule out

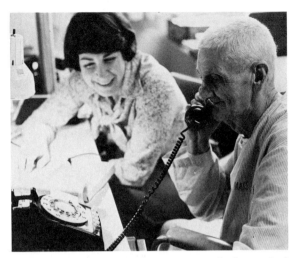

FIGURE 1-3. *Using a large-print telephone dial, the patient practices use of the telephone with the speech pathologist. (Courtesy Massachusetts Rehabilitation Hospital, 125 Nashua Street, Boston.)*

problems that can be corrected by standard measures. They can be obtained from a variety of sources (Table 1-3).

Absorptive aids include different types of sun wear, brim hats, and visors. They protect the eye from excessive rays that might interfere with formation of a clear image. Sun wear may be worn by itself, over a pair of spectacles, or clipped on a pair of glasses. It is available in graded levels of light transmissions, and must be carefully selected to prevent severe loss of acuity because of diminished illumination. It is best prescribed by an ophthalmologist and is easily obtained through a number of sources. The reader is referred to Table 1-3 for suppliers.

Accessory aids include a number of devices that make images larger, clearer, or brighter, or increase contrast. Basically, they can be categorized into 7 groups: communication (Figures 1-1 and 1-3), lighting (Figure 1-1), reading, health management, personal care, leisure, and homemaking aids. Some of the most commonly used devices are listed in Table 1-6, including several designated for the totally blind individual. Suggested sources

TABLE 1-6. *Accessory Aids*

| Communication aids | Personal care aids |
|---|---|
| Envelope guide (see Figure 1-1) | Sock clips |
| Signature guide | Dresser drawer dividers |
| Writing guide | *Leisure aids* |
| Check guide | Large-print cards and bingo |
| Bold-lined paper | Games adapted for visually impaired |
| Bold-lined checks | Large-print tape measures |
| Fiber-tip pens | Self-threading needles |
| Raised-number and large-number watches | *Reading aids* |
| Large-print standard and push-button telephone dials (see Figure 1-3) | Large-print magazines and books |
| Wallets with dividers for coins and bills | Typoscope (reading slit) |
| *Lighting aids* | Book stands |
| Gooseneck or flexible arm lamps | Talking books or cassettes and machines |
| Flashlights | *Homemaking aids* |
| *Health management aids* | Large-print or raised-letter measuring cups, spoons, oven dials |
| Insulin devices | Large-print timers |
| Pill boxes | Large-print cookbooks |
| Bathroom scales with large numbers | |

for obtaining these devices are provided in Table 1-3.

BLIND TECHNIQUES

Several techniques used by the blind may be helpful for the individual with age-related vision problems. Two principal ones involve use of other senses and systematic organization.

Sensory information can be used to aid object identification and orientation to surroundings. The older person may be able to use the sense of touch to identify garments and locate buttons, snaps, and zippers. When making a bed, one can use the folds in the sheets and blankets as guides. Coins may be identified by feeling their size, weight, and texture. Bills folded according to a planned procedure allow discrimination among different denomina-

tions. Touch can be helpful when pouring liquids.

Organization can aid object location and serve as a means of compensation for reduced visual field. The clock pattern can be used in setting up a meal tray. Organization of closets and drawers helps in the locating of clothing and personal items. Equipment used for a specific task can be stored together to compensate for limited vision.

PATHOLOGICAL EYE CONDITIONS

Because of the high incidence of various eye diseases in the elderly, a brief discussion of some common ones is presented with emphasis on the functional implications for the rehabilitation therapist. It is important to keep in mind that these conditions are *not* a part of the normal aging process and are considered *pathological*.

MACULAR DEGENERATION

Macular degeneration (Figure 1-4A) is an untreatable disease that involves changes within the macular portion of the retina. It results in impairment of central vision, but it does not lead to blindness or involvement of the peripheral field. Object identification, reading, and daily activities prove difficult, while vision in familiar surroundings can be preserved [14]. Functional management involves magnification through the use of optical low-vision devices and large-print accessory items, and by decreasing the distance between the individual and the object of view. Use of proper lighting, environmental modification techniques, absorptive aids, and lighting devices, as well as control of glare and contrast are recommended. Eccentric viewing in which the individual is instructed to look off-center may be helpful.

CATARACTS

Cataracts (Figure 1-4B) are a common visual problem in the elderly. With clouding of the lens vision tends to be blurry, and discrepancies exist between near and distant vision, vision indoors and outdoors, and during day and

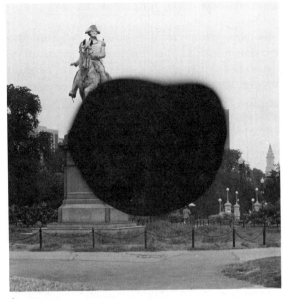

A

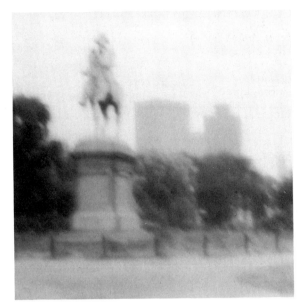

B

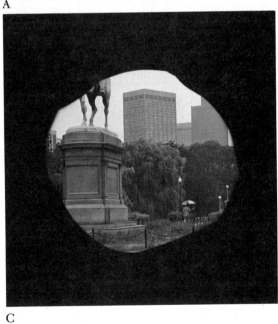

C

FIGURE 1-4. *Functional vision representations. A.
Macular degeneration. B. Cataracts. C. Glaucoma.*

night [15]. Many individuals will benefit from surgical removal of the "ripened" lens, although good sight cannot be guaranteed. Surgery is indicated when the decline in vision interferes with function [48]. Among the devices used following surgery to substitute for the removed lens are cataract glasses, contact lenses, and acrylic intraocular implants.

For the individual who is not a candidate for surgery, control of lighting, glare, and contrast is critical. This may be achieved through the use of environmental modification techniques, accessory aids, and absorptive aids. A well-illuminated work area is important; however, light near the eye must be decreased to allow pupil dilatation and less interference by lens opacity. Where visual acuity is reduced, optical low-vision aids, a reduced viewing distance, or large-print accessory items may be helpful in providing a magnified image.

GLAUCOMA

Another major disease of the eye affecting the elderly is open-angle glaucoma (Figure 1-4C). It develops painlessly, and can damage eyesight with little warning. Glaucoma produces increased pressure within the eye. It is thought to occur frequently in the elderly because of narrowing eye chambers associated with normal aging [35]. If diagnosed in time, the disease can be managed with eye drops that either decrease the production of fluid or increase its outflow. Some drops result in pupils that do not increase in size even in dim light, thereby reducing the light reaching the retina. Surgery may also be indicated.

If left untreated, the increased intraocular pressure may cause damage to the optic nerve, which can lead to impairment of the peripheral field. The central visual field is generally spared [15]. Peripheral field loss can affect most tasks, particularly reading, self-care, and mobility.

Enhancing the visual field through the use of minifying optical low-vision devices (wide-angle lenses, reverse telescopes), and using visual scanning and environmental modifica-

tion techniques can be most useful. Control of lighting, glare, and contrast are important for people using eye drops that reduce the amount of light reaching the retina. Where severe field loss is present, blind techniques may be beneficial in increasing independence and safety in daily tasks.

DIABETIC RETINOPATHY

Diabetes can seriously affect vision. Blood vessels in the eye may hemorrhage, infarct, and proliferate, destroying the retina, and resulting in diabetic retinopathy. With this disease there may be a decrease in visual acuity and in peripheral vision, often with day to day fluctuations. Functionally, there may be difficulty with reading, self-care, and mobility. Magnification is the recommended approach through the use of optical low-vision aids, large-print materials, and reduction in viewing distance. Several low-vision aids may be required because of fluctuations in visual status. Light, glare, and contrast control through the use of environmental modification techniques, and absorptive and accessory aids will also be important. If the visual loss is severe, blind training may be indicated.

It should be noted that some individuals with diabetic retinopathy may benefit from 2 new procedures. Photocoagulation with argon laser may help improve visual acuity by preventing further leakage from hemorrhaging vessels. Vitrectomy, often done as a last resort, involves removal of the cloudy fluid from the eye and replacing it with a clear fluid. This may lead to formation of a clear visual image [55].

MEDICATIONS

In addition to the eye diseases, therapists should be aware that certain medications commonly prescribed for the elderly have side effects that may result in visual dysfunction. This can range from blurring or double vision to decreased accommodation. The reader is referred to *Manual of Ocular Diagnosis and Therapy*, D. Pavan-Langston, editor, for a comprehensive list of drugs and their ocular toxicity.

CONCLUSION
It is clear that the older person with a visual disorder may benefit from many of the same techniques used by those with normal age-related visual changes. Those with a pathological condition, however, may require the services of a comprehensive low-vision service or agency for the blind. The former provides a setting in which an interdisciplinary team offers the opportunity for examination, education, training, and prescription of appropriate aids for the individual. The staff includes an ophthalmologist, optometrist, low-vision assistant, and ancillary services located within the facility or the community. There are approximately 250 such services established in this country. The National Association for the Visually Handicapped and many state agencies for the blind maintain a listing of services according to geographical areas (Table 1-3).

Agencies provide comprehensive rehabilitation programs for the blind or visually impaired. The programs are based on a complete evaluation, and provide specialized training in communication skills, personal management, social and leisure counseling, and orientation and mobility techniques. Rehabilitation counseling and other psychological services are often available. Many of these agencies will provide instruction in the home, which is beneficial for those who may have difficulty transferring techniques to their personal environment. There are more than 400 agencies serving the blind in the United States. Information regarding them can be obtained from the American Foundation for the Blind (Table 1-3).

It is obvious that early identification and referral are essential to permit full benefit from treatment and for the prevention of blindness.

## Psychological Issues
Adult developmental psychology is the study of the progressive sequential patterns of human behavior occurring generation after generation. As each generation matures it nurtures the following one in a circular sense. The life course is continual and an effective effort to deal with any stage must be viewed in the context of all that went on before.

Review of the dominant theories shows a growing trend toward a life span view of psychological development. Assuming there are significant antecedents to each sequential aspect of behavior, resolution of developmental tasks will increase the understanding of late life stages. *Developmental tasks* simply defined are a sequence of social events ordered by age and required as a person goes through life. Havighurst [19] feels a developmental task arises at a certain time, and if successfully accomplished, it will lead to happiness and success in future ones. These tasks may arise from societal demands, pressure of the ego, physical maturation, or a combination of these factors. Zaccaria [57] suggests a given task has a special meaning to every individual, and the variety of approaches and resolutions depends on the individual.

The 2 that are considered most difficult in old age are work and family life. Although the older person has faced adjustments in these areas in previous stages, these are special in many ways at a late point in life.

RETIREMENT
Separation from the world of work has occurred in the lives of aging individuals throughout recorded history, but its form and significance varies for individuals and cultures. In early civilization, the end of productive labor signified approaching infirmity and death. The aged in many agricultural societies, however, enjoyed high status and even reverence. Modern retirement, in which the individual leaves full-time employment and is financially supported from savings or government resources, has emerged in industrial societies during the last half of this century. Kreps [27] points out that one of the major reasons for the establishment of old age benefits in the

United States was the intent to draw elderly persons off the labor market, and thus maintain the balance of supply and demand.

During this century, with increased length of life, retirement has come to be viewed as an expected event within the normal life cycle. Surveys indicate that the majority of Americans expect to retire, and it is reasonable to predict that most will do so by the end of their seventh decade. Thus retirement is increasingly regarded as a legitimate feature of late life. It has been described as an event in an occupational career, a stage in the normal life cycle, and transition from adulthood to old age, and is a role demanding individual adjustment.

Despite the fact that most Americans appear to desire retirement, each must face the problem of economic provision during these years. Low income has been identified as a serious problem of the aged, and prospects for economic security, based on income levels of presently retired Americans, are not encouraging.

Those who are preoccupied with work to the exclusion of other interests dread the time when they are forced to retire. For the work-oriented older person, a job may offer a sense of status and order. Subsequently, for many retirees, more important than additional income is the need to serve, to be occupied, and to remain in the mainstream of life.

The individual facing retirement must cope with a variety of issues associated with the process: cessation of work and the opportunity to associate with others, an implied beginning of old age, an abundance of free time, a changed status in both family and community, and society's perception of the retiree. With retirement, most roles change, and usually at too rapid a pace. One's reference group at work and associations in social and service clubs weaken or disperse. The resultant psychosocial deprivation may cause the retiree to reject the society that brought about this role change, and social disengagement may subsequently occur. For the majority, this means a dramatic change in the pattern of the social life they established during early adulthood and carried on until this point: the elderly person wants and needs social contacts but is deprived of opportunities for them. The result of shrinking sources of contact is dependency on the family circle. The absence of outside contacts may also diminish an individual's sense of prestige based on past accomplishments.

Another difficult adjustment is the change from a scheduled to an unscheduled day. For some, although occupational life may not have been truly satisfying, a compromise was achieved among ambition, opportunity, and ability, and any change might be threatening. Occupational life is the rule rather than the exception, and a way of life that becomes established and comfortable. Retirees, now experiencing a leisure society, maintain a position of little or no status, and find it difficult to cope with an excess of free time.

For the therapist the challenge is in assisting the person to use retirement as an impetus for continued self-exploration and development. Adequate planning in social, psychological, economic, and vocational areas should facilitate adjustment. Situations must be made available in which the person can attain new functional self-identity and establish reference groups. An easier transition will be achieved if we support environments that afford the maximum possibilities for older persons to become involved. Thus we will be able to prevent impending social, emotional, and financial problems. Instead of forcing greater dependency on older people, we should encourage them to remain productive in paid or volunteer work in their communities (Table 1-7). It also seems reasonable to assume that more flexible retirement policies would tend to ease the transition.

Older people have the capacity to learn new skills that, combined with their experience, can permit them to make significant contributions. Initially, they may need guidance in assessing their abilities, generating ideas, renewing self-confidence, and obtaining infor-

**TABLE 1-7.** *Job Options for Older People in Meeting Community Needs*

*Transportation*
Station information aides
Bus drivers
Van drivers
Carpool arrangers
Improved route sign advisors
Service assistance locators

*Cultural activities*
Performers and artists
Programmers
Trainers
Sales and promotion workers
Facilities maintenance workers
Fund-raising counselors and
  assistants
Audience development
  specialists
Arts conservators and
  technicians
Resource and information
  assistants

*Employment*
Job finders
Trainers
Job developers
Career and job counselors

*Neighborhood*
Guards and monitors
Clean-up aides
Repair workers for substandard
  housing
Energy conservation advisors
  and workers

Mediators, conciliators, and
  arbitrators
Fire and safety inspectors
Pest control workers
Translators and communicators

*Health*
Hospital technicians and aides
Home health care providers
  and aides
Rehabilitation technicians and
  aides
Medical equipment operators

*Nonprofit activities*
Fund-raising/membership
  counselors
Bookkeepers and accountants
Government regulations and
  compliance counselors
Coordinators of volunteers
Incorporation advisors

*Environment*
Counselors on pesticides and
  safety
Extended sanitation and special
  clean-up workers
Monitors
Materials recycling aides
Environmental impact analysts

*Employee Relations*
Mediation, arbitration, and
  conciliation specialists (both
  employee/management and
  employer/employee relations)

*Education*
Discipline aides
Tutors and resource specialists
Class administration aides
Library workers
Career and other counselors
Special population education
  programmers and advisors
Fund raisers
Special skill enrichment
  advisors and aides
Financial aid advisors

*Special services to dependent
  persons*
Companions
Nutrition advisors
Form fillers
Eligibility and assistance
  advisors
Readers and communicators
Recreation advisors and
  workers
Meal providers and feeding
  helpers
Day-care providers
Home health aides
Rehabilitation technicians and
  helpers
Representative payees and
  guardians
Homemakers
Shopping assistance helpers

Source: "Older Americans: An Untapped Resource" by the National Committee on Careers for Older Americans. From *Aging: In Agenda for the Eighties. A National Journal Issues Book.* Washington, D.C.: Government Research Corporation, 1979.

mation on existing opportunities (Table 1-8). Assisting them in planning activities to compensate for the loss of a worker's role involves reorganization of personal goals. For example, if a salaried job is high on the list, the person should be encouraged to attempt to place more importance on obtaining some kind of work. For those who were previously active idleness and inactivity can be devastating, and the resulting demoralization can make them ill-equipped to use vast amounts of leisure. It may be necessary initially to help organize and

structure their interests and time. Adult education programs have been developed to encourage interests and skills of older people.

FAMILY LIFE
Adjustment to changes in family life is considered to be a major developmental task for an older person. Patterns established in early adulthood start to change with middle age, and are altered or dropped as appropriate or necessary during progress through life. For parents, the first transition is when the last child de-

TABLE 1-8. *Programs for the Elderly*

| Volunteer/Employment Programs | Purpose | Address |
|---|---|---|
| RSVP (Retired Senior Volunteer Program) | Volunteer programs in public and nonprofit institutions | ACTION<br>806 Connecticut Ave. N.W.<br>Washington, D.C. 20525<br>(800) 424-8580 toll-free |
| SCORE (Service Corps of Retired Executives) | Retired businessmen advising novices in business | ACTION<br>806 Connecticut Ave. N.W.<br>Washington, D.C. 20525 |
| VISTA (Volunteers in Service to America) | Volunteers for 1-2 years in community projects in U.S. with small salary to cover living expenses | ACTION<br>806 Connecticut Ave. N.W.<br>Washington, D.C. 20525 |
| Peace Corps | Overseas service | ACTION<br>806 Connecticut Ave. N.W.<br>Washington, D.C. 20525 |
| IESC (International Executive Service Corps) | Overseas service by executives | International Executive Service Corps<br>545 Madison Ave.<br>New York, NY 10022 |

| Low-Income Elderly Programs* | Purpose | Address |
|---|---|---|
| Foster Grandparent Program | Provide relationship and care to orphans and mentally retarded, physically handicapped, or troubled children and teenagers in institutions; 20 hours per week at $1.60 per hour | ACTION<br>806 Connecticut Ave.<br>Washington, D.C. 20525 |
| SOS (Senior Opportunities and Services programs) | Service in programs to meet needs of older people: nutrition, consumer education, outreach, employment, information, and referral | Office of Economic Opportunity<br>1200 19th St. N.W.<br>Washington, D.C. 20506 |
| Operation Mainstream programs<br>Green Thumb (men)<br>Green Light (women) | Conservation and landscape (men)<br>Community service (women) | Manpower Administration<br>Operation Mainstream<br>Department of Labor<br>Washington, D.C. |
| Senior AIDES | Community service | National Council of Senior Citizens<br>1511 K St. N.W.<br>Washington, D.C. 20005 |
| Senior Community Service Program | Community service | National Council on the Aging<br>1828 L St. N.W.<br>Washington, D.C. 20036 |
| Senior Community Service Aides | Community service | National Retired Teachers Association<br>Senior Community Service Aides Project<br>1909 K St. N.W.<br>Washington, D.C. 20006 |

*Only persons over 60 with income below OEO (Office of Economic Opportunities) guidelines are eligible.

Source: From R. N. Butler and M. I. Lewis. *Aging and Mental Health* (2nd ed.). St. Louis: Mosby, 1977.

parts from home—frequently causing what is referred to as the empty nest syndrome. This event marks the end of daily parental responsibilities and accords couples the opportunity to reshape their life-style and relationship. The next transition can occur with the acquired role of grandparent, which offers the opportunity to develop a new relationship with grandchildren, and a deeper one with adult children. The other major changes in late life are those precipitated by retirement and loss of a spouse.

Retirement may disrupt the framework of marital relations on many levels. Initial difficulties can arise when one or both spouses attempt to adjust to a completely new role. Traditionally before retirement, the marital arrangement is based on the husband's absence from the house during working hours and the wife's self-reliance in making daily decisions for the home. With the husband home primarily in the evenings and on weekends, responsibilities are divided according to this time schedule. With the onset of retirement, these long-standing arrangements are significantly disturbed. The retiree will be spending much more time at home, and adjustment during this period can be influenced by the couple's shared interests and compatibility.

For some couples, marriages are maintained through habit or a limited amount of shared time, making marital tension tolerable. Some remain together to rear children, whose departure from the home increases isolation and makes more time available for viewing the marriage and its problems. Bradford [4] suggests that couples facing retirement approach this transition by openly discussing the potential opportunities and pitfalls of this phase. He encourages a "marital review," or critical examination of past experiences that required adjustment and adaptation. By emphasizing the strengths and coping techniques a couple might have used previously, preparation occurs for joint problem solving in the future. It is important to recognize that accommodations suitable to past conditions may need some adjusting to pressures of this period in life.

## LOSS OF SPOUSE

Death of a spouse, particularly after years of being married, is a major adaptive challenge. Moreover, a spouse's death may add problems of decreased income, which may necessitate reduction of social activities and a move into less desirable living quarters. These, together with a general absence of companionship, all add trauma to a changing role.

The predominant response is grief, particularly during the first few months after the loss [17]. Grief produces initial passivity and inability to cope with the essentials of everyday living. At this time, it is wise to encourage the widowed spouse to make only the most necessary decisions; temporarily the best course of action is inaction. Glick [17] reports that initially, grief is characterized by feelings of shock, disbelief, sadness, and lack of control. As the widowed person moves into intermediate stages and introspective mourning, there is a sense of the dead spouse's continued presence and a compulsive search for meaning. Ultimately, the emotional trauma becomes less extreme and may be resolved.

Loneliness is considered to be a long-term reaction following death of a spouse. Once the initial mourning period is over, widowed persons frequently are not included in heterogeneous groups, and may be forced to limit their socializing to their families and other widowed persons. Occasionally, some become so immobilized by loneliness and desire for the past that they withdraw from old friends and avoid establishing new friendships.

Reluctance to face death inhibits any preparatory discussions between husband and wife of consequences for the survivor. Communication on this subject rarely occurs even when death may be imminent. What appears to occur more frequently is so-called silent consideration, as older people observe their friends and relatives experiencing such loss.

Most newly widowed individuals are overwhelmed, unfamiliar with what to expect, what to do, and what this new status actually means. Grieving cannot be treated on a schedule with stated time intervals for recovery. It is a necessary process, and if avoided, can create negative consequences that may lead to serious mental illness [30]. Frequently, the surviving partner may experience severe depression before adjustment can be reached. Reaction to this status change relates directly to how much the role of being a married person permeated life.

During this period, the therapist can be most helpful by supporting the person in pursuing viable options, encouraging involvement in new activities, providing assistance in learning the skills necessary for daily tasks, and directing the person to available resources.

LOSSES IN OLD AGE

Loss, grief, and concomitant depression are major recurring issues with older people. They experience loss on many levels, and any one loss can affect another. For instance, disability may precipitate functional loss and a change in work capacity. Consequently, economic changes result together with alteration in status.

Depression is the most common response of older people to loss [6]. Unfortunately, it is not always recognized because it may be masked by weakness, apathy, irritability, and passivity, and therefore accepted as "normal" in old age. Depression may be manifested by a sense of anxiety and restlessness. When the condition is allowed to persist, there is usually a lack of capacity to initiate or organize activity.

It should be noted that suicide rates increase with age in both sexes. Resnick and Kantor [45] note that about 10 percent of the 25 percent of all reported suicides are committed by the elderly. There are numerous theories about motivational factors, many agreeing that severe loss in status, control, and possibly decreased finances may precipitate the act.

The usual techniques of suicide are employed by older people. In addition, a long-term process of self-destructive behavior may occur, such as disregarding proper diet, noncompliance with medication schedules, increased risk-taking. Older people must be taken seriously if they threaten suicide, as most are successful in the attempt. Referrals to appropriate resources should be made so that the person can be encouraged to discuss the subject. It is important to be cognizant of sudden lifting of depression; the person may now be energized to enact what was previously only contemplated. Those who are withdrawn, isolated, and aimless need to be assisted in finding meaning in their lives, or this alarming social malady may continue to worsen.

THERAPY PROGRAMS

The elderly face mental health issues related to coping strategies for the normal developmental tasks of aging, together with opportunities for the promotion of a positive self-image. To accomplish this, life, personal, educational, and social skills are essential. Lack of them may impede coping and lead to feelings of low self-esteem, anxiety, hostility, and a general inevitable decline.

Group experiences can be effective in helping them to meet basic needs, to solve problems, and to learn to handle developmental tasks. In addition, a group situation can be an opportunity to learn that peers share similar concerns. Hyams [22] states that the opportunity to use group work "may improve motivation by encouraging interpersonal relationships and by providing instances of other similarly disabled patients making progress toward independence."

Classification of "problem constellations" of older adults is helpful in determining the most appropriate type of group therapy to offer. Classification is as follows:

1. Those who appear to be functioning satisfactorily, but who need assistance in dealing with basic environmental needs and tasks of aging.
2. Individuals who have some serious physical disability in addition to other concerns that impede adaptation to old age.

3. People who are physically or emotionally isolated and withdrawn.

In designing groups for older people, the main objective is enhancement of social, emotional, and physical functioning so that they may achieve their potential. The group may facilitate an opportunity for support from peers, development of a new identity within the context of old age, and improve self-esteem, help define new behavior and expectations, and offer a sense of belonging. The effectiveness of bringing together individuals who share problems is based on the tendency of people to trust and rely on the judgment of those in the same situation, and on the quality of discussion and mutual reinforcement that occurs among participants.

Groups can vary based on their development around such factors as etiology, purpose, structure, content, size, and leadership. Most important for effective work with older people is for the facilitator to have a strong knowledge of the normal changes of old age in addition to well developed group skills.

The following descriptions can be adapted to institutional and community settings. It is the responsibility of the therapist to be sensitive and responsive to the needs of the specific group.

SUPPORT GROUPS

*For the Individual with*
*Age-Related Problems*
The elderly who experience stress from problems of normal aging may not consider their concerns serious enough to require counseling; inherent is their attitude that these feelings of discontentment are to be expected at this time in life. Support groups may be structured as informal workshops to provide a nonthreatening atmosphere; in addition, by designing an open-ended session, personal counseling may be provided when appropriate. A time-limited format is frequently used, although the option for an on-going group may be offered.

The content of these sessions may vary according to the particular needs and objectives of the members, however, health, sensory changes, dependency, mobility, and family relationships are fairly common concerns. Emphasis should be on recognizing age-associated changes while encouraging functional adaption and practical alternatives. It should be an opportunity to help older people become more aware of their strengths, skills, and values; to increase their knowledge of options available to them; and to teach them more effective communication. This type of personal growth group may also be effective in a nursing home setting, recognizing that institutionalized older persons also have the ability to grow and learn. Support groups are helpful in assisting an aging couple to handle functional problems that may occur, such as the strain of living with a hearing-impaired spouse or adjustment to retirement. These groups provide participants a chance to examine, share, and ventilate their feelings about growing older.

*For Families of Older People*
In an institutional setting, groups may focus on the family's fears, guilt, or questions about an institutionalized relative. Working with relatives may help them relieve feelings of remorse or anxiety, as well as establish rapport for future planning.

Support groups can prove useful for those caring for older parents. Some potential sources of conflict can be reduced simply by talking about them. Generating ideas on how to handle even the most mundane matters (i.e., housekeeping, health insurance, bank accounts) between parents and children can defuse more emotionally charged interactions. In later years, parent-child relationships should go beyond attempting to manage old age. This is difficult, because it may mean an alteration in roles as well as accepting a parent as an adult individual. Confronting the physiological and psychological problems of old age can be painful.

It is difficult to be objective when the first occasion to deal with aging is with one's own parents. If a group for people with older parents is designed, it is necessary to consider the obstacles to its success. Initially, this may be measured by the number of participants. To ensure attendance, it may be necessary to consider that many who would benefit from the group may not be able to leave an ailing parent alone. This obstacle can be overcome by organizing alternative care for the ill parent. For example, while offering the sessions for the adult children, an activity or day-care center may agree to offer simultaneous opportunities for the parents. If a parent is homebound, creative options might be explored by asking other older people or students to spend time with the parent while the sessions are going on. This will play a dual role in offering the parent some new stimulation at the same time as allowing the children an opportunity to explore options to help them cope better.

## ASSERTIVENESS TRAINING

Such training can provide a behavioral approach for assisting older persons to cope more effectively with their social environment. As Butler states [7]: "Assertion training is particularly effective in helping older people identify and express their needs explicitly." This communication skill may facilitate closer relationships among the elderly who are so often lonely and isolated. In a model developed by the Continuum Center, participants learn the differences among passive, aggressive, and assertive behavior, develop assertive skills (e.g., making and refusing requests), and practice assertive responses relevant to their situations [9].

## PRERETIREMENT PLANNING

An opportunity for careful planning and increased self-awareness in preparation for the retirement years is provided. The format of short lectures and group discussions provides information on retirement and facilitates sharing of thoughts and feelings about this step.

Topics that should be covered are financial planning, legal issues, physical and mental health, interpersonal relationships, death and grief, and creative use of leisure time. These groups may include spouses, and can be particularly advantageous in increasing a couple's awareness of partners' expectations.

## REALITY ORIENTATION

These are based on the assumption that by the use of repetitive, consistent basic information (e.g., name, date, place, next meal, and so on) the potential exists for overcoming confusion. Formal sessions should be held at both the same time and place at least 5 times a week, at which time visible cues can be used to rehabilitate a confused and disoriented person to increased awareness of self, place, time, and others. It is important to encourage confused persons to make maximum use of their assets. To be most effective, reality orientation must go on informally during all waking hours, repeatedly presenting the same information in a consistent tone and manner. The following methodology was refined at the Veterans Administration Hospital in Tuscaloosa, Alabama in 1974[41]:

1. Remind patients of person, time, and place.
2. Talk distinctly and directly to them.
3. Correct patients tactfully when they ramble in speech and actions.
4. Explain or demonstrate each new procedure one step at a time before asking a patient to do it.
5. Ask for only one response at a time.
6. Allow patients adequate time to respond.
7. Guide patients by giving clear directions.
8. Practice reality orientation consistently.
9. Give immediate praise and recognition for positive responses.
10. Teach alert patients to use reality orientation props and information.

## REMOTIVATION

Remotivation has 3 primary objectives: to assist people to take a renewed interest in their environment, to increase communication skills, and to maintain good personal relationships. Meetings provide an opportunity to share ideas, promote personal interaction, and focus members' attention on subjects unrelated to their problems. Remotivation is based on 5 basic steps that should be followed to create a more stable and durable program[29]:

1. Climate of acceptance: This attempts to establish a comfortable setting. The leader should initially address the group and then greet each person individually by name, with a personal comment to establish further contact.
2. The bridge to reality: This presents a topic in the external world for discussion to focus attention on the environment. The leader should encourage active participation using (a) poetry, quotations, or newspaper articles, (b) trigger questions or ideas, and (c) visual aids.
3. Sharing the world we live in: This specifically directs discussion through the use of objective questions that have been prepared in advance. The therapist should be comfortable with the topics presented so that questions can be answered.
4. Work of the world: This is designed to stimulate the person to consider work in relation to self. To facilitate discussion, past work experiences should be shared, and potential activities in which the person might choose to be involved should be explored.
5. Climate of appreciation: During this wrapping up time, the leader can summarize the discussion, announce the time and date for the next meeting, and express appreciation to participants for attending.

ATTITUDE THERAPY
If consistently used by a rehabilitation team, these groups can help in reinforcing appropriate and discouraging inappropriate behavior. This therapy can be most effective in coordination with reality orientation. The team must decide what attitude would be most helpful when working with an individual, choosing from 5 major attitudes that can be used with 5 types of behavior patterns[29]. It is important that everyone involved with this person be consistent in using the designated attitude. The attitudes are as follows:

1. Active friendliness is supportive, and encourages feelings of self-worth. It is most successful when used with older persons who are withdrawn and apathetic.
2. Kind firmness is especially effective with depressed people who need to have limits set and expectations firmly established and followed. The therapist should attempt to direct focus onto something other than personal unhappiness.
3. Passive friendliness is best used with the older person who is fearful of close and active friendliness. It entails waiting for a friendly or interested overture, and then responding in a concerned but not overly solicitous manner.
4. No demand is the best approach for those who show anger, distrust, and fearfulness. The major expectation that needs to be conveyed is that the person will not harm him- or herself or others. Involvement in activities is a secondary objective.
5. Matter-of-fact attitude is most effective with those who demonstrate character disorders, anxiety reactions, or psychosomatic, seductive, or manipulative behavior. A calm, consistent, and informal response from the therapist is important.

TASK-ORIENTATION
Groups may be designed around functional and avocational activities. The objectives are successful experiences with an activity relevant to the participants together with increased socialization, self-esteem and social awareness, communication skills, peer support, and a sense of affiliation.

## LIFE REVIEW

This technique may be used in a group or individual setting. Reported originally by Butler and Lewis[6], it involves gathering extensive autobiographical information about an older person. Use of materials such as scrapbooks, memoirs, and family photograph albums, as well as discussions with family members will contribute to understanding a patient's background. Any stimulation that facilitates introspection on the part of the patient should be encouraged by the therapist. It is an active listening experience to reflect on unresolved conflicts and gain new understanding and resolution of them. Butler and Lewis [6] state: "The goals and consequences of these steps include expiation of guilt, the resolution of intrapsychic conflicts, the reconciliation of family relationships, the transmission of knowledge and values to those who follow, and the renewal of ideals of citizenship and the responsibility for creating a meaningful life."

Life review need not be formal, but can occur informally and spontaneously; it may be seen in the forms of reminiscence, story-telling, and sharing nostalgia. Therapists working with older people must be skilled in facilitating these moments. It should not be considered a preoccupation with self, but viewed as an important experience, and a necessary, natural process of sorting out a lifetime. It is an opportunity to focus on strengths and skills as older people reflect on their lives and the coping mechanisms that have helped them survive. In offering the chance to articulate past accomplishments, it reaffirms and enhances their sense of self, and can be enriching for both the older persons and the therapists. The skill of listening, in this author's view, is probably one of the most effective but underused tools in many therapy programs.

## PEER COUNSELING

This is an innovative and exciting approach to the delivery of mental health services. It is an opportunity to involve older people who are successfully coping with aging, as role models.

In addition, issues such as loneliness and alienation can be effectively dealt with when people realize that others share these concerns. Peer counselors not only share their ability to handle problems, but demonstrate the possibility of developing new roles. Proper training enables these counselors and staff to communicate positive attitudes about aging, together with a belief that with appropriate support older people can remain in control of their lives. Peer counselors need training only to augment and refine their inherent knowledge and skills.

These descriptions are meant to be illustrative; groups may need to be adapted and expanded creatively depending on the therapist, the client's needs, and the setting. Most relevant is that well-designed experiences create a supportive atmosphere in which positive attitudes about aging may be conveyed. Such an environment will encourage open expression of feelings and thoughts, as well as exploration of new behavior, opportunities, and skills for older persons. Group counseling is an effective remedial and preventive modality when addressing the mental health needs of older people.

## Psychomotor Skills

Psychomotor skills are those necessary to perform tasks that require patterns of finely coordinated voluntary movements of the body. They vary according to 3 elements.

1. The underlying performance of the sensory processes
2. Recognition and integration of incoming signals from the environment and body parts
3. The critical nature of the motor response[2]

As a psychomotor skill develops, the originally perceived elements become integrated into a larger system in which one factor becomes a cue for the next in a sequence of events. Eventually, these skills become automatic. Psychomotor activities are those personal skills that maintain an individual's independence and quality of life, for example, locomotion, self-care, communication, and household and avocational tasks. In later life, these skills, mastered during early development, may become less automatic if sensory losses interfere with the stimulus-response sequence. A simple example of this may be the person who appears to have difficulty walking across a room. The problem may not be inherent in the act of walking, but maneuvering among obstacles may be difficult because of impaired vision.

Psychomotor limitations, otherwise latent, may become apparent in a crisis or emergency situation. A person may be required to climb or jump to escape harm, thus revealing problems in movement not necessarily seen in normal daily living. The agility, sensory capabilities, and general strength of older adults must be taken into consideration, as must their size and weight, when designing safety and escape mechanisms.

Changes in basic motor skills and sensory acuity in persons over 65 contribute to the frequency of accidents of these people. Consideration must be given to the combination of diminished vision, lowered resistance to glare, hearing loss, impairments of movement, and increased reaction time known to occur with age, and the additive impact these can have on appreciable risk. In addition, after middle age, a tendency to general slowing has been observed, particularly with psychomotor activities.

The older person will respond more rapidly if the stimulus is expected, familiar, and clarified, and if the response expected is simple. If there are many elements or irrelevant items to consider simultaneously in a task, the speed with which an older person reacts will be diminished. Individual adaptations are developed so that situations demanding speed, unusual time pressures, or reaction times are frequently circumvented. People may need assistance in developing work methods or approaches that simplify activities of daily living and decrease time pressures.

INTELLIGENCE

It should be noted that former implications of declining intellect with age were results of the methodology used in the studies that reported the implications. More recent findings suggest that intelligence, particularly the crystallized type as opposed to fluid intelligence, can be expected to be maintained or even increased in healthy individuals as they age.

## Theories of Social Gerontology

Gerontologists concerned with social issues have attempted to define consistent patterns of aging based on human behavior in the presence of preconceived social meaning. One such theory is that of disengagement described by Cumming and Henry[12]. They consider the inevitability of disengagement to be a mutual process between an older person and society, resulting in maintenance of the stability of the system. This theory states that society expects older people to step placidly aside to provide places for younger, supposedly more capable people; simultaneously, older people will accept this attitude because they are cognizant of their diminishing capabilities and imminent demise. Subsequently, they experience appropriate shrinkage of social interactions and relationships, and ultimately, disengagement becomes self-perpetuating. In this view, disengagement is seen as a natural rather than imposed process. Controversy surrounding this theory erupted immediately after its initial appearance. Major criticisms focused on the emphasis of natural inevitability; there was presumed withdrawal from the viewpoint of the individual or society, and minimal concern was given to the effects of personality factors on the entire process[33].

Both authors of the original statement have separately made revised comments on the formulation. Cumming retracted her emphasis on societally imposed withdrawal to achieve social equilibrium, but instead concentrated on the role of innate biological and personality differences [11]. She makes a distinction in personality types between "impingers," those who are reactive and assertive in their social interaction; and "selectors," those who are passively waiting for cues to confirm their pre-existing assumptions. In anticipation of disengagement in the later years, impingers are generally considered to be more anxious, while selectors are able to create alternatives that insulate and safeguard their personal orientations.

Henry altered his original view by stressing psychological dynamics [21]. He concurred with researchers concerned with the developmental approach, emphasizing evolving adjustments as individuals make transitions through successive stages during their lives. As do most developmental psychologists, he recognized greater "interiority" over the course of life, or a gradual turning toward inner states with less attention to external events. In Henry's restatement he discussed predisposed personality characteristics during subsequent stages of the life cycle as strong determinants of an individual's ultimate engagement with or disengagement from society.

With the activity theory, in contrast to the disengagement theory, diminished social interaction frequently seen in old age is not viewed as a desired outcome, but as a result of society withdrawing from the person. Proponents of this theory feel that the older person should maintain the activities of middle age as long as possible, and then find substitutes for ones that must be relinquished because of retirement, inability, or death of friends or relatives. Activity theorists contend that the majority of older people who remain active maintain their psychological and social well-being[20], although a small minority of elderly people may affirm the disengagement theory.

An important distinction between these theories is the order in which social and psychological disengagement occurs; social engagement means the visible interactions between an aging individual and other persons; psychological engagement implies behavior that may not be directly observable, but that is indicative of an individual's emotional in-volvement with society. The activity theory assumes that social disengagement occurs devoid of psychological disengagement, with the latter occurring only in response to a changed social climate. In the disengagement theory, psychological disengagement is assumed to precede the social as a developmental phenomenon in aging.

Both of these theories indicate the need for further modification, particularly taking into account our culture's complex value system. The Kansas City study [20A] data confirmed that the diminishing of role activity is regretted although accepted as part of the inevitable process of growing old. The data simultaneously indicated that for some older persons there may occur a strong negative reaction to loss of activity, accompanied by much dissatisfaction.

There are significant numbers of social gerontologists who do not concur with any theoretical framework explaining successful aging patterns. Rather, advocates of the importance of personality characteristics believe that with age, there is increasing consistency of personality, particularly in adaptation to new situations.

Although adjustment is highly individualized, personality types have been described to help identify adaptive patterns seen in aging persons. Neugarten, Havighurst, and Tobin [39] have described 4 major personality types and their patterns of adjustment:

1. Integrated personality: Aging individual who engages in a wide spectrum of activities, effectively substituting new roles for old ones.
2. Armor-defended personality: One who attempts to hold on to old patterns.
3. Passive dependent: The individual who seeks responsiveness in others and maintains a few close friendships with medium activity level.
4. Unintegrated: A person who loses control over emotions and thoughts.

Reichard, Livson, and Petersen[44A] described 5 personality types, and suggest that they do not change appreciably throughout life. Types include:

1. Mature: Those who are well balanced and realistic about the strengths and weaknesses of their age.
2. Rocking chair: Those who are content passively to disengage and depend on others for support.
3. Armored: People who have well-integrated defense mechanisms and frequently rely on activity as a demonstration of their continuing independence. They frequently are aggressive and extremely threatened by aging.
4. Self-haters: Individuals who turn their anger inward and consider themselves failures in most spheres. Aging only adds to their indignities and depressive state.
5. Angry: Those who are bitter and blame others for their failures, and are unable to reconcile themselves with getting older.

These theorists regard personality as the pivotal dimension in predicting patterns of aging. Each pattern subsequently exerts influence on the individual's ability to cope with social and biological changes.

## Sexuality

Many misconceptions and prejudices prevail about the role of sex in the lives of older people, even confusing the elderly themselves. They may feel guilty or ashamed of healthy sexual feelings, particularly if these feelings are considered unacceptable by society.

As life advances, sexuality can be reinforcing for those who otherwise feel physically unattractive because of aging. A study conducted at Duke University Medical Center found that age and sexual activity were not strictly correlated. Although variables such as impaired health often affected sexual behavior, the incidence of activity was maintained at 50 percent at age 80 [43]. Circumstances such as loss of a spouse or physical dysfunction may impede an active sexual life, yet interest continues to exist.

Opposition to sexuality in the elderly population is frequently heard from adult children who are embarrassed by their parents' sexual feelings. This concern has been reflected in the prohibitions commonly found in nursing homes where men, women, and even married couples are assigned to separate wings or floors. Institutions need to preserve the right of personal privacy rather than impose conformity and rigid restrictions. Fortunately, some changes are occurring, especially in facilities where apartment living is available. Nursing homes, institutions, foster care homes, and retirement communities should encourage companionship and intimacy despite physical infirmities or age.

### THE AGING WOMAN

Women in postmenopausal years have significant sexual capacity, although the intensity of response is reduced in later years. Pfeiffer and co-workers [43, 44] found that after age 50, sexual behavior patterns were influenced by marital status. Women attributed the primary reason for cessation of intercourse to their husbands, that is, they were widowed or divorced, or their husbands were physically impaired or had lost interest in sex. Masters and Johnson [37] emphasized the psychic component of aging in determining sex drive in postmenopausal women, noting that many women become more interested in sex postmenopausally. To a great extent, an aging woman's sexual activity depends on the availability of a socially sanctioned, capable partner.

Decrease of tissue elasticity and estrogen deficiency contribute to changes in the size and shape of the breasts [26]. Postmenopausal estrogen deficiency also contributes to atrophy of the vaginal wall and diminished vaginal lubrication. In addition, changes in sexual response occur, including decrease in sex flush and muscle tension, less vaginal expansion and lubrication, and a diminished vasocongestive increase in breast size. If regular sexual activity is maintained, there may be no actual shrinkage in the size of the vaginal barrel or loss of elasticity of the vaginal wall [37].

## THE AGING MAN

Fear of ineffective sexual performance is a very real concern, especially with the widespread acceptance of sexual incompetence as a component of aging. In fact, an older man may turn to a younger woman for a sexual partner in an attempt to establish his sexual potency and attractiveness. Impotence, illness, and loss of interest are reasons given for the cessation of sexual activity [44].

Physiological changes include a decrease in the amount of free testosterone circulation. Although spermatogenesis decreases with age, it does continue into the ninth decade [50]. With loss of skin elasticity there is sagging of scrotal tissue.

Changes in sexual response include delayed nipple erection, loss of vasocongestive flush, and decrease in frequency and intensity of rectal-sphincter contractions. Unless a man over 60 is active sexually, regular recurring contractions of the musculature of target organs are reduced in intensity. Masters and Johnson [37] identify the major change to be the duration of the phases of the sexual cycle. The older man is generally slower in achieving an erection and in ejaculating. Many find they cannot redevelop penile erection for 12 to 24 hours after ejaculation. It should be noted, however, that there is an increase in ejaculatory control.

## CONCLUSION

Therapists must understand that it is natural for older people to maintain their sexual interest; however, even those who have enjoyed sex may need information or alternatives to remain sexually active. Masters and Johnson [36] found that in the absence of physical illness, sexual dysfunction in older couples was related to lack of knowledge of changing physiology and marital difficulties. They should be educated regarding age-related changes in sexual function, and if needed, coital alternatives should be discussed. Informed older people will be less concerned by these changes if they understand that such variants are natural components of aging.

## Environmental Choices

The elderly are not a homogeneous group; therefore the provision of one type of living arrangement for all of them is not appropriate. Differences in health, former life-style, finances, interests, capacity for self-care, and support systems must be taken into account on individual bases. When considering a residence for older people, one should assess the physical environment, services and activities provided, and the potential social interaction the living arrangement may facilitate or impede (i.e., prohibitive price, policies for selection of residents, location, areas designed for socializing).

The personal environment of the elderly is particularly important as it may be the only place left where there is privacy and personal control. It has been noted that when no private space is available for residents in a nursing home, they will find and establish personal domain in a corridor [13]. Private space is essential for the well-being of any individual, and attempting to acquire a niche is a healthy expression of personality. As newly purchased homes will be redecorated according to the new occupants' desires, so should this option be made available to the elderly within their environments.

In studies of spatial preferences of the elderly, it was observed that smaller, somewhat cluttered areas were preferred over more spacious rooms. Delong [13] feels that clutter provides increased perceptual stimulation, particularly in visual, tactile, and kinesthetic senses. Although tactile sensitivity does appear to be somewhat diminished with age, reliance on this sensory input occurs as other senses show even greater decline. Moving about can be facilitated by touching objects that are placed close together, particularly when vision is limited. Placing furniture carefully offers the opportunity for the older person to feel the way through an area.

Bright colors, varied textures, and olfactory, thermal, and auditory cues should be used when designing environments for the elderly; making choices for economic, practical, and convenient reasons is not necessarily giving priority to their needs. Environmental planning must, however, consider the more common physical risks experienced by these people. In addition, provision should be made in furniture design and arrangement that decreases glare and offers tactile, visual, and kinesthetic stimulation.

INSTITUTIONALIZATION
In considering housing for the elderly, institutional living is frequently thought to be the major trend. Presently, only about 5 percent of individuals 65 and over are so housed. The median age of older people in institutions is 82, with 1 percent of those aged 65 to 69, 9 percent aged 80 to 84 years old, and 17 percent 85 years and older. Major gerontological research has shown that the critical determinants of who is admitted to institutions and who remains in the community depend on the social support available, particularly from the family. Poor health is not the primary reason for long-term institutional care. Soldo and Meyers [49] indicated that "each additional child reduces one's chances of being institutionalized in old age." We are now seeing that the longer one lives, the more likely one is to be institutionalized [25]. People in advanced old age often have children who are themselves beginning to age and are not capable of caring for an older parent. Thus the elderly who are living out their remaining years in institutions usually have no other recourse.

Such institutions may vary from custodial care settings to skilled nursing facilities or mental hospitals. Domiciliary care homes offer minimal supervision in a sheltered environment for older people who are capable of caring for themselves. Skilled nursing facili-

ties offer a range of complete to intermediate levels of care, and provide medical, nursing, and dietary supervision. Some institutions may also provide extended-care facilities and serve as a temporary convalescent setting after hospitalization, or occasionally, prior to a hospital stay.

Tragically, a number of elderly may be unjustifiably admitted to mental hospitals. These are often individuals who do not exhibit clinically significant functional or organic disorders, but who may have become slightly disoriented, and for whom no other alternative exists. The increase in community support systems such as mental health clinics, adult day-care centers, and work opportunities for older people may reduce this inappropriate use of mental hospitals.

Many communities now have housing developments designed to meet the particular needs and finances of the elderly. These arrangements include apartments, retirement communities, residential hotels, and group homes (also known as shared living facilities). In some retirement housing there are accommodations for those who are fully independent, as well as for those who may need assistance in meals, housekeeping services, or medical care. These may be in a campuslike setting, including residential and skilled nursing facilities: several types of living arrangements may be housed in one building. The continuum is designed to extend from guarded independence to long-term care for the frail elderly.

Opportunities need to exist in the community that minimize alterations in life-style and relegate institutions to the supplemental role for which they were intended originally. Older people need to be provided with the opportunity to choose the type and degree of assistance they feel they need, and should be directly involved in decision making to continue to control their own lives. Brody [5] says: "The goal should be to provide a complete spectrum of high quality community services and institutions (and other congregate facilities), to iden-

TABLE 1-9. *Organizations for the Elderly*

| Organizations for the Elderly | Comments |
|---|---|
| American Association of Retired Persons<br>1909 K Street N.W.<br>Washington, D.C. 20006 | Age 55 and above, employed and retired |
| The American Geriatrics Society<br>10 Columbus Circle<br>New York, NY 10019 | |
| Association Nacional Por Personas Mayores<br>425 Hedding Street<br>San Jose, CA 95110 | Spanish-speaking elderly |
| Division of Adult Development and Aging<br>(formerly Division of Maturity and Old Age)<br>American Psychological Association<br>1200 17th Street N.W.<br>Washington, D.C. 20036 | |
| Gray Panthers<br>3700 Chestnut Street<br>Philadelphia, PA 19104 | Activist group of older people |
| The Institute of Retired Professionals<br>The New School of Social Research<br>60 West 12th Street<br>New York, NY | Provides intellectual activities for retired professionals |
| The Institute of Lifetime Learning<br>c/o National Retired Teachers Association<br>1909 K Street N.W.<br>Washington, D.C. 20006 | Educational services of the NRTA and AARP |
| International Senior Citizens Association<br>11753 Wilshire Boulevard<br>Los Angeles, CA 90025 | |
| The National Center on Black Aged<br>1730 M Street N.W., Suite 811<br>Washington, D.C. 20036 | Provides comprehensive information to meet the needs of black aged |
| National Council on the Aging<br>1828 L Street N.W., Suite 504<br>Washington, D.C. 20036 | Research and services regarding the elderly |
| National Council of Senior Citizens<br>1511 K Street N.W.<br>Washington, D.C. 20005 | |
| National Interfaith Coalition on Aging<br>298 South Hull Street<br>Athens, GA 30301 | Coordinates the involvement of religious groups in meeting needs of the elderly |
| Sex Information and Education Council<br>of the United States (SIECUS)<br>1855 Broadway<br>New York, NY 10023 | Provides sex information to older people |
| Urban Elderly Coalition<br>c/o Office of Aging of New York City<br>250 Broadway<br>New York, NY | Effort of municipal authorities to obtain funds for urban poor elderly |
| Western Gerontological Society<br>785 Market Street, Room 616<br>San Francisco, CA 94103 | Promotes well-being of older residents of western states |

tify the characteristics of those for whom each arrangement is appropriate and to select the services and the environments that foster maximal well-being for each older person and their family."

## Conclusion

We live in an era that idealizes youth and physical beauty, and thus old age becomes a blot on society. How can the aging person do anything but consider each year a burden while being relegated to the status of third-class citizen?

As therapists, we can present positive concepts about old age to children, as well as encourage middle-aged people to improve the lives of their parents and ultimately their own future old age. Of particular importance is that we include the elderly in this process (Table 1-9). Direct interaction with the community by the elderly will help to dispel negative stereotypes about aging.

Therapists have the opportunity to act as advocates of the elderly. In this century we have witnessed a dramatic increase in their numbers, but not a concomitant increase in our responsibility to them. We must continue our attempts to clarify their needs and priorities, and wipe away the guilt associated with becoming old in America.

## References

1. Bell, B., et al. Depth perception as a function of age. *Aging Hum. Devel.* 3:77, 1972.
2. Birren, J. *The Psychology of Aging.* Englewood Cliffs, N.J.: Prentice-Hall, 1964.
3. Botwinick, J. *Aging and Behavior.* New York: Springer, 1973.
4. Bradford, L. On retirement: Encountering emotional landmines. *Social Change* 9:2, 1979.
5. Brody, E. Women's Changing Roles and Care of the Aging Family. In *Aging: Agenda for the Eighties.* Washington, D.C.: Government Research Corporation, 1979.
6. Butler, R., and Lewis, M. *Aging and Mental Health.* St. Louis: Mosby, 1977.
7. Butler, R. *Why Survive? Being Old in America.* New York: Harper & Row, 1975.
8. Colavita, F. B. *Sensory Changes in the Elderly.* Springfield, Ill.: Thomas, 1978.
9. Continuum Center for Adult Counseling and Leadership Training. Oakland University. Rochester, Michigan.
10. Cristarella, M. C. Visual functions in the elderly. *Am. J. Occup. Ther.* 31:432, 1977.
11. Cumming, E. Further thoughts on the theory of disengagement. *Int. Soc. Sci. J.* 15:3, 1963.
12. Cumming, E., and Henry, W. E. *Growing Old: The Process of Disengagement.* New York: Basic Books, 1961.
13. Delong, A. The Micro-Spatial Structure of the Older Person: Some Implications of Planning the Social and Spatial Environment. In L. A. Pastalan and D. Carson (Eds.). *Spatial Behavior of Older People.* Ann Arbor, Mich.: University of Michigan Press, 1970.
14. Faye, E. *The Low Vision Patient.* New York: Grune & Stratton, 1971.
15. Faye, E. The role of eye pathology in low vision evaluation. *J. Am. Optom. Assoc.* 47:11, November 1976.
16. Gaylord, S. A., and Marsh, G. R. Age differences in the speed of a spatial cognitive process. *J. Gerontol.* 30:674, 1975.
17. Glick, I. O., Weiss, R. D., and Parkes, C. M. *The First Year of Bereavement.* New York: Wiley, 1974.
18. Gordon, D. M. Eye problems of the aged. *J. Am. Geriatr. Soc.* 13:398, 1965.
19. Havighurst, R. J. Flexibility and the social roles of the retired. *Am. J. Sociol.* 59:309, 1954.
20. Havighurst, R. J., and Albrecht, R. *Older People.* New York: Longmans, Green, 1953.
20A. Havighurst, R., Neugarten, B., and Tobin, S. Disengagement and Patterns of Aging. In B. Neugarten (Ed.). *Middle Age and Aging.* Chicago: University of Chicago Press, 1968.
21. Henry, W. E. Engagement and Disengagement: Toward a Theory of Adult Development. In R. Kastenbaum (Ed.). *Contributions to the Psychobiology of Aging.* New York: Springer, 1965.
22. Hyams, D. E. Psychological factors in rehabilitation of the elderly. *Gerontol. Clin.* 11:129, 1969.
23. Johnsson, L-G., and Hawkins, J. E., Jr. Vascular changes in the human inner ear associated with aging. *Ann. Otol.* 81:364, 1972.
24. Kanin, G. To rest is to rust. *Quest* 3:4, 1979.
25. Kastenbaum, R., and Candy, S. The 4 percent fallacy: A methodological and empirical critique of extended care facility population statistics. *Aging Hum. Devel.* 4:1, 1973.
26. Kolodny, R. C., Masters, W. H., and Johnson,

V. E. Geriatric Sexuality. *Textbook of Sexual Medicine.* Boston: Little, Brown, 1979.

27. Kreps, J. M. Economics of Retirement. In E. W. Busse and E. Pfeiffer (Eds.). *Behavior and Adaption in Later Life* (2nd ed.). Boston: Little, Brown, 1977.

28. Leopold, I. H. The Eye. In J. Freeman (Ed.). *Clinical Features of the Older Patient.* Springfield, Ill.: Thomas, 1965.

29. Lewis, S. *The Mature Years: A Geriatric Occupational Therapy Text.* Thorofare, N.J.: Slack, 1979.

30. Lindemann, E. Symptomatology and management of acute grief. *Am. J. Psychiatry* 101(2):141, 1944.

31. Lythgoe, R. J. The measure of visual acuity. *Br. Med. Res. Council.* Special Report Series: 173, 1932.

32. MacNalty, A. S. *The Preservation of Eye Sight.* Baltimore: Williams & Wilkins, 1958.

33. Maddox, G. L. Disengagement theory: A critical evaluation. *Gerontologist* 4:2, 1964.

34. Maddox, G. L. Themes and issues in sociological theories of human aging. *Hum. Devel.* 13:17, 1970.

35. Marmor, M. F. The eye and vision in the elderly. *Geriatrics* 63, August, 1977.

36. Masters, W. H., and Johnson, V. E. *Human Sexual Response.* Boston: Little, Brown, 1966.

37. Masters, W. H., and Johnson, V. E. *Human Sexual Inadequacy.* Boston: Little, Brown, 1970.

38. National Center for Health Statistics. *Vital Health Statistics: Prevalence of Selected Impairments.* Rockville, Md.: Health Resources Administration, Public Health Services, Series 10, No. 99, 1975.

39. Neugarten, B. L., Havighurst, R. J., and Tobin, S. S. Personality and Patterns of Aging. In B. L. Neugarten (Ed.). *Middle Age and Aging.* Chicago: University of Chicago Press, 1968.

40. Neugarten, B. L., Havighurst, R. J., and Tobin, S. S. Adjustment to Retirement. In B. L. Neugarten (Ed.). *Middle Age and Aging.* Chicago: University of Chicago Press, 1968.

41. Nursing Service, Veterans Administration Hospital. *Guide for Reality Orientation* (revised ed.). Tuscaloosa, Ala., 1970.

42. Oyer, H., and Oyer, J. *Aging and Communication.* Baltimore: University Park, 1970.

43. Pfeiffer, E., and Davis, G. Determinants of sexual behavior in middle and old age. *J. Am. Geriatr. Soc.* 22:481, 1972.

44. Pfeiffer, E., Verwoerdt, A., and Davis, G. Sexual behavior in middle life. *Am. J. Psychiatry* 128:1262, 1972.

44A. Reichard, S., Livson, F., and Petersen, P. *Aging and Personality.* New York: John Wiley and Sons, 1962.

45. Resnick, H. L., and Kantor, J. M. Suicide and aging. *J. Am. Geriatr. Soc.* 18:152, 1970.

46. Rosen, S., Olin, P., and Rosen, H. V. Dietary prevention of hearing loss. *Acta Otolaryngol.* 70:242, 1970.

47. Rosow, I. *Social Integration of the Aged.* New York: Free Press, 1967.

48. Snyder, L. H., et al. Vision and mental functions of the elderly. *Gerontologist* 16(6):491, 1976.

49. Soldo, B., and Meyers, G. The living arrangement of the elderly in the new future. Presented at the conference on The Elderly of the Future, sponsored by the Committee on Aging of the National Research Council's Assembly of Behavioral and Social Science, National Academy of Sciences, Annapolis, Md., May, 1979.

50. Talbert, G. B. Aging of the Reproductive System. In C. E. Finch and L. Hayflick (Eds.). *Handbook of the Biology of Aging.* New York: Van Nostrand Reinhold, 1977.

51. U.S. Bureau of the Census. *Current Population Reports.* Series P-20, No. 287. Washington, D. C.: U.S. Government Printing Office, 1975.

52. VanGennep, A. *The Rites of Passage.* Chicago: University of Chicago Press, 1960.

53. Vaughan, D., and Asbury, T. *General Ophthalmology.* Los Altos, Calif.: Lange, 1980.

54. Wallace, J. G. Some studies of perception in relation to age. *Br. J. Psychol.* 57:283, 1956.

55. Ward, B. Sight care and preservation. *Sky* 16: April, 1980.

56. Weale, R. A. *The Aging Eye.* New York: Harper & Row, 1963.

57. Zaccaria, J. *Theories of Occupational Choice and Vocational Development.* Boston: Houghton Mifflin, 1970.

## Suggested Reading

SENSORY LOSS

Carroll, K. (Ed.). *Compensating for Sensory Loss.* Human Development in Aging Project, NIMH Grant #23924. Ebenezer Center for Aging and Human Development, Minneapolis, MN 55407.

Corso, J. F. Sensory processes and age effects in normal adults. *J. Gerontol.* 26, 1971.

HEARING LOSS

Hartford, E. *How They Hear.* Recorded by Gordon Stove and Associates, Northbrook, IL 60062.

Jones, W., and Mittlestedt, D. Surveying speech and hearing problems. *Geriatr. Nurs.* 12, 1967.

Long-term care training program: Hearing impairment/mental health. Kit obtained from Bennett S. Gurian, M.D., Project Director, Aging Services, Massachusetts Mental Health Center, 74 Fenwood Road, Boston, MA 02115.

Maurer, J. F. Auditory Impairment with Aging. In B. Jacobs (Ed.). *Working with the Impaired Elderly.* Washington D.C.: National Council on Aging, 1975.

McCartney, J., and Nadler, G. How to help your patient cope with hearing loss. *Geriatrics* 3:1, 1979.

MyKlebust, H. *The Psychology of Deafness.* New York: Grune & Stratton, 1964.

Services for elderly deaf persons—recommended policies and program. Deafness Research and Training Center. New York University, 1971.


BLINDNESS

Allen, W., et al. *Orientation and Mobility. Behavioral Objectives for Teaching Older Adventitiously Blind Individuals.* New York Infirmary/Center for Independent Living: New York, 1977.

Inkster, W. *Personal Management. Behavioral Objectives for Teaching Older Adventitiously Blind Individuals.* New York Infirmary/Center for Independent Living: New York, 1977.

Paskin, N. *Sensory Development. Behavioral Objectives for Teaching Older Adventitiously Blind Individuals.* New York Infirmary/Center for Independent Living: New York, 1977.

Slater, M. *The Self-Help Community Handbook for Older and Visually Impaired Individuals.* New York Infirmary/Center for Independent Living: New York, 1976.

Yeadon, A. *Toward independence. The Use of Instructional Objectives in Teaching Daily Living Skills to the Blind.* New York Infirmary/Center for Independent Living: New York, 1974.


VISUAL LOSS

Birren, J. E. *The Psychology of Aging.* Englewood Cliffs, N.J.: Prentice-Hall, 1964.

Jolicoeur, R. M., Sr. *Caring for the Visually Impaired Older Person.* Minneapolis: The Minneapolis Society for the Blind, 1970.

Pavan-Langston, D. (Ed.). *Manual of Ocular Diagnosis and Therapy.* Boston: Little, Brown, 1980.

Wolf, E. Studies on the shrinkage of the visual field with age. *Highway Res. Rec.* 167:1, 1967.

Wolf, E. Glare and age. *Arch. Ophthalmol.* 64:502, 1960.

Wolfberg, M. D. *The Role of Vision Care in Society Today and in the Future.* Washington, D.C.: American Optometric Association, 1974.


DEMOGRAPHY

Atchley, R. *Social Forces in Later Life.* Belmont, Calif.: Wadsworth, 1972.

*Guide to Census Data on the Elderly.* U.S. Department of Commerce, Bureau of the Census. Washington, D.C.: U.S. Government Printing Office, 1979.

Siegal, J. *Demographic Aspects of Aging and the Older Population in the United States.* Washington, D.C.: U.S. Government Printing Office, 1976.


GROUPS

Barnes, E., Sack, A., and Shore, H. Guidelines to treatment modalities and methods for use with the aged. *Gerontologist* 13:4, 1973.

Birkett, D., and Boltuch, B. Remotivation therapy. *J. Am. Geriatr. Soc.* 21:8, 1973.

Birren, J. E., and Schaie, W. K. *Handbook of the Psychology of Aging.* New York: Van Nostrand Reinhold, 1977.

Burnside, I. M. (Ed.). *Nursing and the Aged.* New York: McGraw-Hill, 1976.

Corby, N. Assertive training with aged population. *Counsel. Psychol.* 5:4, 1975.

Fink, S., and White, B. Peer group counseling for older people. *Educ. Gerontol.* 1:2, 1976.

Glasser, W. *Reality Therapy.* New York: Harper & Row, 1965.

Goldfarb, A. Group Therapy with the Old and Aged. In H. Kaplan and B. Sadock (Eds.). *Comprehensive Group Psychotherapy.* Baltimore: Williams & Wilkins, 1971.

Harris, P. B. Being old: A confrontation group with nursing home residents. *Health and Social Work* 4:1, 1979.

Klein, W. H., LeShan, E. S., and Furman, S. S. *Promoting Mental Health of Older People through Group Methods: A Practical Guide.* New York: Mental Health Materials, 1965.

Miller, M. *Suicide after Sixty: The Final Alternative.* New York: Springer, 1979.

Petty, B. J., Moeller, T. P., and Campbell, R. Z. Support groups for elderly persons in the community. *Gerontologist* 15:6, 1976.

Waters, E., et al. Strategies for training adult counselors. *Counsel. Psychol.* 6:1, 1976.

Yalom, I. *The Theory and Practice of Group Psychotherapy*. New York: Basic Books, 1970.

## SOCIAL GERONTOLOGY

Hendricks, J., and Hendricks, C. *Dimensions of Aging: Readings*. Cambridge: Winthrop, 1979.

Kalish, R. *Late Adulthood: Perspectives on Human Development*. Monterey, Calif.: Brooks/Cole, 1975.

Zarit, S. H. (Ed.). *Readings in Aging and Death: Contemporary Perspectives*. New York: Harper & Row, 1977.

## RETIREMENT

Atchley, R. Retirement and leisure participation: Continuity or crisis? *Gerontologist* 11:1, 1971.

Atchley, R. *Sociology of Retirement*. New York: Halstead, 1976.

Bolles, R. *The Three Boxes of Life*. Berkeley, Calif.: Ten Speed, 1978.

Bradford, L. It's about time you considered pre-retirement training. *Training J.* 16:6, 1979.

Bradford, L. On retirement: Encountering emotional landmines. *Social Changes* 9:2, 1979.

Busse, E. W., and Pfeiffer, E. *Behavior and Adaption in Later Life* (2nd ed.). Boston: Little, Brown, 1977.

George, L. K., and Maddox, F. L. Subjective adaption to loss of the work role: A longitudinal study. *J. Gerontol.* 32:2, 1977.

Palmore, E. *Normal Aging II: Reports for Duke Longitudinal Studies*. Durham, N.C.: Duke University Press, 1974.

## FAMILY LIFE

George, L. *Role Transitions in Later Life*. Monterey, Calif.: Brooks/Cole, 1980.

## SEXUALITY

Butler, R., and Lewis, M. *Love and Sex after Sixty*. New York: Perennial, 1977.

Christenson, C. V., and Gagnon, J. H. Sexual behavior in a group of older women. *J. Gerontol.* 20:3, 1965.

Comfort, A. Sexuality in old age. *J. Am. Geriatr. Soc.* 22:440, 1974.

Kinsey, A. C., et al. *Sexual Behavior in the Human Male*. Philadelphia: Saunders, 1949.

Kinsey, A. C., et al. *Sexual Behavior in the Human Female*. Philadelphia: Saunders, 1953.

Silverman, A. *Sexuality in the Later Years of Life: An Annotated Bibliography*. Ann Arbor, Mich.: Institute of Gerontology, 1975.

Solnick, S. (Ed.). *Sexuality and Aging*. Los Angeles, Calif.: University of Southern California Press, 1978.

## ENVIRONMENT

Altman, I. *The Environment and Social Behavior*. Monterey, Calif.: Brooks/Cole, 1975.

Annotated International Bibliography on Assisted Independent Residential Living for Older People. International Center for Social Gerontology, 425 13th Street N.W. Suite 840, Washington, D.C., 1977.

Kiernat, J. Adaptive living and accident prevention for the aged. *Allied Health Behav. Sci.* 2:1, 1979.

Langer, E., and Rodin, J. The effects of choice and enhanced personal responsibility for the aged. *J. Personality Soc. Psychol.* 34, 1976.

Lawton, M. P. *Environment and Aging*. Monterey, Calif.: Brooks/Cole, 1980.

Pastalan, L., and Carson, D. *Spatial Behavior of Older People*. Ann Arbor, Mich.: University of Michigan Press, 1970.

# 2 ONCOLOGICAL REHABILITATION

*Martha K. Logigian*

Approximately 675,000 people in the United States develop cancer each year. Of these, approximately one-third survive five years or more [9]. Functional loss resulting from the cancer and its treatment by surgery, radiation, chemotherapy, hormone therapy, or a combination of these, present the rehabilitation team with significant challenges.

Rehabilitation can assist the patient to maintain a productive level of activity, and thus achieve the desired quality of life. In general, rehabilitation problems consist of functional deficits in self-care and mobility, physical weakness, fatigue, pain, weight loss, and emotional distress. Sexual dysfunction, communication difficulties, and cosmetic concerns may also be present. Vocational restrictions and resultant financial burdens can be devastating to the patient and family.

Because of the varying needs and expectations of the patient with cancer, rehabilitation services need to be provided that are appropriate for the individual and the stage and type of cancer. Services include prosthetic, orthotic, or cosmetic devices following surgery; activities of daily living and exercise to help reduce complications following treatment; patient education and psychosocial support for both patient and family to aid acceptance and adjustment; and vocational counseling to assist future plans. In the case of the patient with advanced cancer, methods

The discussion of laryngeal and oral cancer was written by Frances Senner-Hurley and Nancy G. Lefkowitz.

of palliation are of assistance, such as maintaining comfort, and enhancing feelings of self-worth, dignity, and independence. This can be accomplished through the control of pain by proper positioning and medication, emotional support, and participation in appropriate self-care activities.

## Psychosocial Issues

Gates [21] says: "The emotional impact of cancer and its treatment is enormous to the patient and to the family often more than the physical impairments. The diagnosis of cancer brings immediate thoughts of death, usually lingering death, even though many cancers can now be cured and patients survive longer today with many cancers than they did a decade or two ago."

Although the individuality of each patient makes it difficult to generalize about the psychological impact of cancer, there are recurrent emotional issues that these patients frequently share, such as depression, denial, hostility, anger, guilt, despair, and anxiety. There are feelings of helplessness, questions as to why one deserves this fate, loss of self-esteem, and fears of disfigurement or death. There is often a lack of understanding of the illness that serves to complicate the issues. Frequently, as a result of the emotionally charged situation the patient experiences increased marital stress, change in family and societal relationships, and isolation.

The rehabilitation team must be able and

willing to support the patient and family in dealing with these issues. Through honest and open discussions about the diagnosis, treatment, side effects, and prognosis, anxiety can be relieved and the patient and family can arrive at a more complete understanding and acceptance of the disease. This involves communication among patient, family, and team members. The patient must be encouraged to ask questions and discuss feelings, fears, or physical discomfort. Team members need to take the time to find out what the patient has been told, spend time with the patient and family, and in general, demonstrate interest in them. Consequently, the patient is more likely to seek the kind of support that can greatly influence his or her interpretation of and response to the disease.

## The Team
The rehabilitation team consists of physician (oncologist, surgeon), nurse, physical therapist, occupational therapist, social worker, psychologist or psychiatrist, dietitian, and chaplain. The speech pathologist, vocational counselor, recreational therapist, enterostomal therapist, prosthetist or orthotist, respiratory therapist, a variety of physicians (radiologist, pathologist, prosthodontist), and radiology technician may also participate. An interdisciplinary approach is critical to the care of the problems and the emotion-laden issues with which the patient and family must cope. Such organization is necessary to ensure optimal coordination with them.

Although each team member functions primarily within an individual area of expertise, each must be aware of others' specialized abilities. To provide optimum care, cooperative and effective communication must occur, with each member being fully informed of the treatment and information the patient has received. It should be noted that the roles of the members may vary with the type and stage of the disease.

## Nutrition
Cancer and its treatment commonly lead to decreased appetite, weight loss, and in many instances, cachexia manifested by weakness, anorexia, metabolic depletion, hormonal changes, electrolyte imbalance, and altered vital functions. Consequently, nutritional maintenance is of prime concern.

Management must include appropriate assessment, with regular and accurate weight and body mass measurements recorded together with the patients' current intake of nutrients. Patients should be encouraged to eat whatever can be tolerated. Team members can do their part by dealing with the problems of taste abnormalities, nausea, pain, and depression. For example, these patients have increased threshold for sweet tastes and decreased for bitter tastes. Through the use of flavor enhancers and seasoning, the appeal of foods might be improved [41].

Enteral alimentation is indicated when oral intake is inadequate, and is accomplished by a duodenal tube through which feedings are given. If the gastrointestinal tract is nonfunctional, hyperalimentation or parenteral nutrition is a necessity. Through an intravenous line the patient is fed caloric solutions and amino acids with required electrolytes and vitamins. This is accomplished by a hyperalimentation team that consists of the physician who places the catheter; the nurse who is responsible for the explanation and maintenance of the catheter and feedings; the pharmacist who prepares the solutions; the dietitian who determines the nutritional content of the solution; and the physical and occupational therapists who are responsible for mobilizing the patient through exercise and activity [51].

## Pain
Twycross [56] estimates that 40 percent of cancer patients have severe pain, for 10 percent it is less severe, and 50 percent have

none. Although pain could be from nonmalignant causes or the effects of immobilization, it is primarily the result of the disease. Pain associated with the malignancy can arise from nerve compression, nerve tissue infiltration, conduit obstruction, vascular interference, and pathological bone fracture. Infection or the cancer can cause inflammation in pain-sensitive structures, or a sensory neuropathy can result. Dodd and Livingstone [14] note: "Pain occurs most frequently in cancer of the cervix, lung, rectum, and prostate. It may develop in other types of cancer but is not as common."

Spiers [52] recommends management by treatment of the cause rather than the symptom. Examples of this are surgery for removal of an obstruction; radiation therapy directed at painful metastases; hormonal therapy for bone pain in disseminated prostatic cancer; chemotherapy for metastatic breast cancer; antibiotics for infections; or corticosteroids for headache resulting from metastatic brain tumors. When primary pain control is impossible, inadequate, or delayed, modification of neural processing of the painful stimulus or its perception is indicated [18].

Non-narcotic analgesics such as aspirin or acetaminophen used alone or in combination with the narcotic codeine are used for relief of pain. Oral narcotics are available, such as Demerol, Dilaudid, Brompton's solution, Percodan, and Darvon. If they are not sufficient, parenteral narcotic analgesics are used, principally morphine or methadone. Particularly in palliative care [18], "while pain management will be multifactional, it is most effectively built around the regular, time-dependent administration of adequate doses of narcotic analgesics." In addition, pain can be moderated by nonpharmacological measures such as proper positioning, skin care, hot packs, and a supportive environment. Antianxiety and antidepression medications may also be useful, particularly when pain's emotional aspects consume the patient's attention [18].

Anesthetic-neurosurgical procedures, al-though successful in interrupting pain pathways, are rarely used because of the complexity of the pain associated with cancer. For those whose pain is lateralized and nonvisceral, and whose life expectancy is a reasonable period of time, a local nerve block or section, rhizotomy, cordotomy, tractotomy, thalamotomy, or brain stimulation may be indicated [18, 52].

## Bowel and Bladder
Analgesics, particularly codeine and the narcotics, improper diet, and prolonged bedrest can cause constipation. The use of stool softeners and enemas may be indicated. Spiers notes further [52], "Weakness, debility, and sedation promote urinary incontinence in ill patients. The discomforts of such incontinence are accompanied by an enhanced risk of bed sores, and early treatment by condom or catheter drainage is advisable."

## Metastases
Cancer cells that invade the lymphatic and blood vessels allow tumor cells to spread to other parts of the body and set up additional tumor colonies, or *metastases*. The most common metastatic site is the lung. Other sites include the central nervous system (brain metastases or spinal cord compression from epidural or vertebral metastases), bone, liver, abdomen, and pelvis [10]. Some systemic effects of malignancy are anorexia and altered taste, nausea, cachexia, anemia, hypercalcemia, fever, infection, hypercoagulability, and hormone syndromes. Medication and other medical treatments are used in their management. The reader is referred to *Clinical Oncology: For Medical Students and Physicians, a Multidisciplinary Approach* [43], Chapter 24, for more details.

Significant problems face the patient with metastatic disease of the bone, primarily, pain and loss of function of the involved area because of pathological fractures. Most function is lost in bones that bear the most weight, that is, hip, back, and shoulder. Rib fractures can give enough pain to inhibit clearance of pulmonary secretion and lead to pneumonia. Bone pain is treated with hormonal or radiation therapy and analgesics.

To further minimize discomfort and the possibility of pathological fracture, special techniques of handling the patient are recommended. The patient should be carefully supported, with maximal assistance while being moved or turned in bed. A firm mattress and turning sheet can be of assistance. Proper positioning in bed and chair is essential. Small pillows behind the neck, under the elbow, or between the legs are helpful when in bed. Pillows on either side of the trunk while sitting in an armchair help support body weight. Transferring should be done slowly and with maximal assistance required. A back brace may be indicated for support when there is fracture of vertebrae. A shoulder immobilization sling is particularly effective in relieving pain and providing support when there is a pathological fracture in this area. Frequent changes in position are encouraged to prevent skin breakdown, promote circulation, and encourage control over and participation in one's environment.

As pain in metastatic disease may vary from day to day due to sleep loss, fever, nausea, inadequate nutrition, or depression, consideration must be given for individual patient needs on a particular day. Some days the most the patient can accomplish is sitting up in bed and dangling the feet over the side. On another day, wheelchair mobility or ambulation may be possibile, usually accomplished with assistance from the physical therapist and with the use of a walker. Analgesics may be appropriate prior to any activity to help minimize discomfort. Rest periods during ambulation are important to prevent overfatigue. Maintaining conditions as near normal as possible for the patient and family, and allowing and encouraging the patient to do as much as it is possible to do help to retain morale and relieve despair.

Metastatic disease brings the patient closer to death and heralds dealing with issues surrounding it. Depression can often be the biggest problem, and this places additional concern on the family and team. Patience and emotional support are essential. Preparing the patient and family for death can be an extremely valuable experience for all concerned; however, it can be a heavy burden that needs to be shared by all members of the team. As a detailed discussion of death and dying is beyond the scope of this text, the reader is referred to the work by Kübler-Ross and others listed in the suggested reading at the end of this chapter.

## Treatment Methods

To understand the impact of cancer on the patient and to provide needed explanation of the procedures used in its treatment, it is essential to have knowledge of those treatments. Specific functional deficits that occur in reaction to various modalities will be discussed relative to organ system involvement. It should be recognized that oncological treatment frequently involves combinations of the methods described.

### SURGERY

The aim of surgery is total removal of the malignant organ, tissue, tumor, or cells. It is particularly effective following early diagnosis, and is performed to treat most major forms of cancer [55]. The surgery is often radical, requiring removal of the malignant tissue, wide margins of normal tissue, and lymph nodes that drain the area. The last may be necessary to guard against the spread of disease, as bits of malignant tissue can move through the lymph system, become entrapped in the nodes, and establish secondary tumors.

Recovery is facilitated by good nursing care and a well-informed patient. Early mobilization and proper positioning help minimize complications. At times, surgery may be used in combination with radiation therapy or chemotherapy. In addition, if the cancer is advanced, making total removal impossible, surgery may be used to make the patient more comfortable and prolong life by relieving pain, or treating complications such as abscess or obstruction.

RADIATION THERAPY

This involves the use of radioactive substances to damage radiosensitive cancer cells. Radiation can be in the form of x-rays (electromagnetic waves produced by electrons when they strike a metal target), or gamma rays (produced from the breakdown of radioactive isotopes such as cobalt or radium). The latter involves beams of radiation delivered to the body as required, through a shutter. Radioactive isotopes can also be placed directly in or on the body by means of needles, capsules, wires, wax molds, plaques, seeds, or liquid. In general, the dose rather than the type of radiation is the important factor in treating cancer [55].

Radiation therapy is used to cure localized disease if the site is inaccessible for surgical removal, or if surgery would produce extensive damage to vital organs. It is also effective in reducing a tumor to operable size. Radiotherapy is a means of palliation that provides relief from symptoms and prolongs life. It can reduce the size and delay the spread of cancer, heal ulcerating tumors, diminish or stop persistent bleeding, relieve tumor-related obstructions of the blood or lymph vessels, relieve pain, or prevent fractures in the event of bone tumors or metastases [55].

Chemotherapy may be used in conjunction with radiation to increase the effects of the radiation, or to destroy cancer cells that have spread beyond the primary site and are not responsive to localized radiotherapy. When a patient is on combined therapy, the team must be aware of how they interact and whether one enhances the other, as reactions may occur more quickly than with just one treatment modality, and be more severe [45].

Patients receiving radiation therapy need to be made aware of the precautions, contraindications, and side effects.

1. Lines made with red ink may be drawn on the skin indicating the area to be irradiated, and must remain in place until the entire treatment is completed.

2. Extreme temperatures must be avoided on the treatment area, such as hot or cold packs and excessive exposure to sunshine. Skin irritation may follow treatment, and patients must practice proper skin care. Dermatological preparations should be used on skin receiving radiation only after consultation with the radiation therapist [53].

3. Consideration must be given for the fear and anxiety associated with this treatment. As Levene [36] notes, "Most patients faced with undergoing radiation treatment are frightened by the aura of mystery surrounding radiation therapy. They often have been subjected to a variety of upsetting predictions by well-meaning friends and family. A careful explanation of what they may actually expect will usually prove very helpful. Many of the symptoms arising from radiation therapy are controllable with medications. Those symptoms not relieved with appropriate drugs may require a brief interruption of treatment or a decrease in the size of the daily radiation dose. A common misconception among patients receiving radiation therapy is that they or their personal belongings will become radioactive as a result of the treatments. They should be reassured that such is not the case."

4. Because of inherent hazards, precautions must be taken when handling dressings and working with radioisotope applicators or implants.

5. Radiation to large areas of the body may depress bone marrow and result in anemia, low white blood cell count (leukopenia), and a low platelet count (thrombocytopenia), thus leaving the patient susceptible to fatigue, infection, or bleeding, respectively. Antibiotics to treat infection and transfusions to increase red cell count and platelet count are used to combat these side effects.

6. Loss of taste, decreased appetite, nausea, ulcers, and fatigue may be experienced follow-

ing treatment. Other side effects relative to particular organ system include:

a. Dysphagia in patients treated in the oral and upper trunk region
b. Loss of appetite, nausea, vomiting, urinary frequency, diarrhea, and cramps in patients receiving abdominal radiation
c. Myocarditis or pericarditis if the whole heart is irradiated, and pneumonitis if a large area of the lung is involved
d. Reduction of salivary gland activity causing a decrease in saliva and reduction in normal pH, making the patient more susceptible to tooth decay and esophagitis during radiation to the head and neck
e. Hair loss on the face and scalp with radiation to the head and neck
f. Transient myelopathy characterized by paresthesia or permanent paresis, or paralysis with radiation to the spinal cord.

## CHEMOTHERAPY

Chemotherapy is the longest in duration of the treatment methods, and places the greatest physical and psychological stress on the patient [51]. Table 2-1 gives common chemotherapeutic agents and their side effects. The drug used will depend on the type of cancer. The team, patient, and family must be aware of possible side effects and limitations to be placed on the patient, such as isolation in a sterile environment.

As can be seen in Table 2-1, anorexia, nausea, and vomiting are common with most cytotoxic agents. Antiemetic drugs can be helpful in dealing with these symptoms. As mentioned earlier, meals should be appealing and presented in pleasant surroundings. Proper mouth care can help to eliminate the bad taste that may reduce appetite.

Diarrhea is common in patients receiving antibiotics and antimetabolites, and necessitates an increase in fluids and a diet low in roughage. In addition, good oral hygiene must be practiced by patients receiving these drugs because of the common occurrence of stomatitis, or inflamed, painful mouth ulcers.

Bone marrow suppression can cause leuko-penia (low white blood cell count), thus increasing the patient's susceptibility to infection. It has been found [25] that "nasal infections, rectal abscesses, lip ulcers and eye infections cause the patients much suffering." Good body hygiene must be practiced to protect the patient from infection. If the white blood cell count falls too low, the patient may be placed in isolation, or the drug may be stopped to allow the bone marrow to recover. Anemia (low red blood cell count) can cause the patient to fatigue easily, often with decreased exercise tolerance. Thrombocytopenia also results from bone marrow suppression, and may bring on bleeding requiring platelet transfusions. Patients must take care to avoid cuts and bruises.

Plant alkaloid drugs can cause neuropathies and personality changes. The patient must be told to watch for impaired sensation, loss of coordination, unsteady gait, or severe constipation. The patient should be prepared for unusual feelings such as depression, so that if it occurs it can be kept in perspective.

As some investigators suggest [37]: "Alopecia, most often caused by alkylating agents, plant alkaloids and some antibiotics can be devastating to a patient's self-image, especially when it occurs suddenly. Hair follicles proliferate rapidly, so they are damaged as much as, if not more than, the malignant cells . . . . Much hair loss can be prevented by using a scalp tourniquet during I.V. administration to protect the hair follicles from high concentrations of the drug." Ice bags are also being used to control hair loss on the scalp. The use of wigs, scarves, turbans, and hats should be discussed with the patient. They further state that [37], "once the drug is stopped, hair regrows in about eight weeks."

## HORMONE THERAPY

Breast, prostate, uterus, and thyroid are sites known to produce tumors that may respond to changes in concentration of hormones. Steroidal hormones seem to affect growth, division, and function of the susceptible cell. Because of the gradual change of the hormonal

TABLE 2-1. *Cancer Chemotherapeutic Agents*

| Agent | Administration | Indications | Side Effects/Toxicity |
|---|---|---|---|
| *Alkylating agents* | | | |
| Nitrogen mustard (Mustargen) | IV, intracavity (for effusions) | Lymphomas; bronchogenic, heart, and ovarian carcinomas; malignant effusions | Severe nausea and vomiting ½-8 hr after dose; bone marrow suppression |
| Melphalan (Alkeran) | Oral, IV | Multiple myeloma; ovarian, breast, and testicular carcinomas | Moderate nausea and vomiting; little or no alopecia; bone marrow suppression |
| Cyclophosphamide (Cytoxan) | Oral, IV | Lymphomas; chronic lymphocytic leukemia; multiple myeloma; breast, bronchogenic, ovarian tumors; neuroblastoma | Nausea and vomiting 3-4 hr after dose; alopecia 50% of cases; hemorrhagic cystitis; bone marrow suppression; amenorrhea; diminished spermatogenesis appears permanent |
| Chlorambucil (Leukeran) | Oral | Chronic lymphocytic leukemia; Hodgkin's disease; trophoblastic neoplasms; ovarian carcinoma | Minimal nausea and vomiting; bone marrow suppression; dermatitis; hepatotoxicity; gonadal toxicity; alterations of spermatogenesis with variable recovery after cessation of drug |
| Thiotepa | IV, IM, intracavity for effusions | Lymphomas; ovarian and breast carcinomas; malignant effusions | Occasional nausea and vomiting; headache; fever; allergic reactions; GI perforation; mild anemia; bone marrow suppression 5-30 days after dose |
| Busulfan (Myleran) | Oral | Stable phase of chronic myelogenous leukemia; polycythemia vera | Minimal nausea and vomiting; bone marrow suppression; skin pigmentation; gynecomastia; amenorrhea; irreversible pulmonary fibrosis; renal damage; affects spermatogenesis |
| *Antimetabolites* | | | |
| Methotrexate | Oral, IV, IM, intrathecally | Acute leukemia; meningeal leukemia; trophoblastic tumors; head and neck, breast, bronchogenic carcinomas | Nausea and vomiting; diarrhea; ulceration of oral mucosa; GI ulcers; stomatitis; alopecia; hepatic dysfunction; photosensitivity seen early; bone marrow suppression; infertility; dermatitis; headache and blurred vision; menstrual dysfunction |
| Fluorouracil (5-FU) | IV, oral | Colon, breast, ovarian, gastric carcinomas | Nausea and vomiting; diarrhea 2-3 days after dose; stomatitis 5th-8th day; anorexia; bone marrow suppression 9-14 days after dose; some alopecia; darkening of veins; oral effect variable |

TABLE 2-1. *(Continued)*

| Agent | Administration | Indications | Side Effects/Toxicity |
|---|---|---|---|
| Floxuridine (5-FUDR) | Intraarterial | Colon, gallbladder, bile duct carcinomas; liver metastasis | Nausea and vomiting; diarrhea; stomatitis; bone marrow suppression 7-14 days after dose; some alopecia |
| Cytarabine (Cytosar) | IV, subcutaneously, intrathecally | Acute myeloblastic or myelomonocytic leukemia | Nausea and vomiting; gastrointestinal disturbances (stomatitis, esophagitis); bone marrow suppresion 7-14 days after dose; hepatotoxicity; diarrhea; skin rash; crosses blood/brain barrier |
| Mercaptopurine (6-MP) | Oral | Childhood leukemia; chronic leukemia | Oral and GI ulceration; occasional nausea and vomiting; liver dysfunction; bone marrow suppression 4-6 wk after dose; stomatitis; diarrhea |
| Thioguanine (6-TG) | Oral | Acute leukemia | Some nausea and vomiting; diarrhea; stomatitis; skin rash; jaundice; photosensitivity; bone marrow suppression |
| *Natural Products* | | | |
| Vincristine (Oncovin) | IV | Acute lymphoblastic leukemia; Hodgkin's disease; neuroblastoma; Wilms' tumor | Abdominal colic; diarrhea; severe constipation; nausea and vomiting; stomatitis; alopecia; minimal bone marrow suppression; neurotoxicities include: areflexia, peripheral neuropathy, paresthesias, footdrop, weakness, ataxia, mixed sensorimotor and autonomic symptoms; severe skin ulceration with extravasation |
| Vinblastine (Velban) | IV | Hodgkin's disease; MTX-resistant choriocarcinoma | Bone marrow suppression; nausea and vomiting; diarrhea; neurotoxic paresthesias, loss of deep tendon reflexes; constipation; urinary retention; occasional mental depression; local phlebitis; severe skin ulceration with extravasation; diminished spermatogenesis |
| *Antibotics* | | | |
| Doxorubicin (Adriamycin) | IV | Sarcomas; breast, lung, bladder, thyroid, ovarian carcinomas; lymphomas; acute leukemia; neuroblastoma; Wilms' tumor | Nausea and vomiting; fever; stomatitis; gastrointestinal disturbance; bone marrow suppression; severe alopecia; myocardial damage; severe skin necrosis with extravasation; causes red urine up to 12 days after dose |

TABLE 2-1. *(Continued)*

| Agent | Administration | Indications | Side Effects/Toxicity |
|---|---|---|---|
| Daunorubicin (Daunomycin) | IV | Acute lymphoblastic and myeloblastic leukemia | Nausea and vomiting; fever; stomatitis; alopecia; bone marrow suppression; phlebitis; abdominal pain; red urine; cardiotoxicity (sudden CHF) |
| Bleomycin (Blenoxane) | IV, IM, SC | Squamous cell carcinoma of the skin, head, and neck; Hodgkin's disease; cervical, testicular carcinoma | Fever; chills; hypotension; anaphylaxis; nausea and vomiting; skin and nail damage (macular rash); stomatitis; tumor pain; alopecia; acute pulmonary edema; pulmonary fibrosis; pneumonitis; minimal bone marrow suppression |
| Mithramycin (Mithracin) | IV | Testicular carcinoma; trophoblastic tumors; hypercalcemia | Nausea and vomiting peaks 6 hr after dose; hypocalcemia; hypokalemia 24-48 hr after dose; fever; stomatitis; renal damage; liver toxicity; elevated prothrombin time and other clotting abnormalities |
| Mitomycin-C (Mutamycin) | IV | Pancreatic, gastric, cervical, breast, bronchogenic, head, and neck carcinoma; malignant melanoma | Nausea and vomiting; diarrhea; delayed bone marrow suppression 4-8 wk after dose; fever; stomatitis; pruritus; alopecia; paresthesias; renal damage |
| Actinomycin-D (Cosmegen) | IV | MTX-resistant choriocarcinoma; testicular tumors; childhood solid tumors such as Wilms' tumor and rhabdomyosarcoma | Nausea and vomiting 4-5 hr after dose; anorexia last few weeks; stomatitis; diarrhea; gastrointestinal disturbances; alopecia; mental depression; acne; malaise; fever; myalgia; bone marrow suppression; local inflammation |
| Streptozotocin | IV | Carcinoid tumors; functioning islet cell tumors of the pancreas | Nausea and vomiting; renal damage; stomatitis; abdominal cramps; nephrotoxicity; may cause hypoglycemia from sudden relase of insulin; diabetogenic; rapid infusion causing local burning sensation |
| Streptonigrin | IV, oral | — | Bone marrow suppression |
| *Enzymes* | | | |
| L-Asparaginase (Elspar, L-ASP) | IV | Acute lymphoblastic leukemia | Nausea and vomiting; fever; possible anaphylaxis; anorexia; CNS abnormalities; malaise; hepatotoxicity; azotemia; blood dyscrasias; hypoalbuminemia; hyperglycemia |

TABLE 2-1. *(Continued)*

| Agent | Administration | Indications | Side Effects/Toxicity |
|---|---|---|---|
| BCG | Intralesional, intradermal, IV, Heaf-gun; scarification, multipuncture | Acute and chronic leukemia; bronchogenic carcinoma; malignant melanoma; lymphoma | Local inflammation, then necrosis, eschar, and later healing; flu-like syndrome with fever, myalgia, nausea, vomiting, and lymphadenopathy; possible anaphylaxis and syndrome resembling tuberculin shock |
| *Miscellaneous Agents* | | | |
| Carmustine (BCNU) | IV | Primary/secondary CNS tumors; lymphomas; multiple myeloma; malignant melanoma | Nausea and vomiting; delayed bone marrow suppression 3-4 wk after dose; local inflammation; mild hepatotoxicity; crosses blood/brain barrier |
| Lomustine (CCNU) | Oral | Hodgkin's disease; primary/secondary CNS tumors; gastric, renal, bronchogenic carcinomas | Nausea and vomiting; delayed bone marrow suppression 4-6 wk after dose; hepatotoxicity; crosses blood/brain barrier |
| Semustine (Methyl CCNU) | Oral | Primary/secondary CNS tumors; stomach, pancreatic, colon, bronchogenic, squamous cell carcinomas; malignant melanoma | Nausea and vomiting; delayed bone marrow suppression 3-4 wks after dose |
| Dacarbazine (DTIC) | IV | Malignant melanoma; Hodgkin's disease | Nausea and vomiting; delayed bone marrow suppression 2-4 wks after dose; sometimes flulike syndrome with head-ache, myalagia, and malaise; may burn on injection and give metallic taste; protect from light |
| Procarbazine (Matulane) | Oral | Lymphomas; leukemia; bronchogenic carcinoma | Nausea and vomiting; bone marrow suppression; CNS depression; restlessness; some alopecia; skin rash; orthostatic hypotension; crosses blood/ brain barrier; affects spermatogenesis |
| Mitotane (Lysodren) | Oral | Chronic leukemia; malignant melanoma; ovarian carcinoma | Nausea and vomiting; bone marrow suppression; teratogenesis; anorexia; alopecia; rash; pruritus; erythema, buccal, and GI ulcerations; crosses blood/brain barrier |
| O,ṕ-DDD | Oral | Adrenal cortex cancer after excision | Nausea and vomiting; anorexia; diarrhea; gastrointestinal symptoms; lethargy; somnolence; skin rash; CNS depression; dizziness; tremors |

TABLE 2-1. *(Continued)*

| Agent | Administration | Indications | Side Effects/Toxicity |
|---|---|---|---|
| *Hormones* | | | |
| *Estrogens* | | *All estrogens* | *All estrogens* |
| Diethylstilbestrol (DES) | Oral | Prostatic and breast carcinomas | Nausea and vomiting; GI upset; salt and fluid retention; hypercalcemia; libido changes and impairment of ejaculation; uterine bleeding in menopausal women; gynecomastia; polydipsia; polyuria; muscle weakness; lethargy |
| Conjugated estrogens | Oral | | Less nauseating |
| Ethinyl estradiol (Estinyl) | Oral | | Less nauseating |
| *Androgens* | | *All androgens* | *All androgens* |
| Testosterone propionate | IM | Breast cancer; postmenopausal or postcastration | Nausea and vomiting; fluid retention; anorexia; hot flashes; myalgia; libido change and virilization in women; hypercalcemia |
| Fluoxymesterone (Halotestin) | Oral | | Less virilization; fever; increased libido |
| *Progesterones* | | | *All progesterones* |
| 17-α-hydroxyprogesterone caproate (Delalutin) | IM | Endometrial and breast carcinomas | No acute toxicity; minimal fluid retention |
| Medroxyprogesterone acetate (Provera) | Oral, IM | Endometrial, renal cell, and breast carcinomas | |
| *Adrenocorticosteroids* | | *Numerous preparations, the following apply to all* | |
| Prednisone | Oral | Leukemia; lymphoma; breast and multiple myeloma; hypercalcemia; anemia; hyperkalemia; to reduce CNS edema; general debility; fever (noninfectious); anorexia | No acute toxicity; increased appetite; euphoria; long-term treatment causes body changes such as moonface, striae, trunk obesity, purpura, osteoporosis, muscle weakness, psychosis, potassium loss; sodium and fluid retention; hypertension; infection; diabetes; gastric bleeding and ulcers; hyperadrenocorticism or adrenal atrophy possible |
| Dexamethasone | Oral | | |

Source: From R. F. Backemeier, Principles of Medical Oncology and Cancer Chemotherapy. In P. Rubin (Ed.), *Clinical Oncology: For Medical Students and Physicians, a Multi-disciplinary Approach.* New York: American Cancer Society, 1974. R. C. Kolodny; W. H. Masters; and V. E. Johnson. *Textbook of Sexual Medicine.* Boston: Little, Brown, 1979. E. B. Marino, and D. H. LeBlanc. Cancer Chemotherapy. *Nursing '75.* 5(11): 22, 1975.

environment, therapy is usually used initially for one to three months of continuous therapy, with further endocrine manipulations occurring when the first response ends [39].

As can be seen in Table 2-1, fluid retention often accompanies hormone therapy, and requires the use of a low-salt diet and the close monitoring of weight and fluid intake and output. The patient must be observed for signs of edema and congestive heart failure (CHF). As retained fluids stretch and weaken the skin, caution must be taken to avoid decubitus ulcers. The patient who is receiving diuretics should learn to recognize the signs of lowered potassium, and how to deal with this through dietary supplements.

Temporary changes in secondary sexual characteristics may be seen in patients taking androgen or estrogen. These changes should be discussed with the patient, and reassurance given that symptoms last only as long as the drug is taken. Personality changes may occur with patients taking corticosteroids. Again, to avoid a catastrophic reaction, they should be made aware that this may occur.

## IMMUNOTHERAPY

This treatment uses the body's natural defense of its immunological system. The system recognizes and rejects foreign substances or antigens, and produces counter-substances or antibodies and inactivate antigens. There is indication that cancer tissue differs antigenically from normal tissue, and that the body's defenses may be induced to act against the malignancy. This type of treatment is largely experimental.

## SPECIAL CONSIDERATIONS

As part of rehabilitation patients should be made aware of existing organizations and support groups. Organizations that address a specific population are identified according to cancer site and are listed below.

American Cancer Society
National Office
377 3rd Avenue
New York, NY 10017

ENCORE
National Board
YWCA
600 Lexington Avenue
New York, NY 10022

Leukemia Society of America
211 East 43rd Street
New York, NY 10017

National Foundation for Ileitis and Colitis, Inc.
295 Madison Avenue
New York, NY 10017

Office of Cancer Communications
National Cancer Program
National Cancer Institute of the National Institutes of Health
Bethesda, MD 20014

Public Affairs Pamphlets
381 Park Avenue South
New York, NY 10016

United Ostomy Association
1111 Wilshire Boulevard
Los Angeles, CA 90017

The American Cancer Society is one of the largest volunteer organizations in this country, with chartered divisions throughout the United States. It sponsors research as well as provides education and service for patients and practitioners. Workshops sponsored by the Society are excellent means for practitioners to learn specific treatment techniques. In addition, it is a fine source of patient education materials. Action programs such as stop-smoking clinics and breast self-examination demonstrations are provided for the public, as are rehabilitation programs for patients and their families.

The U.S. Department of Health, Education, and Welfare, Public Health Service, and National Institutes of Health have a variety of materials available for the public and professionals, many of which have been prepared by the Office of Cancer Communications. Literature on cancer and other topics is also available through the Public Affairs Pamphlets.

## Common Cancer Sites

The following sections provide information on problems specific to sites. The types of cancer discussed are those most commonly seen in rehabilitation facilities. (Rehabilitation programs for those with lung cancer, and bone and soft tissue malignancy can be found in the pulmonary and orthopedics [Amputation] chapters respectively.) Treatment procedures and references are relative to cancer site as well. Introductory remarks on the psychosocial aspects of the disease and treatment should be kept in mind. The descriptive material for these sections was obtained from Rubin [43] and the American Cancer Society [8].

### BLOOD (LEUKEMIA, LYMPHOMA, HODGKIN'S DISEASE, AND MULTIPLE MYELOMA)

*Leukemia* is a group of neoplastic disorders involving the cells of the blood-forming organs. Most leukemias are characterized by the uncontrolled multiplication and accumulation of abnormal white cells resulting in anemia, increased susceptibility to infection, and hemorrhage. They are usually grouped into acute and chronic categories based on length of survival and degree of maturation of the cells. Leukemias are subdivided according to cell type involved: lymphocytic, granulocytic, monocytic, and unclassified. The incidence of all leukemias in the United States is approximately 9.7 per 100,000 population. Of those, acute leukemias make up 50 percent, with children accounting for 80 percent of the acute lymphocytic leukemia and adults (men more than women) for 90 percent of the acute nonlymphocytic leukemia.

Chemotherapy is the treatment used most frequently for the majority of leukemias, although it may be used in conjunction with radiation therapy in some forms of the disease. Remission can be achieved in 50 to 75 percent of those treated for acute nonlymphocytic leukemia, with a median survival of approximately 1 year. In chronic myelocytic leukemia, the median survival time is approximately 3½ years. Chronic lymphocytic leukemia occurs at the average age of 65 years, in men more than women, with an average survival of 6 to 7 years.

*Malignant lymphomas* are a group of clinically related diseases caused by neoplastic proliferation involving lymph nodes, bone marrow, spleen, or liver. *Hodgkin's disease* and non-Hodgkin's lymphomas are the most common. The incidence of Hodgkin's disease is 2.6 per 100,000 in men, and 2.2 per 100,000 in women. The disease is rare in children, with peak ages occurring at 30 and 70 years. Incidence of non-Hodgkin's lymphoma is 5.0 per 100,000 in men, and 3.4 per 100,000 in women. The median age is 50 years, and incidence increases with age. Radiation therapy is used in early stages of the disease; chemotherapy is combined with radiation therapy in the later stages. Overall response to treatment is approximately 80 percent, with long-term cure of approximately 50 percent.

*Multiple myelomas* are characterized by abnormal growth of plasma cells in the bone marrow. Although leukemias and lymphomas can quickly become widespread, multiple myeloma may remain localized in the bone for a time. The abnormal cells destroy normal bone tissue and cause pain. Back pain, anemia, and repeated infections are common symptoms. It occurs primarily between the ages of 50 to 70 years of age, and more than one-half the patients are men. Survival is approximately 9 to 24 months after initiation of therapy. Chemotherapy is used for treatment, and radiation for relief of pain.

FUNCTIONAL PROBLEMS

Generalized weakness and fatigue are common, and pathological fractures are an indication of advanced disease. The sequelae of chemotherapy pose significant problems for the rehabilitation team (refer to section on chemotherapy for details). Drugs that are toxic to the proliferating cells in the bone marrow also destroy the normal red and white blood cells and platelets. When the red cells are destroyed, the patient may become severely anemic and need frequent blood transfusions. With the destruction of white blood cells, the patient is susceptible to infection, and may require a germ-free environment and antibiotics. Ecchymotic areas, petechial rash, and bleeding gums are symptoms of platelet destruction, and can result in hemorrhaging requiring platelet transfusions. In this situation, the patient must be cautioned to avoid cuts and bruises.

Side effects of chemotherapy are significant and can be catastrophic. Painful mouth ulcers, gastrointestinal and rectal ulcerations, nausea and vomiting, malaise, and hair loss can cause extreme physical discomfort, embarrassment, and depression. Young patients need to be appraised of the sexual and reproductive implications of chemotherapy. With the exception of male infertility, toxic effects can be reversed on cessation of the drugs. Gynecomastia and infertility are common drug-induced phenomena and can lead to problems with body image and self-esteem.

REHABILITATION
As soon as tolerated, active range-of-motion exercises should be initiated. Mobility, activities of daily living, and ambulation begin as soon as the patient is able to participate. For patients with multiple myeloma, efforts to maintain maximal bone function is essential. Bedrest should be avoided and weight-bearing encouraged, with caution taken to avoid stress and strain on the skeletal structure.

Emotional support by the team members and sensitivity to the needs and values of the patient can help the individual through the difficulties of treatment. Sexual issues should be discussed honestly and openly. If sexual dysfunction poses a significant problem for the patient, referral to a psychotherapist is indicated.

Because of higher incidence of the disease in younger age groups, vocational problems are often at issue. Changes in academic or technical training may have to be considered. An employer's lack of understanding of the patient's prognosis can seriously impede present or future employment, and this requires action on the part of the rehabilitation team.

The patient and family must be helped to deal with the remission and regression of these diseases. Educating them and the community is critical.

SPECIAL CONSIDERATIONS
The Leukemia Society of America, Inc. supports research and provides funds for outpatients being treated for leukemia, the lymphomas, and Hodgkin's disease. It also provides referral services and professional and public education.

HEAD AND NECK (LARYNGEAL AND ORAL CANCER)
Cancer of the oral pharyngolaryngeal tract is directly related to tobacco and alcohol abuse, particularly in combination. It accounts for approximately five percent of all malignancies, and is more common in men than women. The disease and its treatment result in profound cosmetic and functional problems and associated social stigma.

LARYNGEAL CANCER
There are approximately 30,000 people who have undergone laryngectomy in the United States, with male-female ratio of 5.5:1. Statistics indicate a narrowing of the sex-based gap over recent years, which may be caused by the increased incidence of smoking-related cancer in women. Patients with localized disease have a five-year survival of 80 percent.

Often the first signs of the disease are noted by the patient. Persistent cough with or without hoarseness is a common initial symptom. If neglected, additional problems such as difficulty swallowing, ear pain, or coughing up blood are likely to develop. Management includes radiation, surgery (partial or total removal of the larynx and surrounding structures), chemotherapy, or some combination of these. When the larynx is totally removed (laryngectomy), the patient is without sound generation for speech because of disruption of the pathway between the oropharynx and trachea, which precludes normal respiration. Therefore a permanent stoma in the neck through which the patient breathes is created to maintain a patent airway.

*Functional Problems*
In addition to the communication problem following radical surgery, the patient with laryngectomy may experience decreased muscular strength, limited range of motion of the upper extremity, and pain. As a consequence of physical alterations, the patient is confronted with numerous life changes that are often related to cosmesis, function, social and emotional issues, and vocation.

*Rehabilitation*
The oncology team provides consistent and realistic preoperative information, including a description of the surgically induced alterations in anatomy and their effects. Having patients verbalize the information received is an effective technique for determining their level of understanding. As a communication specialist, the speech-language pathologist provides information pertaining to the various methods of communication following surgery.

Prior to surgery, with the physician's consent, it is desirable for the patient and family to meet someone who has had a laryngectomy, and who is proficient with one or both methods of acquired alaryngeal speech. This person may use esophageal speech or one of the approximately 15 commercially available artificial devices [6].

General limitations with this form of speech are as follows:

1. Difficulty with manual dexterity because of arthritis, hemiplegia, or quadriplegia
2. Poor articulatory habits
3. Insufficient integrity of articulators
4. Decreased mental status because of senility or confusion; language disabilities; decreased intellectual status affecting memory, attention, understanding, and ability to learn
5. Generalized weakness or fatigue
6. Extensive surgery, including to the oral structures
7. Decreased hearing acuity
8. Excessive saliva
9. Lack of or inaccessibility to a training facility or speech instructor
10. Negative attitudes or psychological maladjustment, including lack of motivation

Whenever possible, the speech-language pathologist obtains preoperative baseline data, including a speech and language sample to assess articulation, prosody, and resonance, an oral peripheral examination (after surgery it is readministered and the surgical report reviewed), and audiometric screening. The results provide information regarding speech skills that may influence the outcome of later treatment.

After surgery it is essential to establish an alternate mode of communication. If the patient is unable to write a message, a picture board or system of gestures can be developed. Some hospitals have intraoral devices available on loan, thus allowing immediate verbal communication. Specific training by the speech-language pathologist is indicated to achieve optimal use of the device.

Medical clearance is required prior to beginning an active alaryngeal speech training program, whether esophageal, with an artificial device, or both.

There are two types of artificial devices: electronic and pneumatic. Electronic devices are further divided into neck and intraoral types, depending on placement. Both have a

TABLE 2-2. *Problems Affecting Acquisition of Alaryngeal Speech*

| Esophageal Speech | Intraoral Device | Neck Device | Pneumatic Device |
|---|---|---|---|
| Stenosis of esophagus | Dentures | Fibrotic tissue secondary to radiation | Pain or tenderness in stoma area |
| Recurrence of cancer | Poor oral hygiene | | Stomaphobia |
| Hernia or ulcers | Excess saliva | Decreased or increased neck sensation | Emphysema or bronchitis |
| Colostomy | Decreased palatal sensation | | Pulmonary insufficiency |
| Edema and secretion in hypopharynx | | Swelling | Cardiac problems |
| Too much tone or inadequate approximation of the pharyngeoesophageal (PE) segment | | Scar tissue | Excessive stoma or secretions |
| | | Insufficient or excessive neck tissue | Decreased abdominal support |
| | | Pharyngeal fistula | |

vibratory source and a sound transmitter, but they differ in the method of sound activation. The pneumatic device is driven by air from the patient's lungs, and requires the use of both hands. The battery-operated electronic device is held in the patient's non-dominant hand. Prior to using this instrument, adjustments in volume and pitch should be made [5].

In addition to the devices available commercially, numerous modifications to improve quality and performance have been described [6]. While it is not necessary for the speech-language pathologist to have them all on hand, a sampling of at least three to four should be available during the selection process [6]. Following a trial of several, one is selected and ordered. Some factors in making the choice are the patient's and family's reactions, the patient's needs, clarity of speech, ease of handling, and finances. Specific contraindications, considerations, and limitations regarding the artificial devices are presented in Table 2-2.

Blom [5] developed the following program with regard to the use of an artificial device:

1. Placement of the device, with initial emphasis on accuracy of voicing, followed by speed with accuracy
2. Timing of accurate onset and termination of voicing so that it corresponds with the speech utterance; stimuli involve a progression from single words to conversational speech
3. Articulation training based on aerodynamic principles; this primarily involves instruction with consonants
4. Normalizing phrasing and rate
5. Incorporating inflection and stress when possible, for example, with pneumatic devices and some neck devices

The approach of Salmon and Goldstein [46] to treatment shows many parallels to that of Blom. They recommend the following hierarchy of speech stimuli for use in training: vowels, consonant-vowels with initial avoidance of stops and fricatives, automatic social phrases, serial speech, questions with known answers, and significant speech. They stress the need to develop and make use of the patient's auditory feedback system at all levels for the patient to make the necessary modifications in verbalizing.

It is the authors' contention that proficiency with the device requires systematic instruction by a speech-language pathologist knowledgeable in anatomy, physiology, speech science, and speech and voice production including suprasegmental features. The importance of helping the patient to achieve the best voice possible cannot be overemphasized; therefore clinicians are cautioned regarding the premature termination of training with the device.

With an artificial device early communication is essential, as it provides an immediate means of verbalizing, which it has been suggested [13, 20, 46] reduces anxiety, improves articulation, and may facilitate the learning of esophageal speech.

Esophageal speech begins with the introduction and trapping of a column of air into the upper one-third of the esophagus. As the air is released and expelled, tissue is set into vibration and acts as a pseudoglottis. A complex sequence of events, which includes changes in air pressure, follows. The end stage is shaping words by the articulators in the oral cavity [12, 13, 20, 30].

Two methods of air intake for learning sound production are commonly recognized: injection (prespeech and consonant-injection), and inhalation. These methods differ in terms of where positive and negative air pressure changes occur during air intake [12, 20]. Esophageal sound thus involves several discrete behaviors, including pressure changes, articulation, articulatory transitions, and voicing. These components must be smoothly integrated to be perceived as a single unit.

Various approaches for obtaining the first sound are reported [12, 13, 20, 35, 42], ranging from a nondirect approach, which selectively reinforces nonvolitional sound, to more direct approaches that involve imitation or specific verbal instruction regarding articulatory placement and movement [17].

The acquisition of esophageal sound as described by Berlin [4], requires 4 basic skills:

1. Ability to phonate on demand
2. Maintenance of a short latency between inflation of the esophagus and vocalization
3. Maintenance of adequate duration of phonation
4. Ability to sustain phonation during articulation

During the early stages of treatment it is critical to extinguish all undesirable and extraneous behaviors that occur with esophageal speech production [26]. Some of the more frequently observed of these are clunking, clicking, lip smacking, facial grimacing, and other accessory movements. Undesirable and inefficient methods of voice production may develop and should not be mistaken for esophageal voice. Pharyngeal and buccal voice ("Donald Duck speech") must be identified and eliminated promptly. Correction of these problems may necessitate change in method of air intake from injection to inhalation [20].

There are numerous publications that contain practice materials [12, 19, 20, 26, 29, 35, 42]. Some [20] include hierarchies of stimuli, with attention focused on phonemic makeup and stimulus length. The best sources for learning specific techniques for initiating and refining esophageal speech are not found in the literature, but at professional continuing education conferences and workshops. Many of these are sponsored by the American Cancer Society.

Once proficiency in basic skills is reached, the focus of treatment moves toward refinement. Objectives during refinement of both esophageal speech and that with an artificial device show notable parallels:

1. Articulation aimed at achieving voice and voiceless and nasal and non-nasal contrasts
2. Normalization of rate, which is less for an esophageal speaker than a normal speaker
3. Increase in phrase length with short latencies between phrases
4. Development of prosodic features aimed at variety in intonation, stress, and intensity [5, 26]

At least six months of active treatment are required, and 17 to 50 percent of patients do not achieve esophageal speech [23, 59]. The postsurgical anatomical and physiological features, in particular the reconstruction of the pharyngoesophageal (PE) segment [59] strongly influence speech acquisition. Those patients with good esophageal speech were found to have a looser PE segment, while patients with a tight PE segment have difficulty achieving esophageal speech and often have swallowing difficulties requiring dilatation. Several researchers [25, 47] have discussed characteristics that good esophageal speakers exhibit.

Total communication is stressed, and preferably the patient is trained in both types of speech production, and will then be able to choose the one that affords the best communication in a given situation [46].

Frequently, because of numerous medical complications and psychological manifestations, successful verbal communication is not achieved. Under such circumstances, alternate modes need to be explored. Possibilities are a gestural system, such as Amerind [50], picture or word boards, and computerized communication systems [54, 57]. If writing is the primary method, some modifications aimed at increasing speed, such as omission of articles, can be taught. Training is required to develop such systems, and necessitates family involvement and support of the team members.

Strategies for compensation of losses in function and methods of work simplification need to be provided by the therapists. Muscle strengthening and range-of-motion exercises, particularly to the shoulder area, are indicated to relieve pain and prevent complications. The nurse gives instruction in stoma care and sterile suctioning to prevent lung infections. The dietitian monitors diet and for side effects from nasogastric tube feedings such as diarrhea and distention, with modifications in feeding as needed.

The patient is likely to require support in adjusting to an altered body image and in dealing with feelings of anxiety, guilt, and shame. The family also need assistance to cope with the diagnosis, the patient's loss of speech and physical alterations, and possible vocational and financial issues. Early inter-

vention of the social worker and other team members, preferably prior to surgery, is recommended while the patient still has a voice for self-expression.

·Team teaching must focus on appropriate instruction of the patient and family with regard to safety precautions. Those who breathe through the neck should be advised to wear a Medic Alert necklace or bracelet, or carry an emergency identification card that details steps in resuscitation. A stoma cover is worn to prevent dust, dirt, and other foreign materials from entering the lungs. Within the home, an air humidification system is useful in maintaining good stomal condition. Showering is possible; however, protection of the stoma is required by a change in the patient's head position, position of the shower head, or use of a commercially available shower guard.

### Special Considerations

The American Cancer Society was instrumental in the inception of the International Association of Laryngectomees (IAL) in 1952, and remains the sole sponsor of the national IAL office [27]. The IAL assists hundreds of local chapters, typically named "Lost Chord" or "Nu Voice" clubs, by providing ideas and information to the clubs and the public. Training institutes are run, and a directory of esophageal speech instructors is published to further the goal of rehabilitation [28]. The individual club activities vary, but may include group speech therapy, counseling, orientation to special equipment, and socialization.

Numerous pamphlets are available at no cost, many through the American Cancer Society, that are geared to the lay person. Some of the issues addressed are mouth-to-neck resuscitation, reemployment, and therapy. *Looking Forward: A Guidebook for the Laryngectomee* [30] is a comprehensive book for patient and family addressing pre- and postoperative issues. In some areas of the country, resource manuals are compiled that provide a wealth of information regarding equipment, literature, and professional treatment.

ORAL CANCER

Among oral cancers, cancer of the lip occurs most frequently, followed by cancer of the tongue. Chronic exposure to irritants, particularly alcohol and tobacco in combination, as well as poor dental hygiene, have been implicated as predisposing factors. There is five-year survival of 67 percent for those treated for localized disease.

Treatments for cancer of the tongue are radiotherapy, surgery (glossectomy), and chemotherapy; they may be used singly or in combination depending on the location and extent of disease. Patients who do not undergo surgery rarely come to the attention of an allied health team. When surgery is performed, the diseased area and wide margins of healthy tissue are removed, the latter in an effort to prevent further spread. Surgery may involve partial or total removal of the tongue. If necessary, other structures such as the mandible or palate may be partially or totally excised. Because oral cancers are most often of the squamous cell type, a rapidly growing cancer, the likelihood of spread to neighboring structures is great. Futhermore, the tongue itself connects to the floor of the mouth, placing the patient at high risk for metastases to cervical nodes [15].

*Functional Problems*

Oral extirpative surgery creates numerous problems in chewing, swallowing, and speech. If the surgery is extensive it can create visible disfigurement, with accompanying psychosocial problems in addition to the physical ones.

*Rehabilitation*

In light of the special problems and needs of these patients, a coordinated team effort is essential to effective rehabilitation. During the preoperative period, the patient and family are provided with information about the nature of surgery, and prepared for the immediate and long-term effects. On physician request, a visit by a rehabilitated person who has undergone glossectomy may further assist in preparing the patient for surgery by providing a good role model and hope for the future. A recorded speech sample is obtained for analyses of articulation, phonation, resonance, prosody, and respiration.

For at least the first two postoperative weeks the patient requires suctioning to avoid the need for aspiration, nasogastric tube feedings, and antibiotics. Training in self-care, including oral hygiene, is important. In addition, involvement of the team with the patient and family to reinforce preparatory efforts and provide emotional support is recommended pre- and postoperatively for continuity of care. The speech-language pathologist explores and establishes with the patient a viable nonvocal system of communication using such alternatives as writing, gestures such as Amerind, picture or word boards, alphabet boards, and written cards of frequently occurring words or phrases.

It is worthwhile to train the patient in the use of an efficient writing system, with a goal of conveying messages in the fewest words. Skelly [48] details specific guidelines for achieving telegraphic writing. Should the patient be unable to develop effective verbal communication, any of the above methods, singly or in combination, could be used on a permanent basis.

Barring complications, speech rehabilitation may begin when the tracheal tube is still in place. By forming a tight seal with a finger, the patient can occlude the trachea and achieve phonation. Skelly [48] developed an approach to sound exploration in which the patient is encouraged to produce various phonemes, often drawing from other languages. Such productions may later be incorporated as sound substitutions for phonemes that can no longer be produced. In addition, training the patient to use tonal patterns to convey intent can be achieved by using those sounds that the patient could fairly easily produce, for example, /m/. By varying inflection, duration, and volume, the patient can then communicate several ideas with a given sound [48]. For example, a brief, low-pitched sound produced twice could be interpreted as "no," while extended phonation with a rising inflection pattern could indicate, "What did you say?"

When the tracheal tube has either been stopped up or removed, and the patient is sufficiently well to participate, formal testing can be initiated. Prior to this it is essential to review the surgical report to determine the extent of excision, as this has implications for testing, treatment objectives, procedures, and prognosis.

In brief, the test battery stimuli [48] include conversational questions and answers, oral reading of a paragraph, production of vowels, and production of glossal and nonglossal sounds arranged systematically across several contexts. The patient's ability to manipulate the remaining oral structures and subsequent effect on speech production are assessed. In addition, the patient's ability to vary suprasegmental features, such as speaking rate, duration, pitch, and intensity, is determined to plan a total treatment program. When the patient is able, swallowing and eating patterns should be examined to determine areas of difficulty that may require therapeutic intervention.

No workup should be considered complete without an audiological assessment, as this patient subgroup is at high risk for hearing loss secondary to radiation, chemotherapy, surgery, or the actual disease [22]. Determining hearing status is important, in that the patient must be able to make fine discriminations among speech sounds to progress in treatment.

Patients who have undergone a partial glossectomy vary in the amount of treatment required, depending on site and extent of tissue removal [48]. There may be minimal distortion detected in a fortunate few, while many may need intensive rehabilitation. Training the patient with a partial glossectomy consists of demonstrating modifications of normal articulation patterns by use of residual tongue musculature [48]. Most patients respond to traditional articulation training.

In contrast, treatment of patients undergoing total glossectomy requires a skilled speech-language pathologist with specialized training. Skelly [48] has determined that treatment should adhere to the progression of establishing consistent articulatory substitutions followed by developing compensatory alternatives. The consistency of substitutions, that is, using a nonglossal for a glossal sound, has been shown to contribute both to early intelligibility and to the foundation for subsequent compensations. For example, a puff of air is used as a substitution for /s/. Later, compensation for /s/ consists of pushing the airstream by way of cheek compression through an extremely narrow slit between the upper teeth and lower lip [48].

Additional consideration throughout the program should be given to manipulation of all possible vocal products, which has been shown directly to improve intelligibility [1, 48, 49]. Vowel prolongation, increase in habitual pitch level, change in speaking rate, and appropriate use of pausing are reported to be among the most effective techniques [1, 48].

Exerting control over the patient's environment is an integral part of speech training. Adequate lighting and limited background noise are important. Face-to-face communication is recommended to allow for visual cues [2]. Family, friends, and team members must become actively involved for any program to be a success, and emotional support for the patient is critical. Of equal importance is listener training [2, 48]. Listener responsibility includes knowing the speaker's specific articulatory substitutions and compensations, as well as how to phrase a response to indicate what portion of a message has been received. Setting the stage for communication, however, is the patient's responsibility as a speaker. Prior to initiating conversation, the patient may need to provide a contextual or topical cue, such as a news headline, photograph, written word, or gesture.

For many patients, prior to and in conjunction with speech treatment, a swallowing program is necessary. This should be carried out as a joint effort by a speech-language pathologist, an occupational therapist, and nursing personnel. It has long been recognized that the vegetative functions of chewing, sucking, and swallowing are precursors to speech. Therefore it may be necessary to train the patient directly in effective swallowing of both food and oral secretions, which will later serve to enhance speech intelligibility. To achieve functional swallowing with some patients it may suffice to develop compensatory mechanisms, such as a quick backward jerk and tilt of the head [1], which may involve many weeks of intensive training. For others, use of adaptive equipment such as a "pusher spoon" or a syringe feeding device [16] is necessary for food to pass into the pharynx, at which point gravity and appropriate head positioning can take over. The most impared patient is unlikely to develop a usable swallowing pattern, in which case surgical intervention, such as gastrostomy, is performed to allow proper nutritional intake.

Improved swallowing and speech using a tongue prosthesis has been reported [1, 11]. In addition, a case of reconstructive surgery resulted in notable improvement in swallowing [1]. Unfortunately, the latter report did not address the effect on speech intelligibility.

The patient with persisting dysphagia has a poor prognosis for obtaining intelligible speech [48]. Factors that have been found positively to influence output are flexibility of remaining tongue musculature, less extensive surgery such as removal of only the lateral aspect of the tongue, and ability to manipulate vocal activity [1, 48]. Even patients undergoing radical surgery have been noted to exhibit some spontaneous recovery [33]. Treatment, however, remains important to develop consistent articulatory habits. Length of such pro-

grams varies; patients having total glossectomy often require more than a year of treatment prior to reaching a plateau [48].

BREAST CANCER

Carcinoma of the breast is the most common cancer in women over 40 years of age. The incidence in white American women is 28 percent, or 72 cases per 100,000 population.

The most frequent treatment is surgery consisting of radical mastectomy, with or without radiation. A modified radical mastectomy in which all breast tissue and axillary nodes are removed (the pectoral muscles are not removed), followed by radiation, particularly in the presence of positive lymph nodes, has replaced the radical mastectomy in many centers, especially in early stages (I and II) of the disease. Simple mastectomy (only the breast tissue is removed) or so-called lumpectomy (excision of the tumor and some surrounding tissue, leaving the breast relatively intact) with radiation is the treatment of choice in more advanced stage (III) of the disease. When distant metastases (stage IV) are present, which occurs in approximately one-half of all patients, hormone manipulation, either surgical or pharmacological, chemotherapy, and local radiation therapy are used to manage the disease. Palliative breast surgery may also be performed.

The 5-year survival for patients treated with radical mastectomy is 50 to 55 percent. Survival is between 38 and 85 percent, depending on the stage of cancer when treated and the study cited. A figure of 70 to 85 percent is given as the 5-year survival for treated localized cancer (stage I), and it is 50 to 55 percent when there is regional spread (stage II). The five-year survival of untreated patients is approximately 20 percent from onset of symptoms.

FUNCTIONAL PROBLEMS

Loss of shoulder motion, lymphedema or swelling of the arm, and posterior shoulder girdle pain are common complications following mastectomy. Wound infection and postoperative radiation therapy can also cause significant complications. The physical, emotional, sexual, and cosmetic problems related to loss of a breast are of critical concern.

REHABILITATION
Emphasis of the rehabilitation program is placed on 4 major areas:

1. Exercise to maintain range of motion and function in the shoulder and arm
2. Restoration of external appearance
3. Emotional support to aid in the psychological adjustment to loss of a breast
4. Patient education pre- and postoperatively on the surgical procedure, exercises, lymphedema, arm care, prosthetic devices, clothing adaptations, and patient and family expectations, fears, and concerns.

The program can be accomplished in a group or on an individual basis, and primarily involves the surgeon, nurse, occupational therapist, physical therapist, social worker, and Reach to Recovery volunteer. In addition to carrying out the procedure, the surgeon discusses the diagnosis, treatment, and follow-up care with the patient. The nurse provides wound and health care and patient education, and is aware of day-to-day patient and family problems, helping support the patient through difficult stages. The occupational therapist assists the patient in functional life activities, arm and hand care, education regarding clothing adaptation, prosthetic devices, and emotional support, as well as reinforcing the exercise program. The physical therapist teaches the patient exercises for the involved extremity and proper positioning to avoid edema, while the social worker assists the family to adjust.

On physician referral, a Reach to Recovery volunteer will also participate. As a representative of this program of the American Cancer Society, she has had a mastectomy and is chosen because of her own healthy adjustment to the surgery and ability to serve as a role model for other patients. She is able and trained to provide emotional support and practical information to the patient and family. A manual, *Reach to Recovery* [34], contains information on exercises, clothing hints, and words of reassurance [38]: "If the patient can see and talk to another woman who has had the same surgery, has successfully adjusted, is carrying on her usual activities, she can perhaps see an improved future for herself."

Shoulder dysfunction may result from inadequate exercise and improper positioning of the arm and shoulder following surgery; to prevent a frozen shoulder and restore its function proper attention to both is critical. The arm should be placed in abduction and slight elevation, and exercises for the forearm and hand should be initiated as soon as possible following surgery to control edema. When permitted, range-of-motion and isometric and isotonic strengthening exercises should commence. These can be done actively such as in wall-climbing, or with the use of a rope pulley. Activities of daily living are encouraged, and should be continued at home. Lymphedema may also have late onset following radiation therapy. Again, proper positioning and regular active use of the arm are essential for successful recovery. Elastic sleeves and pneumo-massage may be helpful.

Brachial plexus injury may occur as a result of axillary dissection, radiation fibrosis, or tumor invasion (refer to Chapter 3). Posterior shoulder girdle pain is common, and may require analgesics for relief.

Prostheses are available in most department stores and corsetieres. The Reach to Recovery program offers a number of suggestions about breast forms, bras, and skin color. In addition, the volunteer will make a temporary form available to the patient. A permanent prosthesis is usually not recommended for wear until sufficient healing has taken place, approximately 8 weeks after surgery. Clothing alterations are usually minimal, and the *Reach to Recovery* pamphlet offers a number of suggestions, including those for the adjustment of night wear, bathing suits, and low-cut or sleeveless dresses.

Reconstructive surgery after mastectomy is a possibility and should be discussed with the surgeon. Although these were previously difficult to achieve, inflatable implants, particularly the silicone gel prosthesis, have improved the situation considerably. This is especially so for women who have received early, adequate treatment, and have undergone less extensive surgery than a radical mastectomy [32].

Many fears and concerns facing the mastectomy patient can be ameliorated with preoperative education and postoperative counseling and care. The understanding and support of the patient's partner can play a significant role in the management of and adjustment to the procedure. She faces issues related to self-image that include her reaction and that of her partner to the loss of a part of her body that is significant in its identification with femaleness and sexuality. The emotional reaction to this loss can leave the woman feeling worthless, incomplete, and with a diminished sense of self-esteem. Klein [31] delineates certain psychological tasks that must be performed to return the patient to a functional and stable way of life. These include acceptance of the loss of the breast and full mourning, including grief with regard to the fears that she might lose her partner or even her life; reintegration of a self-image worthy of love and the rewards of life; and beginning to make peace with the "albatross" of potential recurrence with which she must live for the next five to ten years.

Klein suggests that the team help the patient express her feelings and sort out the real from the unreal, and not give false reassurances. In addition, they can help the patient anticipate the future and consider how and what to tell significant persons in her life. The family must be helped to understand the patient's feelings and to express their own.

The role of the husband or partner is important in the adjustment process. Wellisch and colleagues [58] studied the man's reaction to his partner's mastectomy, and identified several points as critical to adjustment: his involvement in making decisions regarding surgery; frequency of hospital visits; resumption of sexual activity; and viewing his partner's body after surgery. It was suggested [32] that "an in-hospital desensitization program during postoperative recovery with the man viewing the operative site and assisting in changes of dressings might facilitate the development of comfort and involvement."

SPECIAL CONSIDERATIONS

Reach to Recovery is designed to help women with breast cancer meet their physical, psychological, and cosmetic needs [39]. In addition, the American Cancer Society makes available a variety of literature on breast cancer, including self-examination, warning signs, and mastectomy rehabilitation.

ENCORE is the YWCA postmastectomy group rehabilitation program offered at a number of their locations across the country. It includes weekly sessions of exercise and discussion. The latter involves sharing experiences and problems as well as learning about prostheses, clothing, and technical information from professionals.

FEMALE GENITAL TRACT
(GYNECOLOGICAL CANCER)

Malignant neoplasms involving the genital tract, including cancer of the cervix, uterus, ovary, vagina, and vulva, account for one-fifth of cancers in women. They are most common after 40 years of age. Early detection provides the greatest opportunity for cure; surgery and radiation therapy are the usual treatment. Chemotherapy and hormone therapy may be used in inoperable situations, or when there has been a recurrence.

FUNCTIONAL PROBLEMS

Generalized weakness, back pain, leg swelling, and prolonged weight loss are among the physical manifestations of the disease and its treatment. Pathological bone fractures are indicative of advanced disease. Fistulas, postsurgical vaginal bleeding, and postoperative nonhealing wounds may occur, requiring medical, surgical, or nursing intervention. The patient may require an excretory conduit. The reader is referred to the section on cancer of the colon and rectum for more information.

Sexual dysfunction and dyspareunia may be experienced, leading the patient to feeling diminished worth as a woman [61]. Disappointment in the loss of child-bearing ability and marital stress can also be involved.

*Rehabilitation*

A graduated remobilization program and proper positioning following surgery are essential in dealing with weakness and pain. Awareness of the patient's sexual habits and cultural background provide an understanding of the woman, and assist in counseling her and in meeting physical and emotional needs. Support by her partner is critical to adjustment, and he should be included in discussions of the disease and its treatment sequelae. Counseling includes issues related to self-esteem, grief reactions, fear of recurrence, and feelings of anger, guilt, loss, anxiety, and depression.

Gynecological cancers affect sexual functioning in both physical and symbolic manners, creating not only bodily dysfunction that must be coped with, but emotional trauma. Ongoing discussions of sexuality, sexual activity, and the difficulties and fears experienced by the patient and her partner are important to the therapy program. Fear of contagion following radiation therapy, alternative coital positions and coital equivalents following treatment that may limit sexual activity, and emotional feelings such as loss of femininity and worth should be discussed. These discussions are often initiated by the physician or nurse, but can be carried out by any member of the oncology team who feels comfortable and knowledgeable in these areas.

The patient must be encouraged and helped to resume normal vocational and avocational activities without unnecessary fear of rejection or isolation. Maintaining interpersonal social and work relationships is important in dealing with cancer, and may require the team to educate an employer, family, and friends.

## MALE GENITAL TRACT (PROSTATIC CANCER)

Prostatic cancer is typically seen in older men: the median age of incidence is 70 years, and it is found in 14 to 46 percent of men over 50. It is most common in its metastatic form, and once the metastases are present there is two- to three-year survival. Therapy is usually related to life expectancy and general health of the individual, and growth rate of the cancer. Treatment options include hormone therapy, surgery (offering 50 percent five-year survival), radiation therapy (with 60 percent five-year survival), and chemotherapy. Hormone therapy is used primarily for symptomatic metastatic disease.

### FUNCTIONAL PROBLEMS

Generalized weakness is common. Bone pain and pathological fractures occur frequently, and indicate metastatic disease. Incontinence and impotence are often results of treatment.

Issues related to impotence and feelings of an altered body image are of major concern. A further problem can be feminization, which can be a consequence of hormone therapy.

### REHABILITATION

A graduated program of mobilization is initiated as soon as medically indicated. Appropriate orthopedic procedures must be practiced in the case of, or as prophylaxis in impending, pathological fractures. Bone pain is commonly treated with hormone or radiation therapy.

When dealing with issues of impotence or altered body image and its attendant depression, factual, sensitive discussions with the patient and his partner are critical. These discussions can be with the team member who feels most comfortable and knowledgeable in this area, and it is recommended that they occur both pre- and postoperatively for maximum benefit. Such support and encouragement from the team help to prevent withdrawal and isolation on the part of the patient, and anger and resentment of the partner. As 100 percent of patients treated for prostatic cancer experience some degree of impotence, education should include factual information on subsequent sexual function, and coital alternatives. Options such as prosthetic devices should be presented if the treatment will produce permanent impotence. Pain on ejaculation may be experienced following treatment, and should be discussed to avoid inhibition of sexual activity. If incontinence occurs, protective devices such as condoms are made available, and a bladder training program can be initiated.

Vocational counseling may be indicated depending on the age and concerns of the individual.

BLADDER CANCER

This is the most frequent maligant tumor of the urinary tract, is most common in those 50 to 70 years of age, and occurs more often in men than women. Treatment consists primarily of radiation therapy (6 to 33 percent survival at five years) and surgery-cystectomy (18 to 43 percent survival for five years).

FUNCTIONAL PROBLEMS

Generalized weakness is common, amd bone pain may be experienced from metastatic disease. Incontinence and impotence can be serious problems resulting from treatment; however, potency is maintained in approximately 50 percent of patients treated with radiation therapy. Cystitis, ulceration of the bladder, contracted bladder, ileitis, and colitis are among the possible long-term reactions to radiation. Issues relating to altered body image and cosmesis may be particularly devastating to the patient with a urinary conduit stoma.

REHABILITATION

A program similar to that provided for the patient with prostatic or gynecological cancer is indicated. In addition, adjustment must be made to a urinary conduit stoma and urine collection bag if the bladder is removed. Although several different types of bags are available, they all work on the same principle. A plastic or rubber bag is attached with an adhesive disc to the skin over the opening. The bag may be held in place by a belt. It has a drainage tube at the lower end for emptying.

Urinary diversion can be accomplished by a variety of surgical methods—ureteroenterostomy, wet colostomy, or ureterostomy. The last involves insertion of a catheter into the stoma and taping the catheter tube to the leg in its natural position. The catheter is then attached to a drainage tube and leg bag. Appliances worn directly over the stoma are also used. Patients are instructed, usually by the nurse, in skin care around the stoma to avoid irritation, the proper method of applying the appropriate apparatus, care of the equipment, and signs and symptoms indicative of obstruction or infection.

Discussion of the appearance and functioning of the ostomy bag with the patient's partner is encouraged to avoid embarrassment and to aid in adjustment to the appliance. Impotence and other issues related to sexuality should also be discussed.

Vocational concerns may need attention if the patient anticipates difficulty in returning to a previous job or in being hired. Refer to section on cancer of the bowel for further suggestions on ostomy issues.

COLON AND RECTUM (CANCER OF THE BOWEL)

Incidence of this type of cancer is approximately equal in men and women, accounting for about 15 percent for both. It occurs more frequently in persons over the age of 50 years. The most effective treatment is surgery. Radiation therapy may be used with or instead of surgery, and chemotherapy, if used, is primarily palliative. If extensive surgery of the rectum is indicated, a temporary or permanent colostomy is required for elimination of body wastes from a stoma formed from the colon (or large intestine). An ileostomy is performed when the entire colon (or middle part of the large intestine) is removed because of disease, and a stoma is formed from the ileum (or lower part of the small intestine). Early detection of the disease influences survival statistics; less than 50 percent of those diagnosed survive five years.

FUNCTIONAL PROBLEMS

Primarily, the patient faces problems from the surgery and resultant ostomy, such as uncontrollable bowel action, skin irritation around the area, and odor and noise from the ostomy. Patients elect decreased activity because of drainage from the stoma and may be unwilling to travel and socialize. Stenosis, prolapse, retraction, blockage, or perforation of the stoma are of constant concern, and require immediate medical attention should they occur. Low endurance is common, and patients may develop an electrolyte imbalance as a result of the change in activity of the intestine.

Shame, anger, loss of self-esteem, fear of rejection, and altered body image are among the emotional concerns that must be dealt with. Impotence or apprehension about sexual activities can arise, and patients may find difficulty with interpersonal relationships in general. They may also find that vocational problems develop due to a lack of understanding on the part of the employer and fellow workers of the significance of the surgery.

REHABILITATION

For ileostomies and ureterostomies, appliances consist of a rubber or hard plastic disc to which a rubber or plastic pouch is attached. It is custom-fit for the individual stoma. The appliance is attached by an adhesive to the skin; a belt may be used to help keep it in place. It is designed to be comfortable, reasonably priced, nonirritating, inconspicuous, and odor- and leak-proof. In applying the pouch, skin care procedures must be followed, and an appropriate adhesive solvent used when removing it to avoid irritation. The ileostomy bag should be emptied every four to six hours or as needed, and changed every two to three days. At this time it can be washed, and soaked in a weak solution of vinegar or chlorine bleach to control odor and maintain use of the bag for one to two years. For control of odor, special deodorants are manufactured, or a solution of vinegar and water can be used. A diet low in bulk and avoidance of poorly tolerated or gas-forming foods are recommended.

For colostomies, disposable bags are used following surgery for containment of fecal drainage during training in control. This also allows remobilization activities to commence with fewer embarrassing accidents. Care must be taken to select the equipment and technique most useful for the patient.

Management of a colostomy is generally accomplished by irrigation. The degree to which the patient can control the colostomy will vary according to its anatomical location. Some patients are able to function with a dry gauze dressing with a piece of plastic taped in place following regular irrigation. Others may require or prefer to wear a disposable ostomy bag for protection from soiling. Whatever the procedure, instruction in care of the stoma, irrigation technique, and skin care are taught as soon as possible to assist the patient in accepting and adjusting to the colostomy.

Proper diet, adequate fluid intake, regularity of irrigation, and emotional status can affect the function and control of the colostomy, and require patient education while in the hospital and at home. Although the entire team participates in educating and supporting the patient and family, specially trained enterostomal therapists provide valuable instruction and assist in daily practice. Volunteers, who may be representatives of a local ostomy club who have successfully managed an ostomy, are available to help by providing practical information and reassurance pre- and postoperatively. Ostomy clubs are available in many communities for further support following discharge from the hospital.

Problems of stenosis, retraction, or perforation must be handled immediately by surgical intervention. Prolapse, or paracolostomy hernia, requires medical attention. Blockage must be attended to immediately by cleaning the walls of the intestine.

A well-balanced diet is essential to maintain electrolyte balance. Patients are instructed to increase their daily fluid intake, particularly if an ileostomy has been performed. Food should be eaten slowly and chewed thoroughly. Items that cause gas formation, are high in fiber, fried, smoked or highly seasoned, and nuts are omitted from the diet [7]. Odor can be controlled by using special ostomy deodorants, and a variety of ointments and powders is available to prevent excoriation.

It has been noted that [60] "in our society, which places such strong emphasis on early childhood training in complete bowel and bladder control, the sudden deprivation of control is a mortifying experience—perhaps the worst possible insult to one's self esteem." Winkelstein and Lyons further suggest that learning to control the function of the colostomy is vital in renewing self-esteem and minimizing interference of the stoma in daily activities and interpersonal relationships. Reactions of shame, anger, grief, and fear of rejection can be relieved if prior to surgery, the patient and family understand the proposed procedure and its implications, and if self-care is achieved postoperatively. Throughout this time, family understanding and support are critical factors in the patient's adjustment. Apprehension about sexual activities should be discussed between partners. Techniques that may be helpful include extra tape around the bag opening to prevent leakage, and alternate coital positions to avoid pressure on the bag.

In general, most patients are able to return to normal vocational activities unless excessive physical movement is required. Employers may need to be educated regarding the significance of the surgery and the unlikelihood of interference with the job. Supplies must be available at the work site. If travel is involved, simple precautions may be required for air travel, irrigation timing, and fluid alternatives [44].

SPECIAL CONSIDERATIONS

The United Ostomy Association provides comprehensive information with a listing of local groups, distributors of ostomy products, and current publications on ostomy care [24].

The American Cancer Society ostomy rehabilitation program, designed often as local clubs, provides visitors, mutual support meetings, and information on equipment and supplies [39]. In addition, the Society has numerous pamphlets and resource materials on cancer of the colon and rectum, as well as information on colostomies.

The National Foundation of Ileitis and Colitis funds research on inflammatory bowel disease, holds educational seminars for the public, and distributes literature to professionals and the public.

# References

1. Amerman, J. D., and Laminack, C. Evaluation and rehabilitation of glossectomy speech behavior. *J. Commun. Disord.* 7:365, 1974.
2. Anderson, J. D., and Thomas, S. Speech rehabilitation of a laryngectomized-glossectomized patient. *Laryngoscope* 88:1666, 1978.
3. Bakemeier, R. F. Principles of medical oncology and cancer chemotherapy. In P. Rubin (Ed.) *Clinical Oncology: For Medical Students and Physicians, A Multidisciplinary Approach.* New York: American Cancer Society, 1974.
4. Berlin, C. I. Clinical measurement of esophageal speech. I. Methodology and curves of skill acquisition. *J. Speech Hear. Disord.* 28:42, 1963.
5. Blom, E. D. Approaches to treatment: Part B. In S. J. Salmon and L. P. Golstein (Eds.), *The Artificial Larynx Handbook.* New York: Grune and Stratton, 1978.
6. Blom, E. D. The artificial larynx: Past and present. In S. J. Salmon and L. P. Goldstein (Eds.), *The Artificial Larynx Handbook.* New York: Grune & Stratton, 1978.
7. Bouchard, R., and Owens, N. F. *Nursing Care of the Cancer Patient.* St. Louis: Mosby, 1972.

8. Cady, B. (Ed.), *Cancer: A Manual for Practitioners* (5th ed.) Boston: American Cancer Society, Massachusetts Division, 1978.

9. Cassileth, B. R. (Ed.). *The Cancer Patient: Social and Medical Aspects of Care.* Philadelphia: Lea and Febiger, 1979.

10. Deckers, P. J., McDonough, E. F. , Jr., and Shipley, W. U. The physical examination for cancer detection. In B. Cady (Ed.). *Cancer: A Manual for Practitioners* (5th ed.). Boston: American Cancer Society Massachusetts Division, 1978.

11. deSouza, L. J., and Martins, O. J. Swallowing and speech after radical total glossectomy with tongue prosthesis. *Oral Surg.* 39:356, 1975.

12. Diedrich, W. M. Primary stage of teaching alaryngeal speech. In S. Ridgosky, J. Lerman, and E. B. Morrison (Eds.). *Therapy for the Laryngectomized Patient: A Speech Clinician's Manual.* New York: Teachers College Press, 1971.

13. Diedrich, W. M., and Youngstrom, K. S. *Alaryngeal Speech.* Springfield, Ill.: Thomas, 1966.

14. Dodd, M. J., and Livingstone, C. A. Pain and the cancer patient. In B. H. Peterson and C. J. Kellogg (Eds.). *Current Practice in Oncologic Nursing.* St. Louis: Mosby, 1976.

15. Donaldson, R. C. Phases of Patient Care. In M. Skelly (Ed.). *Glossectomee Speech Rehabilitation.* Springfield, Ill.: Thomas, 1973.

16. Dudgeon, B. J., DeLisa, J. A., and Miller, R. M. Head and neck cancer, a rehabilitation approach. *Am. J. Occup. Ther.* 34:243, 1980.

17. Duguay, M. Laryngectomy and esophageal speech. Presented at the Massachusetts Speech and Hearing Association, Hyannis, Mass., 1978.

18. DuPont, G. Pain Management. In B. R. Cassileth (Ed.). *The Cancer Patient: Social and Medical Aspects of Care.* Philadelphia: Lea and Febiger, 1979.

19. Emerson, H., and Witteman, B. *Progressive Steps to a New Voice.* Nashville: Bill Wilkerson Hearing and Speech Center, 1976.

20. Gardner, W. H. *Laryngectomee Speech and Rehabilitation.* Springfield, Ill.: Thomas, 1971.

21. Gates, C. C. Psychosocial Issues in Cancer. In B. Cady (Ed) *Cancer: A Manual for Practitioners* (5th ed.). Boston: American Cancer Society, Massachusetts Division, 1978.

22. Glazer, D. C. Audiological management of head and neck carcinoma patients. *J. Speech Hear. Disord.* 45:216, 1980.

23. Goode, R. L. Artificial laryngeal devices in post-laryngectomy rehabiliation. *Laryngoscope* 85:677, 1975.

24. Harrison, H. Ostomies. In R. M. Goldenson (Ed.). *Disability and Rehabilitation Handbook.* New York: McGraw-Hill, 1978.

25. Horii, Y., and Weinberg, B. Intelligibility Characteristics of Superior Esophageal Speech Presented Under Various Levels of Masking Noise. In B. Weinberg (Ed.). *Readings in Speech Following Total Laryngectomy.* Baltimore: University Park, 1980.

26. Hyman, M. Intermediate Stages of Teaching Alaryngeal Speech. In S. Ridgodsky, J. Leman, and E. B. Morrison (Eds.). *Therapy for the Laryngectomized Patient: A Speech Clinician's Manual,* New York: Teacher's College, 1971.

27. International Association of Laryngectomees. *Laryngectomized Speakers' Source Book.* New York: American Cancer Society, 1975.

28. International Association of Laryngectomees. *The IAL Directory 1980.* New York: American Cancer Society, 1980.

29. Keith, R. L. *A Handbook for the Laryngectomee.* Danville, Ill.: Interstate, 1974.

30. Keith, R. L., et al. *Looking Forward: A Guidebook for the Laryngectomee.* Rochester, Minn.: Mayo Foundation, 1977.

31. Klein, R. A crisis to grow on. *Cancer.* 27:2, 1978.

32. Kolodny, R. C., Masters, W. H., and Johnson, V. E. *Textbook of Sexual Medicine.* Boston: Little, Brown, 1979.

33. LaRiviere, C., Seilo, M. T., and Dimmick, K. C. The pre-therapy speech intelligibility of a glossectomee. *J. Commun. Disord.* 7:357, 1974.

34. Lasser, R. *Reach to Recovery.* New York: American Cancer Society, 1974.

35. Lauder, E. *Self-Help for the Laryngectomee.* San Antonio, Texas, 1977.

36. Levene, M. B. Overall principles of cancer management. III. Radiation Therapy. In B. Cady (Ed.) *Cancer: A Manual for Practitioners.* Boston: American Cancer Society, Massachusetts Division, 1978.

37. Marino, E. B., and LaBlanc, D. H. Cancer chemotherapy. *Nursing '75* 5(11):22, 1975.

38. Markel, W. M. Rehabilitation after mastectomy. In *Rehabilitation of the Cancer Patient.* Chicago: Year Book, 1972.

39. Moen, J. B., and Cady, B. Resources and Rehabilitation. In B. Cady (Ed.). *Cancer: A Manual for Practitioners.* Boston: American

Cancer Society, Massachusetts Division, 1978.

40. Mozden, P. J., Roover, J. E., and Stonberg, M. F. Overall principles of cancer management. V. Hormone Therapy. In B. Cady (Ed.) *Cancer: A Manual for Practitioners*. Boston: American Cancer Society, Massachusetts Division, 1978.

41. Mullen, J. L., and Hobbs, C. L. Nutritional Management. In B. R. Cassileth (Ed.). *The Cancer Patient: Social and Medical Aspects of Care*. Philadelphia: Lea and Febiger, 1979.

42. Rosenstein, A. *Esophageal Speech with Health Concepts and Tips for Laryngectomees*. Long Beach, Calif.: ELOT, 1977.

43. Rubin, P. (Ed.). *Clinical Oncology: For Medical Students and Physicians, a Multidisciplinary Approach*. New York: American Cancer Society, 1974.

44. Rusk, H. *Rehabilitation Medicine* (9th ed.). St. Louis: Mosby, 1977.

45. St. John Elliott, C. Radiation therapy: How you can help. *Nursing '76* 6(9):34, 1976.

46. Salmon, S. J., and Goldstein, L. P. (Eds.). *An Artificial Larynx Handbook*. New York: Grune and Stratton, 1978.

47. Shipp, T. Frequency, duration and perceptual measures in relation to judgments of alaryngeal speech acceptability. In B. Weinberg (Ed.). *Readings in Speech Following Total Laryngectomy*. Baltimore: University Park, 1980.

48. Skelly, M. *Glossectomee Speech Rehabilitation*. Springfield, Ill.: Thomas, 1973.

49. Skelly, M., et al. Changes in phonatory aspects of glossectomee intelligibility through vocal parameter manipulation. *J. Speech Hear. Disord.* 37:379, 1972.

50. Skelly, M., et al. Amerind sign: Gestural communication for the speechless. Presented at the American Speech and Hearing Association, San Francisco, 1972.

51. Smith, E. A. *A Comprehensive Approach to Rehabilitation of the Cancer Patient: A Self-Instructional Text*. New York: McGraw-Hill, 1975.

52. Spiers, A. S. D. The palliative management of cancer patients. In B. Cady (Ed.). *Cancer: A Manual for Practitioners*. Boston: American Cancer Society, Massachusetts Division, 1978.

53. Tealey, A. R. Radiotherapy and Hodgkin's disease. In B. H. Peterson and C. J. Kellogg (Eds.). *Current Practice in Oncologic Nursing*. St. Louis: Mosby, 1976.

54. *Trace Center Resource Book*. Madison, Wisc.: Trace Center, 1978–79.

55. *Treating Cancer*. Washington, D.C.: U.S. Department of Health, Education, and Welfare, U.S. Government Printing Office, 1977.

56. Twycross, R. G. Principles and practice of the relief of pain in terminal cancer. *Update.*:, 1972.

57. Vanderheim, G. C. (Ed.). *Non-Vocal Communication Resource Book*. Baltimore: University Park, 1978.

58. Wellisch, D. K., Jamison, K. R., and Pasnan, R. O. Psychosocial aspects of mastectomy. II. The man's perspective. *Am. J. Psychiatry* 135:543, 1978.

59. Winans, C. S., Reichback, E. J., and Waldrop, W. F. Esophageal determinants of alaryngeal speech. *Arch. Otolaryngol.* 99:10, 1974.

60. Winkelstein, C., and Lyons, A. S. Insight into the emotional aspects of ileostomies and colostomies. *Medical Insight*:, 1971.

61. Wise, T. N. Effects of cancer on sexual activity. *Psychosomatics* 19(12):769, 1978.

## Suggested Reading

### BREAST CANCER

Asken, M. J. Psychoemotional aspects of mastectomy: A review of recent literature. *Am. J. Psychiatry* 132:56, 1975.

*The Cancer Patient: Social and Medical Aspects of Care*. Philadelphia: Lea and Febiger, 1979.

Morris, T. Psychological adjustment to mastectomy. *Cancer Treat. Rev.* 6:41, 1979.

### COLON AND RECTUM CANCER

D'Orazio, M. L. Rehabilitation for ostomy patients. In B. R. Cassileth (Ed.). *The Cancer Patient: Social and Medical Aspects of Care*. Philadelphia: Lea and Febiger, 1979.

Turnball, R. B. Rehabilitation of the stomal patients. In *Rehabilitation of the Cancer Patient*. Chicago: Year Book, 1972.

### HEAD AND NECK CANCER

Catalin, E. The patient who has undergone radical neck dissection. Presented at Workshop to Upgrade Services to Laryngectomees, Washington, D.C., 1977.

Cocke, E. W., and Wang, C. C. Part I. Cancer of the Larynx: Selecting optimum treatment. *CA* 26(4): 194, 1976.

Fust, R. S. Dysphagia. In M. Skelly (Ed.). *Glossectomee Speech Rehabilitation*. Springfield, Ill.: Thomas, 1973.

# 3 ORTHOPEDICS

A comprehensive evaluation of the orthopedic patient is essential to develop an effective rehabilitation program. Before deciding on the best approach, the physician must consider the patient's orthopedic and general medical condition, mental status, age, and premorbid lifestyle, and in conjunction with other members of the team, choose the best mode of treatment.

The program will take into account recommendations of the physician who performed the surgery, the patient's primary physician, and radiological reports. In addition, each facility has certain guidelines that reflect its own philosophy of rehabilitation. The therapist must be sensitive to all these factors.

When discussing such a program, there are certain evaluation and treatment procedures that should be performed regardless of the specific disability. The clinician must first establish the patient's mental status, such as level of consciousness; orientation to name, place, and time; and level of cooperation. In addition, the patient's social, vocational, and recreational history and rehabilitation goals must be established.

## Lower Extremity Orthopedics
*Bess Kathrins*

Most adult lower extremity orthopedic surgery is precipitated by trauma[29]. One general exception to this is the patient who is scheduled for joint replacement surgery. This can be planned days or months in advance [24], and thus preoperative care can be initiated by all members of the team. The patient should be instructed in breathing and coughing exercises and isometric exercises such as quadriceps and gluteal sets, and fitted for crutches or walker and practice ambulation with them. The patient should be familiarized with any equipment that may be used postoperatively, such as traction; precautions to be taken, such as motions to avoid; and proper positioning. Each team member should perform a thorough evaluation preoperatively to establish baseline information.

Postoperatively, team members explain what has occurred and what the patient can expect in the near future. The person with an orthopedic disability can count on a period of immobility varying from days to months, depending on the nature of the disorder. Immobilization can mean traction, a cast, or simply restriction to bedrest. It will take a concerted effort on the part of all staff members to prevent detrimental effects of immobilization such as skin breakdown, pulmonary complications, thrombophlebitis, contractures, and depression.

A common balanced traction assembly is Buck's apparatus with Pearson attachment. It should be suspended to allow gravity-free support and movement. The amount of traction will be determined by the orthopedist. Balanced suspension requires frequent adjustments by a qualified physician, nurse, therapist, or orthopedic technician [25]. Some patients are placed in a cast to achieve immobility. The staff must be acutely aware of skin condition, edema, and nerve entrapment in these patients.

An orthopedic injury may be expected to cause a certain degree of pain, the distribution and effect of which on rehabilitation is individually modulated. Each team member must be concerned about differentiating between pain as a normal response and pain that is a sign of underlying pathology. Astute observation is essential in identifying possible complications. Abnormal clinical signs may include excessive edema, discoloration, drainage, or odor from the wound site or cast, sudden increase in body temperature, and sudden changes in temperature of the extremity, range of motion, strength, or the patient's mental status. Observation of any of these signs must be followed by immediate consultation with the physician.

## EVALUATION
Specific evaluation should include ranges of motion of all extremities, with specific goniometric measurements recorded for the affected one. Muscle testing is included, although guidelines for manual muscle testing can vary greatly with the disability. Generally, the affected extremity should not be tested beyond a fair grade without physician's orders. Certainly, the leg that is restricted in weight-bearing should not be tested or exercised with resistance.

## TREATMENT
A typical exercise regimen may begin with isometric and active assistive exercise, progressing to active and resistive exercise. There are many forms of treatment that can be excellent adjuncts to the program. Decreasing pain is essential for successful rehabilitation; hot packs, cold packs, and transcutaneous electrical nerve stimulation can be used. Hydrotherapy is also effective for decreasing pain, increasing range of motion and strength, and facilitating wound healing. Deep heat must be used with great caution, as metal implants are a contraindication for many of these modalities. Biofeedback can be effective for muscle reedu-

cation. Sling suspension can be used over the patient's bed or in the physical therapy department. The bicycle can be effective in increasing range of motion, strength, and endurance. With all of these possibilities, the patient has a certain degree of control over the activity, which can lead to trusting the therapist and taking an active role in the program.

Strengthening of unaffected extremities is an essential part of the program, as long periods of immobility and premorbid muscle weakness affect the success of rehabilitation. General strengthening can be carried out in a group setting, with an aide, or independently by the patient.

## FUNCTIONAL TRAINING
Proper positioning, bed mobility, transfer training, and activities of daily living should all be included in functional training. Positioning involves a collaborative effort of nursing, physical and occupational therapy, and the patient. Educating the patient is the best means of ensuring success with a program. Remember that no one position can be effective for an extended length of time.

As aids for bed mobility, the bed rails and trapeze are important immediately following surgery, however, long-term use of the equipment should be avoided. The patient who will be returning home will not have bed rails or a trapeze, and should not become dependent on them. Patients can begin rolling onto the affected extremity when stitches are removed, and they frequently need encouragement to accomplish this. Lying prone is also important, although many geriatric patients do not tolerate this position well.

When transfer activities are performed, it is essential that the patient perform proper weight-bearing. If too much weight is being placed on the extremity, the activity should be discontinued and the physician contacted for further orders. In addition, the patient should avoid pivoting on the affected extremity, as the rotary motion can cause injury.

Activities of daily living must be evaluated

TABLE 3-1. *Weight-bearing Classifications*

| Weight-Bearing Status | Description | Assistive Devices |
|---|---|---|
| Nonweight-bearing bed to chair | Affected extremity's foot must never touch ground | No ambulation |
| Nonweight-bearing | Affected extremity's foot must never touch ground | Two-handed device |
| Partial weight-bearing | 50% of body weight onto affected extremity | Two-handed device |
| Full weight-bearing guarded | Total body weight on affected extremity | Two-handed device |
| Full weight-bearing | Total body weight on affected extremity | One- or two-handed device |

at different stages of rehabilitation. For example, beginning weight-bearing or removal of a cast will warrant instructions in self-care techniques. Adaptive equipment, such as a long-handled shoe horn, sock aid, or extended arm reacher, may assist the patient in dressing. To help with toileting, a raised toilet seat, grab bar, or commode may permit independence. There may be difficulty with bathing, and it is useful to assess the need for a tub seat, grab bars, and long-handled sponge. Some patients do best sponge bathing until they have progressed to independence.

## AMBULATION

When the patient is ready to begin ambulation, the physician will assign a certain weight-bearing status based on radiological and physical examination, length of time since onset of disability, age and mental status of the patient, and team member reports (Table 3-1). *Nonweight-bearing bed-to-chair activities* imply an unstable orthopedic condition, and no ambulation should be permitted. *Toe-touch*, or *touchdown weight-bearing*, means the patient may use the extremity for balance only. *Partial weight-bearing* means 50 percent of the patient's weight can be placed on the affected extremity unless the physician specifies otherwise. The patient who is in any of these three categories must use a two-handed assistive device such as a walker or crutches for ambulation. To ensure adherence to the prescribed status, the therapist can place his or her foot under the patient's foot to obtain a subjective measurement. For a more accurate gauge, a boot can be attached to the patient's foot that measures pounds of pressure. When full weight-bearing is allowed, use of a unilateral assistive device should be authorized by the physician. The proper status must be observed during ambulation, transfers, and activities of daily living. Should the patient be unable to adhere to this, the physician should be consulted before the program continues; it should not be assumed that a lesser status will be acceptable. For instance, nonweight-bearing has been shown to be more stressful than toe-touch weight-bearing [17].

When the patient is ready to progress to elevated activities such as walking on stairs or ramps, weight-bearing status must be maintained. Thus if the patient required a two-handed assistive device on level surfaces, the same amount of assistance must be used on the stairs; it is a good policy to consult with the orthopedist before progressing a patient at nonweight-bearing or toe-touch status to stair-climbing.

Gait training should be carried out with the orthopedic patient the same as with one recovering from any other disability, including correcting deviations and increasing endurance. The patient should be evaluated for leg length discrepancy while supine and standing. If an orthotic device is used, it must be evaluated thoroughly with the orthotist and physician. The cast brace is being used with increasing frequency to allow early ambulation. It is essentially a long leg cast with a hinged knee joint. Great skill is required in fabricating the cast brace: hinges should correspond to anatomical axis of the knee, and the foot should be in neutral dorsiflexion with no inversion or eversion [25].

## DISCHARGE PLANNING

Discharge planning should begin as early as possible, as the patient returning home may require community services such as homemaker or home-based therapy that require advanced preparation. The patient should be instructed in a home exercise program. In addition, both patient and family should be familiar with the patient's abilities and restrictions. If necessary, prior to hospital discharge family members should practice functional activities with the patient, such as ambulation and tub transfers. Whenever possible, a home visit should be performed by the physical or occupational therapist to make recommendations concerning safety and efficiency. The recreational therapist will play an important role in preparing the disabled patient for the possibility of being faced with an excessive amount of leisure time. The vocational rehabilitation counselor for adults or the school guidance counselor or physical education teacher for children may need to join the team in certain instances. Education of the patient and family concerning the disability, rehabilitation, and future goals should occur throughout any program, as this is the best guarantee of long-term success. An interdisciplinary team is mandatory for successful rehabilitation. The members may include a physician, nurse, physical, occupational, and recreational therapists, social worker, dietitian, vocational counselor, and psychologist. The team must maintain a constant avenue of communication throughout rehabilitation as no one member has the sole knowledge, experience, and expertise to plan and execute the regimen.

## Fractures

Bone is comprised of two layers: the outer cortical layer is characteristically strong with elastic properties; the inner cancellous bone is spongelike. A break in the configuration of bone constitutes a fracture, which can be open or closed, often referred to as compound or simple, respectively. The category is based on the relationship between fracture site and the skin. The open fracture is often fraught with complications. A fracture can be 2-part, or comminuted, in which the bone is disrupted in three or more places. It can also be displaced or nondisplaced. The latter is inherently more stable.

### HIP FRACTURES

Hip fractures commonly occur at two sites: femoral neck or subcapital, and interochanteric areas (Figure 3-1). The former is often associated with a minor injury. What probably occurs is that a stress fracture precedes a minor torsion injury, which precedes an actual fall [17]. Thus the femoral neck fracture is often pathological as a result of osteoporosis [36].

Femoral fractures have been classified [25] as follows: type I—incomplete; type II—complete with no displacement; type III—partially displaced; and type IV—completely displaced. The femoral neck fracture is intracapsular, resulting in disruption of integrity of the joint. If the ligament of Teres is sclerotic, which is often the case in adults, this, compounded by the disruption of blood supply resulting from the fracture can bring about avascular necrosis for the patient with subcapital fracture. The poor blood supply to this type of fracture must be emphasized, as it can ultimately lead to nonunion.

An intertrochanteric hip fracture occurs between the greater and lesser trochanters (Figure 3-1). This fracture is extracapsular; thus the capsular vessels are salvaged and a good blood supply is present [36]. Despite this, intertrochanteric fractures are inherently unstable. A two-part fracture means one fracture line only, a three-part fracture includes the avulsion of one trochanter, and a four-part fracture includes the avulsion of both trochanters [17].

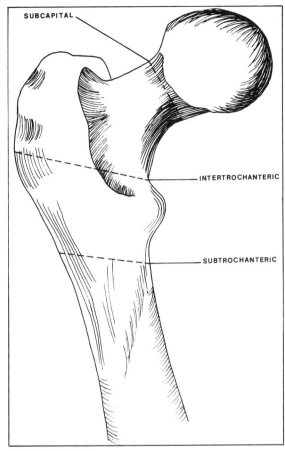

FIGURE 3-1. *Common hip fracture sites. In subcapital and intertrochanteric areas they are always categorized as hip fractures; in subtrochanteric area they can be described as hip or femur fractures.*

Extracapsular bleeding into the soft tissue will cause excessive edema at the injury site [37]. Other complications are malunion that can result in shortening of the extremity, and deformities of the coxa vera and coxa valga [37]. Weight-bearing on the extremity must occur slowly and cautiously in the presence of these conditions.

There are several possible levels of surgical intervention. Prosthetic femoral head replacement is indicated for the markedly displaced femoral head fracture [25]. The advantage of a prosthesis is that it allows early weight-bearing to tolerance and relatively pain-free motion

postoperatively [36]. Prosthetic arthroplasty is the treatment of choice for the geriatric patient with a relatively short life expectancy. Common devices are Austin-Moore, Bateman, and Thompson prostheses. Replacements can loosen in time, thus the patient with a life expectancy greater than ten years who has a prosthesis may be faced with this complication. Postoperative care must emphasize prevention of hip adduction, flexion, and internal rotation to prevent dislocation of the prosthesis [25]. The nursing staff has a difficult task of keeping the confused or bedridden patient in proper alignment, and as a result, spontaneous postoperative dislocation is not uncommon [25].

Internal fixation devices such as sliding screw, nail and plate, or pins are indicated for patients with femoral head or intertrochanteric fractures. Common ones include Knowles' pins, Richards' compression screw, Ender's rods, Smith-Petersen nail and plate, and Jewett nail. Complications include slippage of the device or its protrusion into the acetabulum, poor reduction of the fracture, and shortening of the extremity [17]. Most of the currently used internal fixation devices can be expected to yield satisfactory results. The nail, screw, or pins should sit centrally in the femoral head, with approximately 30 degrees of coxa valga. The compression screw is often favored because it allows conformity to many types of fractures [25].

A total hip replacement is rarely performed solely as a result of a hip fracture, but is indicated for persons with severe rheumatoid or degenerative arthritis [17]. Goals of the procedure are to decrease pain, increase range of motion, and improve function and ambulation [2]. It is often voluntary surgery, which means that candidates can be chosen with respect to potential for rehabilitation. Complications include dislocation, ectopic bone formation, nonunion of the greater trochanter, loosening of the prosthetic component, and infection [14].

A review of the literature unanimously favors surgical treatment for hip fracture [9, 17].

The goal is to restore patients to their preoperative status as soon as possible. Early and effective rehabilitation can best be achieved by reduction, internal fixation, and early ambulation [36]. If a patient is a poor operative candidate for medical reasons, nonoperative treatment is skeletal traction generally maintained at 10 to 12 pounds with the hip slightly abducted and externally rotated. Traction must be maintained at least four to six weeks with frequent radiological studies [36], as it is a difficult means of obtaining and maintaining proper alignment.

Evaluation and treatment of hip fracture should be carried out in the standard manner, with few restrictions. The clinician must be careful to prevent dislocation of any hip arthroplasty (total replacement or prosthesis). For such patients the goniometry examination should exclude hip flexion past 90 degrees, hip adduction past neutral, and internal rotation while the hip is flexed in the sitting position. Manual muscle test for flexion and internal rotation should not be performed in sitting position, and adduction should not be tested past neutral. Side-lying abduction should be tested, but with great caution. If the patient is nonweight-bearing or has an avulsion fracture of the greater trochanter, side-lying abduction should be avoided. Premature exercise of the gluteus medius in side-lying can cause complications; a physician should be consulted if doubt exists. The exercise program will typically begin with active assistive exercise, isometrics, and gentle passive range-of-motion exercises, gradually progressing to active and resistive exercise.

Proper positioning must be enforced. When the patient is supine, the involved extremity should be positioned with the hip in slight abduction, extension, and neutral rotation. A towel roll may be helpful in preventing external rotation at the hip. The head of the bed should not be kept elevated for long periods of time to prevent hip flexion contractures. A pillow under the knee should be avoided, as it can result in a knee flexion contracture. A foot board can be used to maintain the ankle in proper position. Special precautions must be taken for the patient with an arthroplasty. As preciously stated, the motions to avoid are a combination of hip flexion, adduction, and internal rotation. Thus when a patient rolls or is positioned on the uninvolved extremity, a pillow must be placed between the legs for proper alignment.

Sitting activities must be gradually introduced postoperatively. A patient with an arthroplasty must never sit on a low surface so that the hip would be flexed past 90 degrees. When sitting it is not necessary to elevate the extremity at all times, rather, the leg's position should be frequently altered.

Restrictions must be applied to daily living. Arthroplasty patients must avoid excessive bending during such activities as dressing and homemaking. A raised toilet seat or grab bar may be required to prevent excess flexion at the hip. Adaptive equipment such as a long-handled shoe horn, sock aid, or extended reacher may assist the patient. To prevent excessive bending, it may be necessary to reorganize contents of drawers and closets.

Surgery may help the patient achieve early ambulation. Thus gait training will begin within two to five days postoperatively for the uncomplicated hip fracture [17]. If a leg length discrepancy exists, the patient should be evaluated for a lift.

FEMORAL FRACTURES

The femur is the largest and strongest bone in adults. A femoral fracture is thus the result of a forceful trauma. It can occur at any age, and a long period of treatment and rehabilitation is necessary. These fractures include injury to the subtrochanteric, shaft, and supracondylar areas.

The subtrochanteric fracture is often seen in the age group younger than 60 years [17]. Internal fixation is certainly the treatment of choice. The Zickle device, and more recently Ender's rods, have been used to allow a simplified surgical procedure. Nonsurgical treatment in the form of traction is only used for severely comminuted subtrochanteric fractures. Balanced suspension traction is needed until there is radiological evidence of union [36]. The patient is then placed in a single spica cast with restricted weight-bearing until further callus formation is noted. Unlike with hip fracture, nonunion and avascular necrosis are rare complications for a subtrochanteric insult, however, external rotation and shortening of the extremity are common [9].

The femoral shaft fracture is often accompanied by massive bleeding at the time of injury because of the exceptional force required to cause the break. Surgical treatment is often accomplished with intermedullary rods. Internal fixation allows more rapid rehabilitation than nonsurgical treatment. The procedure is difficult, however, and common complications include comminution of the femur and infection. Children and young adults are usually treated by closed methods [25]. Adults are less tolerant of long periods of immobility and are treated surgically whenever possible. If the shaft fracture is comminuted, open, or located at the distal one-third of the femur, nonsurgical traction may be indicated [9]. Continuous skeletal traction is required for 12 to 20 weeks [9]. Balanced traction is preferred over fixed traction. A Thomas' splint with hinged Pearson attachment will allow motion at the knee. Skin traction is not suitable, as the large forces that are required would cause skin necrosis [25].

Frequent radiological studies must be obtained for femoral shaft fractures. When callus formation is noted, the patient can progress to a cast brace or hip spica cast. The former has great advantages in its ability to allow early weight-bearing and improved motion at the knee, and is ideal for simple fractures of the middle and distal femur; it should be worn for six to eight weeks [25]. The hip spica cast is used with simple fractures of the proximal one-third of the femur and comminuted fractures. The cast is waist-high, with a long leg portion on the involved side and a short or long leg portion on the uninvolved side. It may be designed for bedrest or ambulation. Complications of shaft fractures include nonunion, malunion, infection, and complications from fixation devices.

The supracondylar fracture is often accompanied by displacement of the fragments. The great forces of the gastrocnemius muscle pull the distal end posteriorly while the hamstrings and quadriceps muscles cause shortening of the femur [6]. Supracondylar fractures that are displaced or comminuted are best treated nonoperatively. Traction for three to seven weeks followed by a long leg cast, or a cast for the entire 12 to 16 weeks, is required for proper healing [9]. Surgical treatment usually occurs when nonoperative techniques have proved unsuccessful [25]. Nail and plate or compression screw is the device commonly used. The supracondylar fracture is often intracapsular, thus interfering with the mechanisms of the knee joint. Popliteal vein, popliteal artery, and sciatic nerve injuries can result from this fracture [9].

Whether the patient has been treated operatively or not, traction will probably be indicated at first, and can be used for a few days to a few months. A study of the literature indicates that early exercise while the patient is still in traction is essential [25, 37]. Generally, quadriceps sets are initiated immediately. When tenderness at the fracture site diminishes progressive active assistive and active exercises can be performed with the Pearson attachment and Thomas' splint in place [17]. Early intensive strengthening of the quadriceps muscle and range of motion of the knee can not be overemphasized inasmuch as limitation at that joint is a common complication.

For the patient in a cast (hip spica, long leg, or cast brace) the physician must determine if exercise is permissible. If it is indicated the patient should be instructed in quadriceps and gluteal sets, and ankle range-of-motion exercises. The patient in a cast brace may be able to incorporate gentle knee exercises as well.

When the period of immobility ends, active

intensive rehabilitation is imperative. If the patient was at home for the period of immobility admission into a rehabilitation facility or outpatient therapy should be considered. The emphasis of the postimmobility period is regaining range of motion and strength at the knee, and the patient should be exercising constantly. Miniature quadriceps arcs, straight-leg raising, constant quadriceps sets, and hold-relax are all necessary. Passive range-of-motion exercise is rarely indicated during this stage. Hydrotherapy, bicycle, and sling suspension permit the patient to exercise without the therapist being constantly present. Whether the patient is in a health-related facility or at home, an exercise program should be carried out independently. Family members and home health aides can all be instructed to assist the patient.

As more callus formation is noted on roentgenogram, the physician will order resistive and passive exercise. Progressive resistive exercise, proprioceptive neuromuscular facilitation, and resistive bicycle maneuvers are all examples of successful resistive programs. Passive range-of-motion exercises may be painful, and the therapist can perform these and hold-relax techniques in the whirlpool to decrease pain. The patient will require at least 90 degrees of knee flexion to carry out many activities of daily living, and that should be the goal whenever possible.

The time to initiate gait training will fluctuate significantly for the patient with femur fracture. The patient with an internal fixation device may begin ambulating days after surgery, while for one with a comminuted supracondylar fracture this may take months. Measuring for leg length discrepancy and obtaining a lift is important, as shortening of the femur is a common complication. The amount of weight-bearing permitted will be ascertained by the stability of the fracture on roentgenogram and physical examination [25]. The physician may order a long leg brace to be worn during ambulation to decrease the amount of weight placed on the femur. The therapist, orthotist, and phy-

sician must work closely to obtain the proper type and fit for an orthotic device. When gait training, it is important to have the knee motion gained on the mat carried over into gait by encouraging flexion through the swing phase of walking.

The occupational therapist will have to evaluate the patient through various stages of rehabilitation. For instance, the reacher that was necessary when the patient was in a spica cast may prevent the patient from gaining knee motion once the cast has been removed.

The social worker must work closely with the family and other members of the team to determine how and where the patient's needs can best be met during many months of rehabilitation. The goal is to return the patient to the premorbid life-style in the shortest time possible. With the femur fracture, long periods of immobility cannot be avoided, and it takes a concerted effort on the part of the team to prevent detrimental complications.

TIBIAL FRACTURES

The tibia is the most common site for long bone fractures [25]. They can be categorized as occurring in the plateau, shaft, and malleoli. Indications for open reduction and internal fixation include irreducible intraarticular fractures, irreducible epiphyseal injuries in growing children, concomitant neurovascular injury where emergency intervention and osseous stabilization are necessary, certain unstable or comminuted metaphyseal and diaphyseal fractures, and nonunions [25].

Fractures of the tibial plateau can usually be treated by nonsurgical methods. The patient will be immobilized in a cast, splint, or cast brace. Occasionally, traction will precede the period of immobility [25]. Should the tibial plateau be severely depressed or irreducibly displaced, surgical fixation may be necessary.

Tibial shaft fractures are associated with an injury such as with a moving vehicle [37]. Incidence of open fractures of the area is high [37]. Closed fractures can be treated with closed reduction followed by immobility in a plaster long leg cast or cast brace, and early weight-bearing [25]. When the fracture is unstable, a rigid external device such as a Hoffman apparatus or internal fixation with pins or intermedullary rods may be required.

Fracture of the malleoli can involve the medial or lateral malleoli, or posterior margin of the tibia, often called the third malleolus [37]. Treatment can involve closed reduction followed by a short leg cast and a period of nonweight-bearing. If the malleolus cannot be reduced surgical fixation may be necessary.

Whether the treatment is operative or not, the patient is often immobilized for many weeks. The treatment program may begin with gentle isometric quadriceps exercise and active ankle motions while the patient is in the cast. Frequent radiological studies will determine when the patient should begin active knee flexion and extension exercises. The patient must often remain nonweight-bearing for many weeks, followed by weight-bearing in a cast, cast brace, patellar tendon-bearing cast, or splint.

The tibial fracture is riddled with complications. It can result in knee and ankle stiffness, and occasionally, related ligamentous injuries. Early effective rehabilitation of knee and ankle motion is imperative in preventing a stiff joint. The therapist must be astute, looking for signs of lateral popliteal nerve damage. Should it exist, electromyographic studies and electrical stimulation may be indicated. Chronic edema can be combated with elastic stockings and active exercise. Other complications may include popliteal artery injury, degenerative joint disease, delayed union, nonunion, malunion, infection, and shortening of the extremity [9].

## Knee Disabilities

The knee is a complex joint that creates a challenge for the health care team when pathology is evidenced. Disability in the form of advanced rheumatoid arthritis or osteoarthritis can have a devastating effect on the patient's life-style. When medication and a conservative physical rehabilitation regimen prove unsuccessful, surgery should be considered.

TOTAL KNEE REPLACEMENT
When procedures such as synovectomy, debridement, and osteotomy have been ruled unfavorable by the surgeon, total knee replacement often becomes the treatment of choice [7]. The primary indication for this is relief of pain [21]. In addition, knee arthroplasty can restore stability of the joint, increase range of motion, and improve deformity and function [21]. Contraindications include a history of intraarticular infection, osteoporosis, severe laxity of ligaments surrounding the knee, neurogenic arthroplasty, arthrodesis or fusion of the joint, and uncorrectable genu recurvatum. Situations that would caution against the procedure include obesity, poor motivation, young active person, poor general health, and anyone with an active systemic disease [33].

There are many types of prosthetic devices presently being used. They can be categorized according to the degree of constraint they impose [33]. The fully constrained, or hinged, prosthesis has the femoral and tibial components locked together. Thus the fully constrained knee allows flexion and extension with little or no rotation. This type of prosthesis causes great stress at the knee because of the lack of rotation, and requires a large amount of bone resection for implantation [21], which means that alternative treatment of joint fusion is eliminated should the prosthesis prove unsuccessful. Therefore it should be used for the patient with marked instability and who lives a fairly sedentary life. Walldius, Shiers and Guespar, Kaufer, Matthews, and Sontsgard are common varieties of the fully constrained knee arthroplasty [21].

The partially constrained prosthesis is most widely used at the present time. The geometric, UCI, and total condylar arthroplasty are examples [33]. The femoral and tibial components are not linked; thus internal and external rotation can occur at the knee.

The minimally constrained or nonconstrained prosthesis relies on the ligaments and joint capsule for stability [33]. It should be considered for the patient who has mild instability yet may have severe pain. Examples include Gunston, Charnley, Freeman-Swanson, and Duo-condylar [21]. These polycentric replacements most closely simulate the normal human knee.

Rehabilitation begins preoperatively. All team members should perform a complete evaluation of the patient to obtain reference information. Prior to surgery, the patient should be thoroughly familiarized with the procedure, and instructed in quadriceps and gluteal set exercises and the use of crutches or a walker.

Immediate postoperative care should commence on day one, when the physical therapist begins isometric quadriceps exercise with the patient. On the second day, the dressing is replaced by a bandage. The patient is placed in a resting knee splint to be worn at all times except when exercising. Exercise is now broadened to include active assistive straight-leg raises, and active assistive knee flexion and extension in side-lying.

Early goals of the program are to obtain functional range of motion and strength of the knee as quickly as possible. It is important to confer with the surgeon to determine realistic goals. Typically, landmarks for functional use include flexion to 90 degrees, complete active extension or a knee lag no greater than 10 degrees, and the ability to perform active staight-leg raising [24]. A rigorous program is required to meet these goals, with the patient, therapist, and nurse actively working toward them. The therapist should have the patient perform isometric quadriceps exercise, and active assistive exercise leading to active exercise of knee flexion and extension two times per day. In addition, the patient must begin taking the initiative for performing these exercises when the therapist is not present. The patient gradually progresses to the sitting position at the edge of the bed to increase knee flexion. The bicycle can be useful at this time. By gradually lowering the height of the seat the patient will gain more flexion. Should it not be possible to achieve 90 degrees of knee flexion, manipulation is performed under anesthesia [11].

Proper positioning is important and cannot be overlooked. The nursing staff sees the patient 24 hours a day and plays a key role here. The patient should not sleep with a pillow under the knee, but rather under the ankle to encourage knee extension. The patient should be encouraged to lie prone as early as possible, and the knee should never be flexed or extended for more than one-half hour at a time.

Functionally, the patient may begin transfers with the splint at three to five days postoperatively. When active straight-leg raising is achieved with good control, the splint is discontinued. When active straight-leg raising is performed and knee flexion is 90 degrees, partial weight-bearing ambulation is begun [24]. A three-point gait (in which the patient was instructed preoperatively) should be initiated and the patient must be encouraged to flex the affected knee through the swing phase. Crutches or a walker will be needed for at least 4 to 6 weeks, after which a unilateral weight-bearing device can be used [21]. The occupational therapist should evaluate activities of daily living, the various stages of the patient's rehabilitation, and supply the necessary assistive devices such as grippers, raised toilet seat, and long-handled shoe horn. In addition, the patient with rheumatoid arthritis should be instructed in joint protection and proper body mechanics [24].

Discharge planning should begin preoperatively. The patient may require continued physical therapy at home, and a proper referral should be completed. Patient and family should be proficient in the home exercise program prior to discharge.

Complications resulting from a total knee replacement can be mechanical or nonmechanical. Instances of the former include loosening of the prosthesis, dislocation of the device, and fracture of the femur or tibia in osteoporotic bone [21]. Nonmechanical complications include infection, thrombophlebitis, contracture of the knee requiring surgical manipulation, knee extension lag greater than 15 degrees, and peroneal nerve injury [21, 33].

## LIGAMENTOUS INJURY

The ligaments surrounding the knee provide stability to the joint. The cruciate ligaments prevent shearing motions at the knee and excessive rotation between the tibia and femur [7]. The medial and lateral ligaments provide stability when the knee is positioned in extension [44].

Trauma to the knee, as commonly seen in sports injuries, can cause ligamentous injuries. Acute treatment includes first aid, stress tests, and application of compression dressings. After thorough evaluation the degree of ligamentous injury can be classified into mild, moderate, or severe sprain [6].

A mild sprain preserves the integrity of the ligament and joint [7]. Treatment involves the application of a long leg cylinder cast or semirigid knee immobilizer for one to three weeks, with the patient permitted full weight-bearing [23]. For the patient who is reliable and willing to follow explicit instructions immobility may not be necessary. Moderate sprains result in weakening of the ligament while joint stability remains intact [7]. The patient is placed in a cylinder cast from three to six weeks, and allowed to ambulate with partial or full weight-bearing after the acute stage. Severe sprains involve a torn ligament with joint instability [7]. The treatment of choice is immediate surgical repair of the ligament and capsule. The extremity is then placed in a cylindrical cast for four to six weeks. If the medial and lateral ligaments are repaired, a cast brace follows the casting for four weeks [37].

The ligamentous injury can mean the patient is involved in a health care program for weeks or months. For the athletic or work-related injury outpatient therapy may be appropriate. For the geriatric patient, a home health care program will be important, including homemaker, home-based therapy, and social service.

During the period of immobility exercise is restricted to isometric quadriceps exercise, straight-leg raising, and hip abduction. The involved extremity may be casted in knee flexion depending on the ligament injured. After the cast is removed intensive rehabilitation must be initiated on outpatient, inpatient, or home basis. Hydrotherapy will decrease pain and swelling and increase range of motion. Gentle active exercise is begun with the goal being 120 to 160 degrees of knee flexion [5]. The bicycle can be an excellent adjunct to treatment at this time for increasing range of motion and endurance. A resistive exercise program can commence when 70 to 80 degrees knee flexion is obtained [44]. Exercises for the hamstrings and quadriceps muscles may include progressive resistive exercises, proprioceptive neuromuscular facilitation, or isokinetics. The goals at this stage are to increase strength, endurance, and speed.

Ambulatory status can vary significantly with this disability. The cast brace can be helpful in allowing early weight-bearing and knee mobility during gait. Knee cages are often discouraged, as they supply little support [23].

As strength, range of motion, and muscle bulk improve and as pain decreases, the patient is encouraged to begin swimming and bicycling. The physician must determine when the patient can begin running, and return to work or to competitive sports.

Rehabilitation following a knee ligament injury can be hampered by knee lag, decreased range of motion of the joint, pain, swelling, and snapping of the knee. Instability can occur as a result of improper diagnosis or limited results from ligamentous repair [44]. Chronic instability can cause degenerative changes, pain, and loss of function.

# Lower Extremity Amputations

*Richard J. Kathrins*

Amputations are performed for a variety of pathological trauma, malignancy, and congenital abnormalities of bone, tendon, and joint. Arterial reconstruction is used as a means to preserve the integrity of the extremity or enable amputation at a lower level.

An amputation secondary to trauma does not allow the surgeon to decide stump length or, in many cases, the shape of the stump, although revision may be made to eliminate infection or obtain a better shape or contour [26]. In elective amputation, the site is preselected. The surgeon keeps in mind the prostheses available and what type of stump would best conform to the device chosen. In addition, the amount of disability the patient can endure, expected increase in energy, age, sex, and premorbid life-style are considered.

## PROSTHETIC EVALUATION

When determining if the patient is a candidate for a prosthesis, a variety of factors must be assessed including desired life-style, prior ambulation status, and mental and physical status. An amputee who receives a prosthesis must have motivation, dedication, and the ability to endure a rigorous rehabilitation program before and after receiving the device. In addition, one must be prepared to tolerate the increased physical demands, particularly energy expenditure.

The patient who is disoriented, confused, or uncooperative may not be a prosthetic candidate. This would apply also if gross muscle weakness is present in either extremity and is not improving. Joint contractures of the hip greater than 30 to 35 degrees, or knee flexion contracture greater than 15 degrees may preclude an artificial aid. Joint contractures in the unaffected extremities may also produce complications for fitting. Poor skin condition must be remedied, and the patient must be medically stable before a prosthesis can be ordered. It should be noted that a patient may not want a prosthesis, and may be satisfied with functional independence with a wheelchair or other assistive device such as a walker.

If the patient is to have a prosthesis, a decision must be made whether to choose a permanent or temporary one. When looking at normal locomotion, it becomes clear that something cosmetically acceptable and mechanically efficient is needed. It must be suspended from the stump so as to be comfortable, and able to communicate the stress forces efficiently from the body to the ground [26].

Comfort is a major consideration. The socket or the suspension device must not rub, bind, or pinch during rest or motion. Pressure points and tender areas demand attention. Ease of putting on and taking off the article often depends on the patient's age and level of disability; it is difficult to put on a prosthesis if there is decreased mobility, balance, or strength. The weight of the unit is important, as it must be heavy enough to give security but light enough to avoid the sensation of heaviness. A secure and appropriate suspension device aids in maneuverability [32]. It should be noted that there is no standard device for any one level of activity. It is up to the team to determine the ideal prosthesis for each patient.

## PROSTHESES

The preparatory or temporary prosthesis is less expensive and can be fabricated more quickly than a permanent one can. It can be used to aid in rapid shrinkage of the stump and to prevent contracture. It can be used for the more debilitated patient, or during assessment of the patient's suitability for a more intricate and costly device [26]. The preparatory prosthesis may also be indicated for patients unable to benefit from training with a permanent one because of senility or general physical disability. Preparatory aids are usually made of plaster of Paris, plastic adjustable molds, or adjustable leather with laced sockets and a long leg brace attached to a foot. Major disadvantages include discomfort, lack of cosmetic appeal, and inadequate simulation of normal gait [32]. These factors may have to be overlooked if the patient has to be mobilized quickly.

The permanent prosthesis offers a wide array of advantages for the patient who can benefit from the rehabilitation program. With the development of total contact sockets, the patient is better able to duplicate gait patterns. The prosthesis aids in the difficult task of proper distribution of weight, enhances proprioception, and eliminates the restrictions of stump length. It helps to reduce the problems of distal edema, ischemia, and ulceration. It has been shown that the total contact socket promotes healing [32].

The knee joints newly devised for amputations above the knee allow better simulation of normal gait. The shaft of the prosthesis can be made to look skinlike. Cosmesis, comfort, security, sensory feedback, and psychological adjustment are all additional benefits. The major disadvantage is that it is difficult to alter once it is made, particularly the socket. The socket can be shaved down, built up, or the patient can alternate the number of stump socks worn, but these are limiting factors. It should be noted that the contour of the stump often changes after wearing a total contact socket for prolonged periods.

A team approach is used in treating amputees. Members must be aware of psychological needs so that support can be provided. In addition, a prosthetic clinic provides a means of organizing activities and communication among a number of people, and enables contact between various specialties involved in rehabilitation. The clinic is often composed of the physiatrist, prosthetist, physical therapist, and occupational therapist, who make the recommendation for the type of prosthesis that is to be ordered. The clinic is also a good place for patient and staff education.

EVALUATION
Range of motion and muscle strength are evaluated, and significant abnormalities noted. Measurement is made of the length and cir-

cumference of the stump. The below-knee area is measured from the medial tibial plateau to the end of the tibia. The extra soft tissue is not measured, but will make the stump appear longer. For the above-knee stump, measurement is from the ischial tuberosity to the end of the femur. Circumference is measured by marking the stump vertically every two inches, and noting the circumference horizontally at each two-inch marker.

Evaluation of the condition of the stump should include information on the shape, scar, skin, musculature, sensation, and phantom sensation, and if present, a discussion of rashes, inflammation, abrasions, or adhesions. This initial record will give the therapist a guide against which changes over a period of time can be noted.

The patient's functional status is also assessed, including ability to transfer and ambulate, mobility in bed and wheelchair, and ability to perform activities of daily living.

TREATMENT
The program involves therapy for the patient's amputated extremity as well as the uninvolved extremities. Preprosthetic training consists of exercise and functional techniques. Goals are to improve circulation, muscle tone, strength, and joint mobility, and decrease hypersensitivity if present, all directed toward preparing the patient to accept the prosthesis.

Exercise begins as early as possible and is designed to help the patient coordinate the stump with the rest of the body parts and facilitate body symmetry. Dynamic stump exercises [9A] are used with most, if not all patients, but may have to be modified depending on age and general ability. Proprioceptive neuromuscular facilitation patterns may be incorporated into the program, as can a developmental mat sequence. These exercises may be performed in conjunction with progressive resistive exercise and a sling suspension program. Whatever technique is used, the objective is increased muscle strength and coordination.

Bed mobility and positioning should be

stressed. Without instruction, the patient is likely to keep the stump in flexion, abduction, and external rotation, possibly resulting in deformity or muscle contractures. Pillows should not be used beneath the knee in a below-knee amputation, or under the stump in an above-knee amputation. If elevation is required, the entire extremity must be supported evenly for the below-knee amputee, and the pelvis must be elevated evenly for the above-knee amputee. The patient may also lie prone twice daily to maintain and increase range of motion of the hip or knee.

Edema must be treated early in the prepros-thetic stage, as if it is allowed to continue it can lead to pain, joint contractures, or adhesions. Edema can be treated with bandaging or stump shrinkers. Desensitivity techniques are instituted if the extremity is hypersensitive. The stump that is too sensitive will cause the patient difficulty in the prosthetic socket. Desensitivity procedures include rubbing the stump with textured materials or cloths, slapping, vibration, and tapping.

If pain is a problem, careful evaluation of its etiology is necessary. When the trigger point is a neuroma, ultrasound may be used. This may have to be given under water to avoid pain from the pressure of the sound head.

Gait and functional training activities begin early in the preprosthetic program with emphasis on gait pattern and balance activities. Once good balance is achieved the sequencing of the gait pattern is taught. Endurance may need to be improved, as the energy expended is greatly increased when walking with a prosthetic device. Transfer training and bed and wheelchair mobility must be accomplished early. When ordering a wheelchair, attention must be given to keeping the below-knee stump straight. With a bilateral amputee, care must be taken with regard to the center of gravity of the chair, as it must be more posterior than normal.

HIP DISARTICULATION
The hip disarticulation, or hemipelvectomy, is

rare, accounting for less than two percent of amputees [30], and is often done as a life-saving measure [22]. In dealing with the patient preprosthetically, similar problems are encountered as with an above-knee amputee, with the only difference that there is usually no stump. In this situation the therapy program concentrates on the remaining extremities and trunk for strengthening and mobility. If there is musculature remaining in the hip region, the therapist can work to maintain its integrity. Balance and gait training are initiated as soon as possible.

Although a number of prostheses have been developed for hip disarticulation [14, 30], the Canadian type is most frequently used. This unit is functional, comfortable, and cosmetically more acceptable than others. It is a socket-waistband constructed of continuous laminated plastic. The plastic is rigid over weight-bearing areas such as the ischial tuberosity and the gluteal tissues, and flexible elsewhere to allow ease in putting it on. It permits increased stability in stance, as the hip joint is located anterior to the knee, ensuring the knee's stability. Knee flexion is performed by contact of the extension bumper on the socket against the superior posterior portion of the thigh. A hip flexion control strap limits flexion during swing to about 15 degrees between the thigh and socket. The hip joint and socket are attached to a thigh shaft and mobile knee. This is attached to a lower shaft and solid ankle and cushioned heel, or SACH foot.

Preprosthetic training is vitally important to promote confidence in strength, balance, gait pattern, and functional activities. The therapist should work with the prosthetist in fitting and adjusting the prosthesis. This is particularly important when discussing the hip bumper, flexion control strap, and foot-ankle characteristics [35].

Once the patient is instructed in donning and doffing the prosthesis, pregait activities begin. These include weight-shifting from side to side and front and back, and foot placement. The patient should get a good feel for the stability of the knee at heel contact, which is imperative for normalization of gait. The more weight that is transmitted through the prosthesis, the greater the knee stability [35].

The patient must be trained to maintain the medial and lateral support of the torso. The socket is contoured to prevent excessive mediolateral motion. The tendency during stance is to allow the body's center of gravity to extend toward the medial aspect of the vertical support of the prosthesis. This is prevented by one of the diagonal forces exerted by the waistband over the sound hip, and the minimal distance between the center of gravity and the vertical support of the prosthesis [30].

The patient must be encouraged to have good extension of the trunk over the shaft, thus preventing forward flexion. If forward flexion is a continuing problem because of pain, the prosthetist may have to be consulted about providing reliefs or padding. Finally, considerable emphasis is placed on timing and use of the pelvis to propel the prosthetic knee forward in swing. The amputee has to sit backward to flex the knee, exerting a pressure on the bumper; circumduction or rotation should not be used to accomplish this maneuver [35].

Major problems with this prosthesis are with fit, balance, foot placement, and knee stability. The patient must be able to get weight over the prosthesis and compress the heel. If the unit fits poorly or there is pain, the patient will shift weight unevenly. If weight is not placed on the unit, knee extension cannot be maintained and mediolateral support will be compromised.

ABOVE-KNEE AMPUTATION
Above-knee amputation is usually performed with an anterior skin flap. A musculofascial flap may be done over the bone, securing the muscles. This procedure will increase stability and strength, and also reduce chances of distal pressure necrosis [32]. The distal end of the stump should be no more than four to five inches from the knee axis; ideal length is 10 to 12 inches, allowing adequate space for the knee device [30].

Increase in muscle strength and range of motion, suppression of edema, and control of pain are part of the postoperative program. In addition, preprosthetic training includes stump wrapping on a 24-hour basis. It should be removed every few hours to let the area breathe and to observe for any skin breakdown or reddened areas. Wrapping is done in such a way as to avoid hip flexion and promote hip extension.

The top of the above-knee socket is in the shape of a quadrilateral brim, and contours to the stump at the level of the ischium. The adductor tendons are anteromedial, the ischial tuberosity posteromedial, and the greater trochanter is lateral: these boundaries form the quadrilateral brim. The ischial tuberosity and the tendons of the hamstring support the majority of the weight. Most amputees with above-knee stumps are fitted with this type of socket, as it provides good support and permits good use of remaining musculature. The distal end of the socket usually provides total contact and thus helps to prevent edema, enhance venous return, provide improved sensory feedback and weight dispersion, and aid with shin problems [30].

The suction socket is a means of attaching an above-knee prosthesis to the stump without the use of a pelvic belt or other type of suspension apparatus. This socket is often used by an amputee who has a well-shaped strong stump. It has a valve on the distal surface that allows air to be expelled from it during stance and does not allow air entry during swing. With the swing stage, the prosthesis has a tendency to fall off but the suction keeps it in place. Although it is put on with a sock to help get the stump into the socket, the sock is removed through the valve opening [18, 30]. The patient then screws the valve in place from the outside of the socket. The prosthesis is usually put on while standing. This type of socket offers many advantages including improved cosmesis, greater freedom of movement, increased use of remaining musculature, decreased pistoning action between the stump and socket, and comfort. It is, however, difficult to put on, and requires a certain degree of mobility and balance [30].

If the patient feels insecure or has difficulty keeping the prosthesis in place, a silesian bandage is used. This is a belt that attaches to the lateral aspect of the socket, passes around the body to the opposite iliac crest, and down to the center of the anterior wall of the socket. The band will help prevent rotation and maintain the prosthesis in adduction. If this is found to be insufficient, a pelvic band can be applied. There are two types of pelvic belt: rigid and flexible. The former is made of metal curved to fit the patient's waist. It contains a joint between it and the prosthesis that is usually located one-half inch anterior to the greater trochanter. The flexible belt gives support but also permits some mobility. Its pivot point is similar to that of the rigid joint, but slightly superior to it. The flexible belt passes around the body in a manner similar to the rigid band [1].

The knee assembly on these units can be either fixed or flexible. The fixed joint is more commonly used with a temporary prosthesis. It allows no motion at the knee during gait and can be released when sitting. The flexible knee unit provides stability during stance, particularly early to midstance, and allows knee flexion during late stance into swing. The stability of the knee may be accomplished by muscle force. In this way the knee is held into extension at heel strike and at midstance. The knee axis may be placed posterior to the weight-bearing line of the prosthesis, thus promoting extension. A locking mechanism is also incorporated into many prosthetic legs to prevent or restrict motion [30].

Knee joints are available with a single axis plus friction device (Table 3-2), and polycentric axis joints. With the latter there is rotation around more than 1 axis, with friction to movement applied with weight-bearing [30]. A myoelectrically controlled knee monitors movement by impulses picked up from the stump musculature. Hydraulic and pneumatic

TABLE 3-2. *Friction Devices at the Knee*

| Device | Action During Locomotion |
|---|---|
| Constant friction | Constant braking during swing phase |
| Constant friction with friction brake | Stability on stance and constant friction during swing phase |
| Variable friction | Increased friction at beginning of swing and minimal during midswing |
| Variable friction with friction brake | Same as above, except resists flexion on weight-bearing |

Source: Adapted into tabular form from New York University. *Lower Extremity Prosthetics.* New York: New York University, Post-Graduate Medical School, 1973.

knees are mainly used to control the swing phase, and can adapt to varying rates of walking [12, 30]. The lower shaft connects the knee unit and the foot/ankle assembly (usually a SACH foot).

Once the prosthesis has been fabricated, it should be checked out with the patient standing, sitting, and ambulating, and the stump should be examined after the prosthesis has been worn. The rehabilitation team watches for stability, comfort, fit, and energy expenditure. When standing, palpation or visual inspection of the adductor longus tendon should be made to ensure it is in the channel that is built into the socket medially to accommodate it. The patient should be resting on the ischial tuberosity, which should rest one-half inch behind the inner surface of the posterior wall [30]. At this time, the length of the prosthesis should be reviewed. The suspension device is also checked and evaluated for stability and the amount of mobility it allows. The patient then sits down and the prosthesis is observed to make sure that it does not fall off. If it does, there may be a problem with the suction socket or pelvic joint.

With the patient walking, the therapist should check for any gait deviation or pistoning in the stump. The patient should have a

TABLE 3-3. *Common Gait Deviations Following Amputation*

| Gait Deviation | Possible Cause |
|---|---|
| *Above-knee* | |
| Lateral bending of the trunk to the amputated side on stance | Pain in the groin area Abducted socket Pain on the lateral aspect of the distal stump |
| Circumduction of the prosthesis laterally | Insecurity; excessive knee friction leg length discrepancy |
| Medial or lateral whip at swing corresponding to whether the heel moves medially or laterally at toe-off | Incorrect rotational forces at the knee bolt |
| Uneven heel rise | Poorly adjusted friction mechanism at the knee |
| *Below-knee* | |
| Jack-knifing during early stance | Long lever arm Firm cushioned heel |
| Rotation of the prosthesis around the stump | Space between the lateral of the socket and the stump because of malalignment |
| Lateral bending of the trunk during stance | Abductor weakness Short prosthesis |
| Inversion or eversion of the foot | Loose fit requiring additional stump socks |
| Early knee flexion during late stance; circumduction during swing | Soft cushioned heel Weak quadriceps muscle |

Source: Adapted into tabular form from New York University. *Lower Extremity Prosthetics.* New York: New York University, Post-Graduate Medical School, 1973.

sensation of continuous contact during stance and swing phases [30].

Once the prosthesis is removed, the skin is examined for irritation, pressure points, edema, and specific areas of pain or tenderness. There should be some redness over the poste-rior brim around the area of the ischial tuberosity.

Instruction in the use of stump socks is important if the prosthesis has anything other than a suction socket. Socks must be worn over the stump for a good fit, and the number will depend on the tightness of fit.

Gait activities begin with weight-shifting and balance exercises, and is important for the patient to be comfortable and confident with the device. If gait training is initiated too soon, the patient will have problems later with cadence. Placement activities such as abduction and adduction of the leg are stressed, followed by weight-shifting with swing and walking in place. Gait training is often started using the parallel bars. It is important to stress a correct pattern in the program, however, and patient should not be allowed to gain a false sense of security with any assistive devices.

Some key points to emphasize are stability with the knee mechanism in early to mid-stance, and flexion of the knee at late stance and swing. The patient must be able to pull the prosthesis into extension at heel strike. During midstance there should be good hip extension over the prosthesis.

Some gait deviations (Table 3-3) may be observed because of improper alignment, pain, tightness of the socket, pinching, uneven leg length, timing, loss of sensation, muscle weakness, decreased range of motion, faulty knee mechanism, or even a SACH foot that is too soft or too hard. Most if not all of these problems are interrelated and often noticed at the time of evaluation or check-out, when they can be altered by the prosthetist.

BELOW-KNEE AMPUTATION
The length of below-knee amputation should be five to seven inches below the tibial plateau. A musculofascial flap is not always indicated. The end of the fibula is rounded and cut one inch shorter than the tibia. The program begins with wrapping to shape the stump, and exercise, with emphasis on the knee joint.

The prosthesis is usually made of a socket, a

shaft of either wood or metal alloy, and the ankle-foot assembly. The most common type of below-knee socket is a patellar tendon-bearing socket (PTB). As the name suggests, most of the weight is placed on the patellar tendon. This socket is usually a closed-end, total contact unit made in slight flexion to allow the tendon to bear the weight. The anterior wall contains the patellar shelf, which lies between the tibial tubercle and the patella's inferior surface. The socket contains a relief to encompass one-half of the patella, and the medial and lateral borders contain the femoral condyles. Distal to the medial femoral condyle relief is the medial flair of the tibia, which also supports a large percentage of the weight. The posterior wall contains the popliteal bulge, which forces the stump against the patellar shelf anteriorly for weight-bearing. The fibular head, peroneal nerve, and the distal end of the fibula are all encased in reliefs. Most of the sockets are made of a plastic laminate with a soft synthetic insert; stump socks are used.

Because of its total contact design, this socket helps prevent edema, provides additional areas of support for the stump, and gives better sensory feedback. In most instances a suspension system is required, some variants of which are supracondylar, supracondylar-suprapatellar, and the air-cushioned sockets. The air-cushioned socket was fabricated to allow increased weight-bearing distally. It is made of a rigid outer shell and an inner elastic sleeve [30]. There is an air chamber between them, compression of which provides distal support.

The supracondylar cuff suspension uses a cuff that goes around the thigh just above the femoral condyles and patella. The other type of supracondylar suspension system has high medial and lateral walls that encompass the femoral condyles completely. To make it easier to put on, a removable wedge is used between the socket wall and the medial epicondyle to ensure an intimate fit [30].

The supracondylar-suprapatellar prosthesis also has a high medial and lateral wall, but it does have a higher anterior wall to encompass the patella as well. There is no wedge, but there is a removable compressible insert for donning. The prosthesis is usually put on while sitting with the knee flexed. The compressible insert is put on first, then slid into the prosthetic socket. This socket design with the supracondylar wedge socket offers increased mediolateral support.

The other suspension system is a thigh corset with a knee joint that can either be mobile or rigid, with a release lock. The decision to use a locked knee will depend on how much stability is required. The advantage of this system is that it supports the prosthesis on the stump during stance as well as during swing, but it does not allow for polycentric mobility. A fork strap with an elastic strap may be used as well. This unit attaches from the shaft of the prosthesis to a waist belt. This again helps to support the prosthesis and aid in knee extension during swing. An extensor strap may be used posteriorly to limit overextension at the end of swing and during stance.

The prosthesis has to be checked out, and static and dynamic alignment evaluated before gait training begins. The patient is evaluated sitting, standing, and walking, and the cosmetic appearance assessed for acceptability. Leg length and suspension are observed while standing. There should not be any pistoning between the stump and socket. The patient should be able to flex and extend the knee without pain. Once the prosthesis is removed the stump is examined to note any areas of redness or tenderness. Some redness over the patellar tendon and the medial tibial flair is to be expected. The prosthesis is then put back on and the patient ambulates. Stride length should be the same, with no jack-knifing during early stance, and good alignment at mid-stance.

The actual training in ambulation of the below-knee amputee is usually easier than with the above-knee amputee. Before gait training begins, balance, weight-shifting, and placement activities are started. The patient must gain confidence before continuing. After walking in place and stepping with weight-shifting are accomplished, forward walking begins. Timing and rhythm are encouraged. Advanced gait activities can then be instituted, such as stepping backward and to the side, and getting up from the ground.

## SYMES AMPUTATION

The Symes procedure is designed for full end weight-bearing. With this procedure the medial and lateral malleoli are removed, as is the lower inch of the tibia. The end weight-bearing flap is brought up from beneath the heel of the calcaneus [15]. This amputation is usually performed only where there is a loss of the foot, or when the foot stump is too short and there is an adequate heel flap to accept the weight. The ends of the tibia and fibula are contoured but left quite bulbous. The stump is usually painless and trouble-free.

Prosthetic care is essentially that of the below-knee amputee; the only exception is that these patients usually have less of a problem with edema and pain. The prosthesis most frequently used is a total-contact, plastic laminated socket. There is a posterior or medial opening for donning. Its sides reach as high as the medial and lateral tibial plateau. The unit usually encompasses a SACH foot.

Although this prosthesis allows for almost complete end weight-bearing, some weight is carried between the socket and the sides of the stump. No suspension is required because of its design.

Check-out is similar to that of the below-knee unit. Gait training is not usually required in great detail. The only thing to keep in mind is that the patient has no ankle. Thus there must be appropriate concentration on the fabrication and alignment of the SACH foot. If the heel cushion is too soft or hard the patient's hip and knee will not be able to line up appropriately.

## BILATERAL AMPUTATION

Bilateral below-knee amputees do well with PTB prostheses, but the bilateral above-knee patient has more difficulty. Because of the increased lack of the sensory input essential for balance, there is diminished awareness of self in space, and significant restriction in mobility. The patient may have one stump that is stronger than the other and therefore is used as the more normal side.

Pre- and postprosthetic training is similar to that with unilateral involvement, although more time is needed with balance activities and weight-shifting exercises. It should be emphasized that proficiency in these two areas must be achieved before gait training begins. These patients will require increased external support through such devices as parallel bars, walkers, or crutches.

# Upper Extremity Orthopedics

*Elaine LaCroix and Judith G. Helman*

From the first moments of medical intervention, restoration of maximum functional use must be promoted because of the complexity and precision required to perform vocational and avocational tasks. Therapy must be comprehensive and address all upper extemity joints. For example, the shoulder is one of the keys to hand function. Disability of the shoulder can limit the effectiveness of the hand as readily as hand involvement can result in shoulder restriction. The total person, and not just one small portion, is treated.

## EVALUATION

When the patient first arrives for therapy, rapport is established and the goals are fully explained. The patient should understand that the aim of therapy is to improve function not cause pain; knowing this can help lessen anxiety and encourage cooperation.

Assessment includes the areas outlined as follows:

Background: Diagnosis, cause, surgery (date

and type), old injuries, age, dominance, employment

Attitude: Orientation, ability to follow directions, cooperation, expectations for recovery

Trophic: State of the wound, dressings, cast (removal date), coloration, edema, temperature

Range of motion: Active, passive, tips to distal palmar crease

Prehension: Gross grasp, lateral pinch, three-pad pinch, three-tip pinch

Manual muscle testing: Group strength, individual muscles

Sensation: Pain, light touch, temperature, two-point discrimination, Tinel's sign, numbness, pins and needles, hypersensitivity

Functional status: Ability to perform common one- and two-handed daily tasks

Whenever possible, the therapist who performs the initial evaluation should carry out follow-up assessments. Sessions last as long as is feasible for the patient; generally, more than one hour at a time is too taxing.

## ATTITUDE

The success of any treatment program will depend on the patient's understanding, cooperation, and compliance. All too frequently the patient does not ask questions, but decides that the physician is too busy or the questions are too trivial, or simply feels too overwhelmed to think of questions while the physician is available. Answering some of these concerns is another way of beginning therapeutic rapport.

Trauma can cause personality changes that may be noticed by the therapist or the family. At times a spouse may comment on such a difference, and be relieved to find that this is common and usually reversible. As the treatment program progresses, a more positive, less irritable individual evolves, and the family regains its original member. In some cases, however, it is the family's changed attitude toward the injured person that has to be dealt with because it interferes with the patient's progress.

## SKIN CARE

As soon as the cast or splint is removed, the patient should learn to touch the injured extremity again. One beneficial way is through skin care. First, the body part is bathed. If sutures are still intact, an antiseptic soap is used. Whirlpool is helpful, but may be contraindicated for the edematous extremity. The arm is never allowed to hang in a dependent position during cleansing. Warm water is used as hot can lead to increased swelling. Some surgeons prefer that cleaning of the area wait until all of the sutures are removed, although this may cause limitation of early motion.

Once the sutures are removed and the wound is closed, lotion is applied to the area. Longer-lasting results are found with those creams containing cocoa butter, lanolin, or mineral oil. If edema is a concern, the lotion is applied using gentle circular motions going distally to proximally. This technique is sometimes referred to as *gentle retrograde massage*.

## EDEMA

Liquid, soft congestive, or pitting edema can occur in varying degrees after any injury in which blood and lymph circulation are obstructed. This fluid is rich in protein and provides a good nutrient medium for fibroblast formation [46]. The exudate can penetrate between the muscles and the gliding surfaces and cause them to become adherent. Basically, the longer edema remains, the more particles are left behind to hamper motion. The amount of edema can be assessed objectively by a volumeter or tape measure [16].

The interplay between edema and scar formation and between scar formation and active and passive motion must be understood and respected by both therapist and patient. Edema is excessive body fluid, and is generally present during the intial stage of wound healing, acutely from three to five days [8]. Eleva-

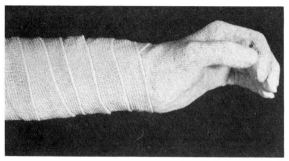

FIGURE 3-2. *Glove with Ace wrap. This technique may be used with an edematous extremity. The bandage should be applied using even tension, and overlap the end of the stretch glove.*

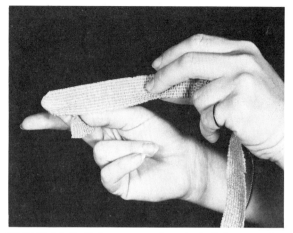

FIGURE 3-3. *Coban wrap. One-inch Coban can be wrapped distally to proximally, using even tension as a control for digital edema.*

tion of hand or arm above the heart is commonly regarded as initial control, whether the person is sitting, standing, or supine. If possible, the hand should be held on the chest when sitting or standing. If there is a heavy cast, slings can be useful for daytime wear. Care must be taken to ensure that undue stress is not placed on the opposite shoulder or neck as a result of inadequate fit or padding. The elbow is usually flexed to 90 degrees or more, and the hand must be fully supported in the sling. During rest, whether supine or side-lying (the affected side up), the hand or arm should be elevated. The forearm should be inclined, with the hand higher than the elbow and the elbow above the shoulder.

Active motion is considered the most effective approach for increasing venous and lymphatic outflow from the extremities. As soon as medically indicated, isometric and active motion should be encouraged. External compressions can be used if edema persists.

A JOBST pressurized compression sleeve can be applied once the cast has been removed, to maintain the size of the area. A customized JOBST garment may be ordered, or a Futuro Aris or other elasticized glove can be used on an interim basis. If the forearm is involved, an Ace bandage can be applied. The patient or family member should learn to wrap the arm going distally to proximally with even pressure. The bandage should overlap with the end of the glove. One must never apply pressure only to the arm, as the hand is likely to swell (Figure 3-2).

When involvement is only one or more fingers compression can be given through individual digit wrapping, thus avoiding loss of sensory input to uninvolved areas. Coban or string wrap may be used for the fingers (Figure 3-3). Coban is a nontacky self-adhering product that can be easily applied by the patient. It gives external pressure while allowing active motion. String wrap using three-ply cotton rug yarn [16] is harder to apply, and restricts motion to some degree. With both of these materials, the patient has to be taught not to wrap the finger too tightly, causing a tourniquet effect. With all external compression garments, the best results are achieved when the garments are worn at all times except for bathing and other activities that might get them wet.

Contrast baths of hot and cold water have also been found to help in controlling edema [16]. Contrast baths and compression garments are not indicated for the patient with a peripheral vascular disorder such as Raynaud's phenomenon. Also, with any extremity trauma smoking is not advised as it decreases peripheral circulation [27].

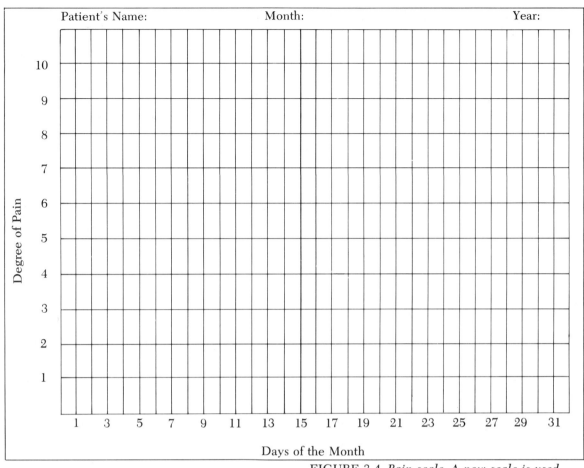

Patient's Name:          Month:                    Year:

Degree of Pain

10
9
8
7
6
5
4
3
2
1

1   3   5   7   9   11   13   15   17   19   21   23   25   27   29   31

Days of the Month

FIGURE 3-4. *Pain scale. A new scale is used each month. Pain should be plotted on a daily basis at the same time each day. An X indicates pain level prior to treatment; a dot (•) indicates posttreatment pain level.*

## RANGE-OF-MOTION EXERCISES

Active exercises should be attempted first, as they are important in controlling edema and in keeping muscles strong and tendons gliding. The patient should learn to appreciate the difference between discomfort and actual pain when exercising, and go to the point of discomfort and a little beyond. Activity that causes pain can lead to increased edema and soreness that will make the person less likely to want to exercise again. Frequent and brief sessions are advised, rather than a few prolonged attempts. Pain or the fear of it may interfere with at-

tempts at motion. Pain must be respected and investigated, as its presence could indicate remaining infection or a foreign body. Constant throbbing pain suggests that the patient is using aggressive passive movement rather than gentle active exercise.

Heat modalities such as paraffin, warm water soaks, or hot packs prior to exercise may help to lessen pain and stiffness [8]. The patient should record the perceived level of pain before and after movement, using a scale from one to ten, ten being maximum pain (Figure 3-4). Responses often become fairly consistent with each individual. It should be noted if pain medication has been prescribed as this may be a factor in changes observed in the extremity.

If complete active motion is not possible, gentle active assistive ranging is introduced. The joint is actively moved as far as it can go, and using the other hand, the patient pushes the joint just beyond the point of discomfort. This position is held while the affected extremity relaxes a few seconds. The patient then contracts the muscles in the affected area, and tries to maintain the new position while the support from the uninvolved hand is removed. With an injured finger, active assistive exercise exercise can be accomplished by taping the finger with an adjacent digit or wearing a buddy strap [16].

Once sutured or fractured structures are stable, active resistive exercise is advised. Resistance can be provided by the other hand, various grades of exercise putty, weights, or functional activities. The patient needs to know that an increase in swelling or persistent aching are signs of attempting too much too soon and either the number of repetitions or the degree of resistance requires a decrease. The diagnosis will indicate if an increase in endurance or strength is the primary goal.

The second phase of wound healing is the laying down of scar tissue. Fibroblasts synthesize collagen, which increase the area's tensile strength. For complicated injuries, up to 12 months may be needed for preinjury strength to be regained. This phase begins in the second or third week after injury. It is followed by the third phase in which fibroblasts, capillaries, and new collagen remodel along the lines of stress. Gentle passive stretch is believed to be the only clinical way to remold scar [47]. Passive range of motion is thought to tear scar and cause it to bleed, thus creating additional scar formation [10]. Slight tension over a prolonged period is more beneficial than a great amount for a brief time. A sustained gentle pull can be provided by weights, for example, and elbow flexion contracture can be treated by means of wrist cuffs. With the elbow sup-

ported, a cuff that gives slight stress is worn for increasing periods throughout the day, beginning with five to 15 minutes and working up to approximately an hour. Gains in range of motion of the elbow or other joints can be achieved and maintained by serial or dynamic traction splinting.

STRENGTH
During immobilization, muscle strength decreases as much as 7½ percent per day [28]. Thus isometrics are taught while the cast or splint is on [45], and proprioceptive neuromuscular facilitation patterns [19] and progressive resistive exercises are started as early as medically indicated. Exercise may be viewed as boring; a motivating factor is the use of appropriate daily tasks, through which strength and range of motion improve and a result is achieved.

Objective measurement of strength is recorded at regular intervals, through use of either dynamometer or pinch meter.

SENSATION
During initial evaluation, patients are asked about altered perception of light touch and temperature. Ojective measurement follows, with particular attention to areas of suspected impairment. Precautions with regard to sensory loss are reviewed. If hypersensitivity to cold exists, the person must learn of the potential for frostbite and the need to wear mittens, not gloves, when hands are exposed to cool or cold air. Mittens allow body heat to pass from finger to finger and permit better motion.

SPLINTING
Splints can be designed to stabilize joints, maintain and improve function, protect structures, and prevent deformities. They may be static or dynamic, prefabricated or custom-made. No matter what the function or design, the wearer must be aware of the rationale for its use, proper care, wearing precautions, and the desired wearing schedule to aid in its achieving the desired results.

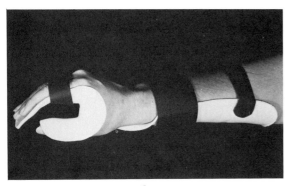

FIGURE 3-5. *Resting splint.*

A solution of 70 percent alcohol or a mild household cleaner can be used daily for cleaning the splint surface. The patient must be taught to check periodically for signs of edema and compression of skin, nerves, and blood supply, and know who and where to call if a problem develops.

If more than one splint is indicated, a wearing schedule for each should be clearly written to avoid confusion and possible complications; diagrams can also be helpful. The desired wearing time may not initially be possible because of lack of tolerance. The wearer must understand that this can occur and know gradually to increase wearing time. Within a few days after receiving the splint, the patient should return to the clinic for a check.

The position a relaxed hand assumes naturally when the arm is at the side is the position of function, and is commonly used for resting (supportive) splints, although it may not be the best one in which to immobilize a traumatized hand. With the tendency of ligaments to shorten, corrective or preventive splinting, including immobilization of the hand during healing of a fracture, places the wrist in 30 to 60 degrees of extension, the metacarpophalangeal (MP) joints of the fingers in 60 to 90 degrees of flexion, and the interphalangeal (IP) joints of the fingers in 0 to 15 degrees of flexion. The thumb is abducted and extended, and volar to the index finger (Figure 3-5). For fine manipulation the hand uses variations of this position, but for larger grasping, the MP joints extend and the terminal joints flex.

Before the affected extremity can begin daily activities, instruction in one-handed techniques takes place. As strength and coordination improve, normal grasp patterns are encouraged. Occasionally, dominance has to be changed.

HOME PROGRAM

All gains may not be made during therapy sessions. Time has to be spent on a home program, and the person's motivation can greatly affect results. Compliance can be promoted by providing a written regimen that coordinates exercise, activity, and splint-wearing. It should include frequency of the program components, sequence of the tasks, and the therapist's name and telephone number. Linking the sessions with regular activity, such as before meals or at bedtime, can make it easier to remember to do them. Making a name and number available is a sign of support and interest.

## Shoulder Orthopedics
### ADHESIVE CAPSULITIS

The terms *frozen shoulder* (glenohumeral and scapulothoracic joints) and *adhesive capsulitis* (glenohumeral joint) refer to a painful stiff shoulder that has limited active and passive range of motion. Pain is usually diffuse [6, 34, 37]. The best treatment of adhesive capsulitis is not to allow it to develop. It usually lasts three to six months, although two years of therapy may be required to regain full range of motion. Medication may be used to reduce inflammation and prevent pain.

Evaluation should include measurement by goniometry. Passive range of motion may be too painful to assess. Neck and elbow range should be recorded to be sure that pain is not causing a decrease in motion of uninvolved joints. Strength need not be assessed at the first visit, as it will be diminished by pain. Pain, however, should be assessed using the scale previously described, with location and precipitating factors noted. In the early phases of this syndrome, edema of the hand may not be a problem, although it may occur in later phases because of the posture of the arm.

The program includes instruction in active range-of-motion exercise performed while the patient is supine. This position is used to stabilize the trunk and avoid compensatory motion. The patient moves the arm to the point of discomfort. Often, abduction is the most painful motion. Hot packs may be used prior to movement to reduce pain and stiffness.

Use of a dowel may be helpful for shoulder flexion, and also to keep the arm in the proper plane. Wall-walking for shoulder flexion can be used to give the patient feedback on progress. It can be done sitting or standing, and the patient can mark and date a place on the wall to keep a record of gains. Pendulum and internal and external rotation exercises are also indicated.

The next step in therapy is to progress the patient to active assistive motion to increase strength.

## DISLOCATION

Anterior dislocation of the humeral head is frequently seen, and often occurs from trauma to an abducted, externally rotated arm [34]. After dislocation, closed reduction is generally possible and the arm is supported in a sling for three to six weeks.

On physician's orders, the patient may begin pendulum exercises. Care must be taken not to overstretch the capsule during the early post-reduction period. Active exercising is guarded at first. Depending on the patient's condition and the physician's assessment, external rotation may not be permitted or only performed within a limited range. Strengthening exercises are started as soon as medically indicated.

## ROTATOR CUFF TEARS

Rotator cuff tears most often occur as a result of indirect trauma to the shoulder during elevation of the arm, as to break a fall or maintain balance, and rupture, as with an older person who has had several attacks of bursitis. Anterior dislocation or a degenerative process may also lead to rupture of the supraspinous tendon. Of the rotator cuff muscles, this is the one most often ruptured [34, 42].

During the initial stages there can be a great amount of pain in the shoulder. Injection of an anesthetic and steroid combination may reduce inflammation and pain. Treatment is to immobilize the arm in a sling until pain subsides enough for the patient to begin gentle exercise. Therapy starts with pendulum exercises and progresses to active assistive and active exercises. Conservative management continues for two to threee months. If the patient has not improved, surgical intervention may be indicated to repair the tendon [34].

# Upper Arm, Elbow, and Forearm Orthopedics

## HUMERAL FRACTURES

Fractures of the humerus can occur at the head, along the shaft, or at the condyles. Shoulder stiffness may be the result of a malunion of the head of the humerus. Generally, exercise can reduce the stiffness, but a decrease in abduction may require surgery at the acromion [42].

Fracture of the humeral shaft usually does not require surgical correction, but can result in entrapment of the radial nerve. When there is involvement of the radial nerve, dorsal support of the wrist is provided in extension, and the thumb and fingers in slight flexion. This prevents joint pain, extensor overstretching, and ligament tightening. A conventional outrigger splint design can be used, or a dorsal shell with elastic straps for the fingers and thumb can be fabricated. Both allow finger flexion and functional grasp, but the latter is easier to deal with, particularly when putting on and taking off clothes.

A supracondylar fracture can affect the trunk of the median nerve or the anterior interosseous nerve. Immobilization continues until the site is pain-free. Although motion begins early, it can take up to two years before results are realized. If the fracture is into the joint, open reduction may be indicated and results can be limited. Volkmann's ischemia has been known to develop with condylar fractures, causing severe forearm edema that critically reduces circulation. If it is not identified and corrected early, sensation and motion are reduced or even lost. Malunion of condylar fractures may affect elbow motion. The valgus and varus deformities that occur from condylar malunion cannot be corrected therapeutically [42].

In addition to a splint supporting the hand, another may be worn at the fracture site [3, 41]. Once the initial pain and swelling have subsided, the cast may be replaced by a custom-molded, circumferential, thermoplastic splint for closed shaft reductions. Sarmiento's design allows full shoulder and elbow range, and Bell's splint limits shoulder abduction slightly.

The humeral splint is worn until roentgenograms show healed bone. As this can take up to six months, it is important for the patient to be examined periodically. As the upper arm changes size with decreasing muscle bulk and edema, the splint will need to be altered so that it is always snug. Frequently, a strap over the opposite shoulder is needed to keep the splint from shifting and sliding. Moleskin lining may be enough to prevent motion.

To lessen disuse atrophy, isometric exercises are started immediately. Hand elevation and pumping are critical for reducing swelling. One to two weeks after the thermoplastic cuff has been applied, limited active motion should begin for all upper extremity joints [41]. Sitting or standing, the patient leans forward toward the affected side so that pendular motion can be performed. Stress on the humerus will be reduced if the elbow remains slightly flexed. Full elbow flexion can be stimulated by beginning hand-to-mouth activities. Incorporating the hand in simple lightweight activities of daily living and recreation can help maintain wrist and hand range and strength. Once complete healing has been determined, traditional therapeutic techniques can be pursued.

EPICONDYLITIS

The term *tennis elbow* (epicondylitis) can be misleading. It implies that the injury is incurred through playing the sport. As stated by Bowden [4], most studies have shown that tennis elbow occurs in the nonathlete more than in the athlete, as a result of direct or indirect trauma. Tennis elbow is also applied to any one of a number of complaints of discomfort, usually at the lateral and occasionally at the medial epicondyle of the elbow [4, 31].

Treatment appears as diverse as the causes. During the acute active phase, rest and immobilization are important. There are several ways to immobilize the arm, choice of one is often based on what has already been tried.

A common method is a wrist cock-up splint, which can be effective if pain is from resistance to the wrist extensors. It is designed in 25 to 30 degrees of extension, and is ideally made of a moldable thermoplastic material. Some commercially available items do not offer complete immobilization of the wrist. As in any wrist splint, it should not come over the distal palmar crease, should allow complete metacarpal joint flexion, and should be molded to preserve the palmar arch. The patient is instructed to remove the splint several times a day and take the wrist and elbow through a complete range of motion. It is worn during daytime functional activity to eliminate resistance to the wrist extensors.

Immobilization can be achieved by the use of a wide elastic band (tennis elbow strap) around the proximal forearm. This reduces stress on the extensor muscle mass and tends to distribute force evenly [20]. The third method is to splint the elbow in 90 degrees of flexion with the forearm in neutral (position of the forearm may vary according to the location of the pain), and the wrist in 25 to 30 degrees of extension. The splint is worn continuously until discomfort subsides, and is only removed for hygiene purposes. While the splint is off the patient takes the shoulder, elbow, forearm, and wrist through a comfortable range of motion.

## FOREARM FRACTURES

Colles' fracture, or fracture of the distal radius, is the most common forearm fracture seen by therapists. It usually occurs in women over 50 who have fallen on an open, radially deviated hand and extended wrist [42]. Depending on the patient's age, the cast is on for three to six weeks with the forearm pronated, wrist flexed, and hand ulnarly deviated. Generally, the elbow and finger joints are allowed full range of motion, however, edema can limit this. Thus the patient must elevate the forearm and put all unrestricted joints through complete range-of-motion exercises several times a day. With older patients, shoulder, elbow, and MP joints often become stiff. The greatest limitation is in forearm supination, wrist flexion and extension, and MP flexion.

Once the cast has been removed, a plastic or plaster wrist support may be used while strength is improving. As strength and range increase, wearing time for the support decreases. The splint should not restrict motion of uninvolved joints, so that simple daily activities can begin. Exercises with putty and functional activities help to improve hand strength and range, which in turn will be reflected in increase in wrist strength. Gains can also be made by the use of graded weights. The amount of weight used in the beginning will depend on the patient, generally 1 pound to start, with an additional pound each day. Typically, a can weighing 16 ounces is placed in a canvas or shopping bag. The patient sits in an armchair with the forearm supported, but wrist and hand free. While holding the bag, the wrist is extended, flexed, and then radially deviated. In each motion the forearm position is changed so that the hand moves against gravity. The number of repetitions for each direction will depend on the patient.

The position in which the forearm bones are reduced can influence function. Whether one or both bones are involved, the position of the head of the radius must be maintained to allow adequate forearm rotation and elbow extension. If both bones are fractured, radioulnar synostosis may result and prevent rotation [42]. The level of injury will determine position in the cast. With proximal fractures, the forearm is placed in supination; with midshaft, in neutral; and with distal, in pronation. Except for Colles' fracture, the wrist is placed in slight extension. After the initial pain and swelling have subsided, the cast may be replaced by a thermoplastic splint [39]. Even with the cast on, therapy can take place [13].

To control edema, elevation of the hand and forearm is stressed; gentle retrograde massage and pumping the fingers can also be useful. If swelling persists, external compression with a glove or Coban should be tried. Reflex sympathetic dystrophy is a complication, especially with Colles' fracture. Persistent edema and other signs of circulatory and sensory changes must be watched for by the therapist and reported to the physician.

Forearm fractures can result in nerve damage, therefore hand motion and sensation are assessed routinely. With a fracture of the proximal radius requiring open reduction, the posterior interosseous nerve can be damaged. This can also occur with a fracture between the upper and middle two-thirds of the radius. With a midshaft radial fracture, both the anterior and posterior interosseous nerves can be affected. Distal radial and ulnar fractures and some carpal fractures and dislocations result in ulnar nerve impairment. Finally, de Quervain's disease is often seen with forearm and wrist injuries, especially in cases where the cast compresses the first dorsal compartment of the hand.

Sarmiento [40] has promoted the application of a thermoplastic splint within the first few days of a closed forearm fracture. When fabricating the forearm and carpal splint, the therapist must position the forearm as it was placed in plaster. A Meunster-type elbow limits the last 20 to 30 degrees of extension, but allows full flexion. Supination and pronation are eliminated by making the forearm portion elliptical and snug against the volar and dorsal forearm. The hand and forearm parts are connected by flexible hinges, thus only wrist flexion and extension are allowed. The forearm portion must not be tight enough to cause hand swelling.

When roentgenograms indicate that the fracture is well-healed, splinting is frequently discontinued. In distal fractures, a wrist support splint may be indicated for a time because of pain with motion and muscle weakness. As activity progresses the patient gradually discontinues its use, wearing the splint at night and outdoors is usually given up last. It should be noted that none of the splint designs should interfere with finger or thumb motion.

## Wrist and Hand Orthopedics
### FRACTURES
Fractures can occur in all bones and joints of the hand. Although these structures are small and a minor fracture may not seem critical, even a slight problem can reduce hand function. Important features of treatment are to reduce the fracture and immobilize the injured part properly. Closed reduction is attempted first, and if the results are not satisfactory open reduction may be required. Failure of union or osteoarthritis occasionally necessitates prosthetic replacement.

Reduction of the fracture should restore proper alignment, rotation, and length of the bone [38]. The position of immobilization during healing is 30 to 60 degrees of wrist extension, 60 to 90 degrees MP flexion, and 0 to 10 degrees IP flexion, to maintain the length of the collateral ligaments. A complication of immobilization is the intrinsic plus hand. Thus intrinsic stretching exercises are begun as soon as the fracture is stable. The period of immobilization varies with each injury [16].

With MP and IP shaft fractures, gliding structures may adhere to the fracture site, but with intraarticular fractures motion may be lost with ligamentous shortening resulting from immobilization, joint incongruity, or secondary osteoarthritis. Following a complicated joint fracture in an adult, normal range of motion may never be achieved [38].

Therapy may begin as soon as the site is stable. As in most hand injuries, early treatment is to control edema and begin active range-of-motion exercise, and progresses to active resistive exercise. If the patient continues to have joint stiffness or limitation, sustained gentle, passive stretch may be required to loosen adhesions or lengthen collateral ligaments. This can only be done when the fracture is well healed [16, 38].

The most common fracture of the carpal bones is to the scaphoid, often injured in trauma to an extended hand. This fracture is difficult to diagnose, and is often treated with a short arm/thumb spica cast for at least 2 weeks despite negative roentgenograms. Immobilization can last eight to ten weeks or longer if the proximal one-third of the scaphoid is fractured [38]. Fractures of this or other carpal bones may not heal and will require an implant. The treatment goals after carpal fracture or implant surgery are to increase range of motion and strength of the hand and wrist, as well as monitor edema.

### THUMB INJURIES
Intraarticular fracture of the first metacarpal, or Bennett's fracture, is frequently referred for therapy after it has healed. Pain may occur with gross and fine prehension and with the development of secondary arthritic changes [42]. Joint motion may remain limited.

The ligamentous tear most commonly referred for rehabilitation therapy is that of the ulnar collateral ligament of the MP joint, *gamekeeper's thumb*. Whether surgically corrected or not, the patient is to avoid active and passive abduction and extension while healing is taking place. A splint is designed to restrict abduction and extension. Pressure on the thumb during prehension should not cause radial movement at the joint. The splint extends across the dorsum of the hand so that the piece cups the ulnar border. The Velcro strap is pulled across the palm and attaches to the ulnar border so that the fit of the splint is more stable. When the splint is removed, such as for bathing, abduction and extension of the thumb are to be avoided.

Immobilization in a splint may be indicated if there is persistent joint pain from arthritic changes or trauma. A thumb splint that does not restrict the wrist may be needed to allow functional use of the hand. Joint range will be limited with the immobilization. Techniques used to increase the amount of motion will depend on the diagnosis.

One of the most common sites of tendinitis is at the first dorsal compartment of the hand. Here the abductor pollicis longus and the extensor pollicis brevis become restricted, and use of the thumb for pinch leads to pain. This is frequently referred to as *de Quervain's disease*. Conservative treatment is to avoid such movements by splinting the wrist and entire thumb. The thumb spica splint holds the wrist in slight extension, and the thumb in the neutral resting position. The distal joint's flexion should be limited, as the extensor pollicis longus moves through the same area of the wrist. The splint is worn for one to three weeks and removed only for bathing, at which time only slight flexion is recommended. Antiinflammatory medication may be used during the period of immobilization. This disease is commonly seen after a pregnancy or a Colles' fracture.

The patient with decreased sensation in the thumb should be instructed to guard against injury, but out of necessity will probably return to use of the thumb spontaneously. When hypersensibility is present, use is avoided and the thumb is not incorporated into the grasp pattern. Desensitization should be attempted.

## LIGAMENTOUS INJURIES AND THE STIFF HAND

The stiff hand can result from ligamentous involvement following injury. In addition to direct trauma to the ligaments, a stiff hand can develop from improper immobilization following a fracture, or lack of exercise to the digits when a forearm or wrist fracture is casted. Ligamentous injuries to the hand and wrist require a long time to heal because of limited blood supply. Whatever the cause of the contracture, therapy is similar [16, 47].

The goal of therapy is to gain maximum flexion and extension at each joint, accomplished with gentle sustained stretch. Great care must be taken that the traction applied does not cause increased pain or swelling. Swelling may remain in the area of injury for six to 12 months, and should be treated as mentioned previously. Prior to applying traction on a stiff hand, it is helpful to use massage or hot packs to loosen structures.

For wrist stiffness, serial splinting in extension, flexion, or both is the best method for gaining motion. Accompanying wrist exercises provide traction for passive stretch. The patient can do this by working with a weight such as a soup can in a canvas bag, similar to active resistive wrist exercises. The forearm is stabilized and the weight is hung from the hand. This can be done in either extension or flexion of the wrist.

The MP joints usually become stiff in extension. There are a variety of commercially available splints and patterns for dynamic splint fabrication. General considerations for splinting are that the wrist is stabilized, pull of the fingers is toward the scaphoid bone, and tension on each finger is individualized (Figures 3-6 and 3-7).

Proximal interphalangeal (PIP) joints generally stiffen in flexion, and both flexion and extension are limited. Gaining PIP joint extension is probably one of the biggest problems in therapy. There are many commercially available splints to accomplish this. The safety pin design provides slow sustained stretch and is

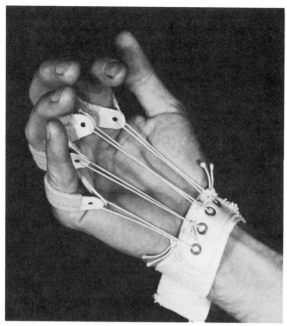

FIGURE 3-6. *Flexion cuffs. Whether used with or without a wrist support splint, finger cuffs of this type can be used when gentle sustained pull is desired for individual MP joints.*

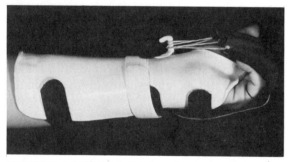

FIGURE FIGURE 3-7. *The plastic wrist support shell should be as contoured as possible in order to reduce the amount of distal displacement caused by the tension from the leather cuff.*

readily accepted by patients. When splinting, the proximal phalanx is immobilized for a concentrated stretch on the PIP joint. The line of pull should be toward the base of the thumb. In all splinting for the stiff hand, tolerance is increased gradually with the eventual goal of nighttime wear so the hand can be free during the day for active use.

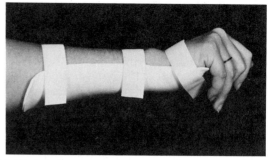

FIGURE 3-8. *Wrist support and resting splint. Many variations of this splint can be fabricated in order to meet the patient's needs.*

NERVE LACERATION AND COMPRESSION

Nerve compression and laceration can occur to the peripheral nerves resulting in temporary or permanent loss of function. Restoration of function by nerve grafts, tendon transfers, or release of the compressing force requires surgical intervention. Splints are applied to maintain proper position and function, and prevent deformities. Manual muscle testing is needed to establish baseline function and note progress.

Sensory reeducation is an integral part of the treatment program. Additional therapy includes increasing range of motion, improving hand function, and increasing strength; biofeedback may also be useful.

Carpal tunnel syndrome is compression of the median nerve in the carpal tunnel of the wrist. Symptoms include pain in the hand, wrist, and forearm radiating up to the shoulder. There is tingling and numbness in the median nerve distribution usually at night, although it may occur during the day. Thenar atrophy may follow. The use of a wrist cock-up splint in neutral to slight extension is recommended at night and when symptoms are noted during the day (Figure 3-8).

Cubital tunnel syndrome is pressure on the ulnar nerve at the elbow. A splint with 90 degrees of elbow flexion and the forearm in slight pronation will relieve stress on the nerve. The splint must be bowed out at the elbow to be

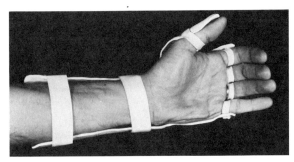

FIGURE 3-9. *Radial nerve splint. Patients have found it to be less bulky, more cosmetic, and therefore more acceptable than the conventional outrigger.*

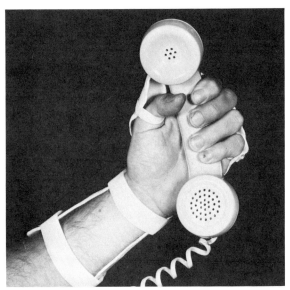

FIGURE 3-10. *This dorsal design offers support while allowing functional grasp.*

sure that no more pressure is placed on the nerve.

Radial nerve compression is treated with a dynamic splint with the wrist in 25 to 30 degrees of extension. Thumb and fingers should be in slight flexion (Figures 3-9 and 3-10). The goal is to maintain proper hand position and function during recovery.

## SENSORY REEDUCATION

Sensation can be the most important factor in hand function. Its ability to discriminate position, hot and cold, pain, deep pressure, light touch, and stereognosis aids in functional tasks. It is interesting to note that two terms are used when discussing the sensory-impaired hand: *sensibility* and *sensation*. Sensibility is identifying an object, while sensation is identifying its properties. After nerve injury, treatment is to improve sensibility, not sensation [16].

When evaluating the sensory-impaired hand, baseline information is needed prior to establishing a retraining program. Using a combination of tests, the therapist can gain a clear understanding of the patient's sensibility and sensation (see suggested reading at the end of this chapter). The Moberg pick-up test, Ninhydrin sweat test, Weber two-point discrimination test, and tests for pressure-sensitive monofilament, pin-prick, temperature, graphesthesia, stereognosis, proprioception, and sensory nerve conduction are most useful. Active and passive range of motion, manual muscle testing, prehension, and trophic status should be assessed.

The purpose of sensory reeducation is to teach the patient to interpret correctly the different impulses. Treatment is a series of graded stimuli such as constant pressure, movement, light touch, and vibration, with the least stressful to the patient introduced first. The hand should be pain-free. As this kind of treatment can be taxing, sessions should take place in a quiet area with a proper amount of time scheduled. Training sessions are short, and sensibility exercises are performed throughout the day [16]. The patient completes the exercises on the unaffected side and then the affected side, first with eyes open and then closed.

Areas of hypersensitivity are noted, and sensory stimulation is used as part of the therapy program. This includes stroking, deep pressure, rubbing, and maintained touch using different textures and shapes. Transcutaneous electric nerve stimulation is also used. It should be noted that hypersensitivity is difficult to treat.

## TENDON LACERATION

About 70 percent of all flexor and extensor tendon lacerations occur in the area distal to the distal palmar crease [47]. Lacerations of the volar surface from the distal palmar crease to the PIP joint crease are the most difficult to repair and rehabilitate. When the flexor digitorum profundus and superficialis are severed, their repair can cause a great deal of scar tissue in a small area, which can result in the tendons adhering to each other. Frequently, the superficialis is not repaired but excised, and only the profundus is repaired in an attempt to regain flexion in the fingers.

Flexor tendons are most commonly severed, especially at the wrist and digital levels as a result of falling on or grasping sharp objects. With injury at the wrist, median and ulnar nerve involvement can result, necessitating sensory precautions and positional splinting. For functional and protective reasons, digital nerves when severed are usually repaired on border fingers.

Repair of severed tendons of the fingers is difficult, particularly when both tendons are affected. Although wrist scarring can limit full return of tendon excursion, scar build-up in the volar finger can be more difficult to overcome. Tendolysis may be indicated if decreased range of motion occurs after repair. If there is a limitation of motion because of scarring prior to the tendolysis, complete range may not be seen following surgery.

Laceration of extensor tendons is seen less often. Laceration or rupture at the terminal joint results in a *mallet finger,* or flexed distal interphalangeal (DIP) joint. Nonsurgical treatment is to splint the joint in hyperextension for several weeks. An imbalance in the central tendon and lateral bands can result in either a *swan neck deformity* (PIP joint hyperextension and DIP joint flexion), or the

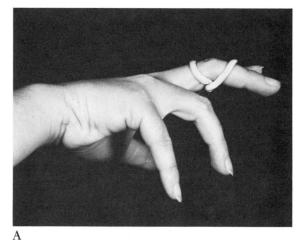

A

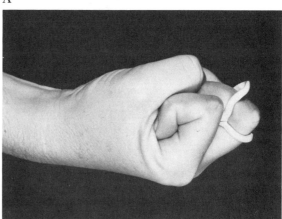

B

FIGURE 3-11. *Swan neck splint. A. PIP hyperextension should be restricted, but B. full finger flexion should be allowed.*

opposite, a *boutonnière deformity.* The former can be splinted in a small figure eight splint that restricts PIP hyperextension but allows flexion (Figure 3-11). Both may require surgical intervention. Severance of the extensor tendon at the MP level will result in loss of IP joint extension.

Timing, precautions, and type of motion indicated for optimal results are individualized according to the patient, surgeon, and therapist. Traditionally, in flexor tendon repairs active and protective passive range-of-motion exercises begin three to four weeks following surgery, and graded active resistive activities about five or six weeks later [47]. This schedule is delayed one week for flexor tendon grafts or extensor tendon repairs, and two weeks for extensor tendon grafts. If a two-stage repair is done, passive joint motion must be maintained for the period that the rod is in place and the graft is to be attached [16].

In all cases, the therapist can only guide the exercise program, as the patient is ultimately his or her own therapist. Self-motivation is needed to continue active range-of-motion exercises, and therefore promote good tendon gliding and the desired reorganization of the developing scar tissue.

An edema control program is an essential part of therapy. In addition, as soon as the sutures are removed, lotion can be applied to the suture line. Only light pressure should be used initially, so as not to stress internal repair and encourage scar formation. Generally, six to eight weeks after the repair, the patient is instructed to lift light items, for example, spice cans or one-inch blocks, as a part of the therapy program. This helps demonstrate that the hand will indeed regain some functional use. Once active resistive exercise has been allowed for a few weeks, strength measurements can begin in case earlier prescriptions were too strenuous for the repair. All joints can be taken through their ranges with gentle passive movements if great care is taken to slacken the tendon through positioning of the other joints. Frequently, this is not attempted until the repair is strong enough to allow active motion.

From one to four weeks after repair, the surgeon may order active motion. Active and passive flexion and active extension are usually allowed for the first three weeks. During the first week, all movements are done with the patient's wrist held in flexion. In the second week, the wrist is in neutral, and in the third week it is in extension. These positions must be carefully followed to prevent possible rupture. In gaining active control, flexion of the DIP joint may be the last to return. Passive

extension is generally not recommended for the first seven to eight weeks.

Extensor repairs are immobilized longer than flexor repairs. Following a wrist program, the reverse cited for the flexor repair, movement can begin with active and passive extension and gentle active flexion [47]. With both types of injury and repair, full active tendon excursion is forced within the first few weeks. There is a delicate balance, however, between doing this safely without rupture yet before scar tissue adhesions become too binding. If the latter does occur, once the repair is well healed, passive stretch with retrograde massage can be used to stretch adhesive areas. Splinting can be used to maintain scar tissue in the newly elongated position.

Initially, plaster or plastic protective positioning splints are worn at all times. They are discontinued when potential for rupture from passive stretch subsides, although even then the patient may find that wearing the splint for an additional week of protection (for example, to bed or in crowds) is comforting. As the wrist motions for exercising change, so should the position of the wrist in the splint.

Serial or dynamic splinting is often indicated during rehabilitation. If extension of the fingers or thumb is desired, before a splint is fabricated the therapist must identify whether the problem is with decreased tendon gliding or joint stiffening. If lack of active extension is caused by joint contracture, a dynamic splint, PIP joint serial cast, or safety pin splint is appropriate. Serial splinting is effective for stretching a shortened or adhered tendon; all of the joints that the tendon crosses have to be included. Extension of the MP joints should be last, to lessen the possibility of ligamentous shortening.

When further proximal or distal interphalangeal joint flexion is sought, a modification of a Bunnell block can be used. A splint is fabricated that covers the palm, wraps around the thumb for security, and extends just proximal to the joint to be ranged (Figure 3-12). The MP joint is splinted in extension.

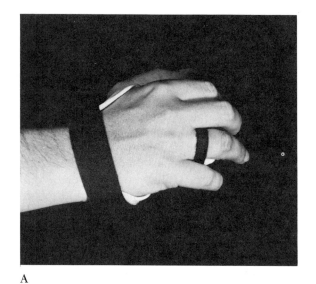

A

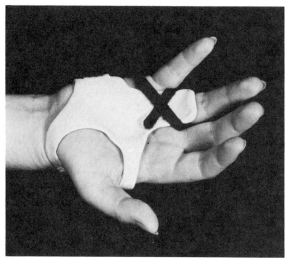

B

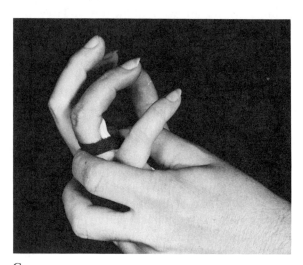

C

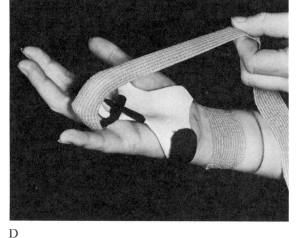

D

FIGURE 3-12. (A, B) *MCP block splint.* (C) *When attempting to increase PIP flexion through active motion, secure the splint against the proximal phalanx with the opposite hand.* (D) *Coban can be used to provide passive stretch for prolonged periods throughout the day.*

While the other hand holds the splint securely on the affected hand, the patient tries actively to flex the joint. This splint can also be used to give prolonged passive stretch. Coban can be used to wrap the finger in flexion against the splint. Intrinsic stretching can also be done using this combination.

It should be noted that treatment of tendon repairs requires time and understanding by both the therapist and the patient.

## CRUSH INJURIES

These are complicated and difficult to manage because of multisystem involvement. The physician's primary concerns are to maintain structural alignment and vascularity, and to decrease the risk of infection [16]. Control of edema must begin promptly. The therapy program starts with active range of motion to maintain tendon gliding and reduce stiffness and edema. Passive range of motion is contraindicated because it may risk anastomosis of structures and increase edema and pain. Therapy should be initiated at the physician's order, and can begin within the first few days.

An attempt is made to decrease pain at the same time as edema is controlled. Ice, heat, or transcutaneous electrical nerve stimulation will be helpful in an effort to reduce pain, with care taken that none of these modalities leads to increased edema. The next steps are to reeducate the remaining muscles and repaired tendons, restore muscle balance, maintain tendon gliding, influence scar modeling, and begin sensory reeducation. In later stages, if deformities do develop, they can be treated with dynamic splinting and active resistive and gentle passive exercise. As with all therapy programs, the ultimate goal is function.

## Upper Extremity Amputation

Amputation of an upper extremity may be the result of congenital anomaly, medical problem, or trauma. Elective amputation can be the result of vascular, neurological, muscular, or skeletal conditions.

Amputation can be at any level on the upper extremity, and generally, stump length is long enough distally or short enough proximally to the nearest joint so the prosthesis will not be too long compared to the uninvolved arm, or too unstable to be functional. Every joint that remains makes the prosthesis easier to operate and lighter to wear. Typically, prostheses are operated by a cable and strap system (Figure 3-13). When indicated, myoelectric contacts or electrical switches can be used to activate the device. The conventional design is lighter than

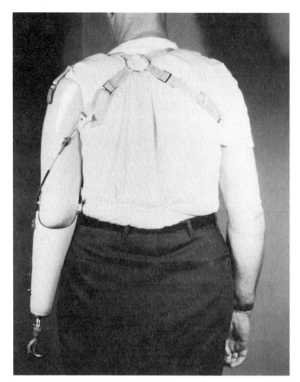

FIGURE 3-13. *A standard above-elbow prosthesis with a figure eight harness. (Courtesy Liberty Mutual Medical Service Center, Boston, Mass.)*

the other two, and requires fewer trips to the prosthetist.

If a temporary prosthesis is not applied in the operating room, the stump should be bandaged using a figure eight pattern distally to proximally. Within a few days, as indicated by the physician, compression Ace wrapping can be applied over the bandaging, with the figure eight pattern repeated in an attempt to decrease edema. Active exercise to all joints proximal to the amputation will also help control both edema and joint stiffness.

A compression wrap, either an Ace or elasticized sock, should be worn until the stump size has stabilized circumferentially for five or more days, at which time the prosthetist can take measurements and begin fabrication. Compression should be continued during the prosthetic training period if there are signs of edema when it is removed. When learning to tolerate the device, wool or cotton stump socks are usually worn.

Often there is initial fear and rejection of the operation and its result that requires support and understanding from the rehabilitation team. Looking at and touching the stump are encouraged from the beginning, as this can help in adjustment to the amputation. Even before the prosthesis arrives, therapy can begin with a program of edema control, skin care, joint motion, one-handed techniques, stump desensitization, dominance change (if necessary), and psychological support. Also, time can be devoted to learning the prosthetic parts, which aids in understanding operation of the device and enables the person more easily to discuss problems with the prosthetist and therapist. Detailed training programs can be found in a number of publications listed under Suggested Reading at the end of this chapter.

In the majority of cases, a voluntary opening hook terminal device is ordered for training and functional use. The hook is smaller and lighter and requires much less energy to operate than the prosthetic hand. Hook and hand can be easily interchanged at the wrist, thus a hand may be worn for cosmetic reasons. When a cosmetic hand is first discussed, the therapist should tactfully explain what it will and will not be able to do. This can be emotionally distressing for the patient, but is necessary with regard to expectations and ultimate adjustment. Although the outer covering of the prosthetic hand is flesh tone, it does discolor with time and exposure to light and soil.

PARTIAL HANDS
Loss of part of a hand has an emotional impact. It may also affect a person's ability to continue employment, although surgical reconstruction often enables a person to return to work or to an alternative job. For some patients, a palmar hook or partial hand prosthesis may be indicated.

The therapist can be instrumental in assisting the patient and prosthetist in the develop-

ment of a design for such a device. One of the more moldable thermoplastic splinting materials can be used to form a prototype. Alterations can be made and friction surfaces accurately located if the wearer demonstrates the grasps required. Once the prototype is finalized, a more permanent device can be made by the prosthetist.

No matter how functional the partial hand may be, for some patients a static cosmetic glove may be most appropriate. The patient and family may require support in learning to accept the device.

THUMB AMPUTATION
Fine prehension can be accomplished using only the fingers, but manipulation is quite difficult and gross grasp may be impossible when the thumb is missing or very short. Altered motion or sensation of the thumb can also affect the hand's use. Because of its functional significance, every effort is made to maintain thumb length.

Complete amputation may require transposition of a finger, deepening of the web space, creation of a thumb post, or grafting of a toe. With any of these procedures, the therapist helps the patient adjust to the altered grasp pattern and increase strength and coordination. A prototype prosthetic thumb can be molded out of a thermoplastic splinting material and fit to the patient. Functional retraining is needed, with the possible exception of the person with a partial thumb amputation.

# Reflex Sympathetic Dystrophy
Reflex sympathetic dystrophy is a complex syndrome, also known as shoulder-hand syndrome, that can occur in an extremity when the hand is the primary source of trauma with the arm becoming involved later. Shoulder-hand syndrome often refers to an injury to the shoulder and subsequent stiff hand. Steinbrocker [43] identifies five components of the syndrome and delineates three stages of dysfunction:

1. Pain: Usually excruciating and may be excessive for the severity of the injury
2. Vasomotor changes: Diffuse nonpitting edema; abnormal sweating response may also be present
3. Range of motion: Loss of motion in the involved extremity
4. Trophic changes: Thickened and shiny skin, excessive sweating
5. Function: Delayed return of function after injury

Stage 1: There is soft edema. The hand may appear dusky pink or red, and increased temperature and sweating are usually noted. Pronounced pain is present in the extremity. At this stage there are no fixed contractures.

Stage 2: The hand may appear cyanotic; edema may or may not be present. Joint contractures begin to develop, and trophic changes of the skin may begin to appear. Pain begins to decrease in this stage.

Stage 3: The hand is pale and cool; the skin becomes glossy, and the hand is stiff.

The mechanism that causes reflex sympathetic dystrophy is difficult to describe and it is hard to know how long the syndrome will last. The best treatment is prevention; therapy, however, addresses all of its components.

Active range of motion of the affected extremity is recorded, although passive range of motion is usually too painful to assess. In the hand, the distance between the finger tips and palmar crease may be measured if goniometry causes too much pain. Edema is evaluated and treated as previously outlined.

Early treatment of reflex sympathetic dystrophy does not require increasing strength. If hypersensitivity is noted, techniques are begun to desensitize the hand. If no hypersensitivity is noted, sensation must be checked to ensure that it is within normal limits. Location and description of pain as well as what triggers it must be documented. Techniques to decrease pain include the use of transcutaneous electrical nerve stimulation, stellate ganglion block, and medication.

Active range of motion to the involved joints to the point of discomfort is part of early intervention. As pain decreases therapy can become more aggressive. If contractures develop, dynamic splinting and gentle passive range-of-motion exercises may be used to gain motion. Paraffin, contrast baths, warm water soaks, and hot packs may be helpful to reduce pain and stiffness. If the hand is edematous, caution must be used not to make it more so with therapeutic techniques. There is no set rule when to begin strengthening exercises, however, endurance should be increased before strength.

# References

1. American Academy of Orthopedic Surgeons. *Orthopedic Appliances Atlas*, Vol. 2. Ann Arbor, Mich.: Edwards, 1972.
2. American Rheumatism Association Section of the Arthritis Foundation. *Primer on the Rheumatic Diseases* (7th ed.).
3. Bell, C. H., Jr. Construction of orthoplast splints for humeral shaft fractures. *Am. J. Occup. Ther.* 33:114, 1979.
4. Bowden, B. W. Tennis elbow. *J. Am. Orthop. Assoc.* 78(1):97, 1978.
5. Burri, C., et al. Functional Postoperative Care After Reconstruction of Knee Ligaments, An Experimental Study. In Ingwersen, et al. (Eds.). *The Knee Joint: Recent Advances in Basic Research and Clinical Aspects.* New York: American Elsevier, 1974.
6. Calliet, R. *Shoulder Pain.* Philadelphia: Davis, 1966.
7. Calliet, R. *Knee Pain and Disability.* Philadelphia: Davis, 1973.
8. Conolly, B. W., and Kilgore, E. S. *Hand Injuries and Infections.* London: Arnold, 1979.
9. Derian, P. S. *An Outline of Orthopedic Surgery.* Springfield, Ill.: Thomas, 1968.
9A. Eisert, O., and Tester, O. Dynamic exercises for the lower extremity amputee. *Arch. Phys. Med. Rehab.* 35:695, 1954.
10. Flatt, A. *The Care of Minor Hand Injuries* (4th ed.). St. Louis: Mosby, 1979.
11. Fortune, W. P., and Adams, J. P. Geometric Total Knee Arthroplastics: A Report of Fifty Cases. In Ingwersen, et al. (Eds.). *The Knee Joint: Recent Advances in Basic Research and Clinical Aspects.* New York: American Elsevier, 1974.

12. Fulford, G. E., and Hall, M. J. *Amputation and Prostheses*. Bristol, Engl.: Wright, 1968.
13. Grace, T., and Eversmann, W. Forearm fractures—Treatment by rigid fixation with early motion. *J. Bone Joint Surg.* 62A: 433, 1980.
14. Gschmend, N., and Debrienner, H. V. *Total Hip Prosthesis*. Baltimore: Williams and Wilkins, 1976.
15. Harris, R. I. The History and Development of Symes Prosthesis. In *Selected Articles From Artificial Limbs*. New York; Krieger, 1970.
16. Hunter, J. M., et al. *Rehabilitation of the Hand*. St. Louis: Mosby, 1978.
17. Iversen, L. D., and Clawson, D. K. *Manual of Acute Orthopaedic Therapeutics*. Boston: Little, Brown, 1977.
18. Klopsteg, P. E., and Wilson, P. D. *Human Limbs and Their Substitutes*. New York: Hafner, 1968.
19. Knott, M., and Voss, D. E. *Proprioceptive Neuromuscular Facilitation: Patterns and Techniques*. New York: Hoeber, Harper & Row, 1956.
20. LaFreniere, J. G. Tennis elbow: Evaluation, treatment and prevention. *Phys. Ther.* 59:742, 1979.
21. Laskin, R. Total knee replacement. *Orthop. Clin. North Am.* 10:223, 1979.
22. Loon, H. The Past and Present Medical Significance of Hip Disarticulation. In *Selected Articles From Artificial Limbs*. New York: Krieger, 1970.
23. Marshall, J. L., and Rubin, R. M. Knee Ligament Injuries—A Diagnostic and Therapeutic Approach. In J. Nicholus (Ed.). *Symposium on Injuries in Sports: Recent Developments*. Philadelphia: Saunders, 1978.
24. McCann, V. H., Philips, C. A., and Quigley, R. T. Preoperative and postoperative management, the role of allied health professionals. *Orthop. Clin. North Am.* 6(3):881, July, 1975.
25. Mears, D. C. *Materials and Orthopedic Surgery*. Baltimore: Williams and Wilkins, 1979.
26. Mital, M., and Pierce, D. *Amputees and Their Prostheses*. Boston: Little, Brown, 1971.
27. Mosley, L. H., and Finseth, F. Cigarette smoking: Impairment of digital blood flow and wound healing in the hand. *Hand* 9(2):97, June, 1977.
28. Nagler, W. *Manual for Physical Therapy Technicians*. Chicago: Year Book, 1974.
29. Naylor, A. *Fractures and Orthopedic Surgery for Nurses and Physiotherapists* (6th ed.). Baltimore: Williams and Wilkins, 1968.
30. New York University. *Lower Extremity Prosthetics*. New York: New York University, Post-Graduate Medical School, 1973.
31. Nirschl, R. P. Etiology and treatment of tennis elbow. *J. Sports Med.* 2(6):308, Nov.-Dec., 1974.
32. Pederson, H. E. *The Geriatric Amputee: Principles of Management*. Washington, D.C.: National Academy of Sciences, 1971.
33. Peterson, L. F. A., Fitzgerald, R. H. J., and Johnson, E. W., Jr. Total joint arthroplasty of the knee. *Mayo Clin. Proc.* 54:564, 1979.
34. Post, M. *The Shoulder: Surgical and Non-Surgical Management*. Philadelphia: Lea and Febiger, 1978.
35. Radcliffe, C. Biomechanics of the Canadian Type Hip Disarticulation Prosthesis. In *Selected Articles From Artificial Limbs*. New York: Krieger, 1970.
36. Rockwood, C. A., Jr., and Green, D. P. *Fractures*, Vols. 1 and 2. Philadelphia: Lippincott, 1975.
37. Salter, R. B. *Textbook of Disorders and Injuries of the Musculoskeletal System*. Baltimore: Williams and Wilkins, 1970.
38. Sandzén, S. C., Jr. *Atlas of Wrist and Hand Fractures*. Littleton, Mass.: PSG, 1979.
39. Sarmiento, A., Pratt, G. W., Berry, N. C., et al. Colles' fractures—Functional bracing in supination. *J. Bone Joint Surg.* 57A(3):311, Apr., 1975.
40. Sarmiento, A., Cooper, J. S., Sinclair, W. F., et al. Forearm fractures—Early functional bracing: A preliminary report. *J. Bone Joint Surg.* 57A(3):297, Apr., 1975.
41. Sarmiento, A., Kinman, P. B., Galvin, E. G., et al. Functional bracing of fractures of the shaft of the humerus. *J. Bone Joint Surg.* 59A(5):596, July, 1977.
42. Shands, A. R., Jr., and Raney, R. B., Sr. *Handbook of Orthopaedic Surgery* (7th ed.). St. Louis: Mosby, 1967.
43. Steinbrocker, O., et al. The shoulder-hand syndrome in reflex dystrophy of the upper extremity. *Ann. Intern. Med.* 92:22, 1947.
44. Trickey, E. L. Ligamentous injuries around the knee. *Br. Med. J.* 2(6050):1492, Dec., 1976.
45. Trombly, C. A., and Scott, A. D. *Occupational Therapy for Physical Dysfunction*. Baltimore: Williams and Wilkins, 1977.
46. Usoltseva, E. V., and Mashkara, K. I. *Surgery of Diseases in Injuries of the Hand*. St. Louis: Mosby, 1979.

47. Weeks, P. M., and Wray, R. C. *Management of Acute Hand Injuries—A Biological Approach* (2nd ed.). St. Louis: Mosby, 1978.

## Suggested Reading

AMPUTATION

Bender, L. F. *Prostheses and Rehabilitation After Acute Arm Amputation.* Springfield, Ill.: Thomas, 1974.

*Upper Extremity Prosthetics* (1971 Revision). New York: Prosthetics and Orthotics, New York University Post-Graduate Medical School, 1973.

FRACTURES

DePalma, A. F. *The Management of Fractures and Dislocations: An Atlas.* Philadelphia: Saunders, 1970.

Holstein, A., and Lewis, G. B. Fractures of the humerus with radial nerve paralysis. *J. Bone Joint Surg.* 45A:1382, 1963.

Muckle, D. S. (Ed.). *Femoral Neck Fractures and Hip Joint Injuries.* New York: Wiley, 1977.

HAND

Boyes, J. H. *Bunnell's Surgery of the Hand* (5th ed.). Philadelphia: Lippincott, 1970.

Campbell Reid, D. A., and Gosset, J. (Eds.). *Mutilating Injuries of the Hand.* New York: Churchill Livingstone, 1979.

Chapchal, G. (Ed.). *Injuries of the Ligaments and Their Repair: Hand–Knee–Foot.* Littleton, Mass.: PSG, 1977.

Jebson, R. H., et al. An objective and standardized test of hand function. *Arch. Phys. Med. Rehabil.* 50:311, 1969.

Kellor, M., et al. Hand strength and dexterity. *Am. J. Occup. Ther.* 25(2):77, 1971.

Landsmeer, J. Anatomy of the dorsal aponeuroses of the human finger and its functional significance. *Anat. Rec.* 104:35, 1949.

Lister, G. *The Hand: Diagnosis and Indications.* New York: Churchill Livingstone, 1977.

Littler, J., et al. *Symposium on Reconstructive Hand Surgery,* Vol. 9. St. Louis: Mosby, 1974.

Mittelbach, H. R. *The Injured Hand—A Clinical Handbook for General Surgeons.* New York: Springer, 1977.

Nichlas, J. S. The swollen hand. *Physiotherapy* 63(9):285, 1977.

Sandzén, S. C., Jr. *Atlas of Acute Hand Injuries.* New York: McGraw-Hill, 1980.

Semple, C. *The Primary Management of Hand Injuries.* London: Pitman, 1979.

Smith, R. J. Balance and kinetics of the fingers under normal and pathological conditions. *Clin. Orthop.* 104:92, 1974.

Smith, R. J. Intrinsic Muscles of the Fingers: Function, Dysfunction, and Surgical Reconstruction. In *Instructional Course Lectures.* St. Louis: Mosby, 1977.

Smith, R. J., and Dworecka, F. Treatment of the one-digit hand. *J. Bone Joint Surg.* 55A(1):113, 1973.

*The Hand: Examination and Diagnosis.* Aurora, Colo.: American Society for Surgery of the Hand, 1978.

Verdan, C. (Ed.). *Tendon Surgery of the Hand.* New York: Churchill Livingstone, 1979.

Wolfort, F. G. (Ed.). *Acute Hand Injuries: A Multispecialty Approach.* Boston: Little, Brown, 1980.

Wynn Parry, C. *Rehabilitation of the Hand* (3rd ed.). London: Butterworth, 1973.

MODALITIES

Bowden, R. E., and Napier, J. R. Assessment of hand function after peripheral nerve injuries. *J. Bone Joint Surg.* 43B(3):481, 1961.

Dellon, A. L., Curtis, R. M., and Edgerton, M. T. Evaluating recovery of sensation in the hand following nerve injury. *Johns Hopkins Med. J.* 130(4):235, 1972.

Dellon, A. L., et al. Re-education of sensation in the hand after nerve injury and repair. *Plast. Reconstr. Surg.* 53:297, 1974.

Levin, S., et al. Von Frey's method of measuring pressure sensibility in the hand: An engineering analysis of the Weinstein-Semmes pressure anesthesiometer. *J. Hand Surg.* 3(3):211, 1978.

Licht, S. *Therapeutic Exercise* (2nd ed.). Baltimore: Waverly, 1965.

Moberg, E. Evaluation of sensibility in the hand. *Surg. Clin. North Am.* 40(2):357, 1960.

Spinner, M. *Injuries to the Major Branches of the Peripheral Nerves of the Forearm* (2nd ed.). Philadelphia: Saunders, 1978.

Tappan, F. *Healing Massage Techniques—A Study of Eastern and Western Methods.* Reston, Va.: Reston, 1978.

Vasudevan, S., and Melvin, J. Upper extremity edema control: A rationale of the techniques. *Am. J. Occup. Ther.* 33(8):520, 1979.

Wynn Parry, C. B. Sensory re-education after median nerve lesions. *Hand* 8(3):250, 1976.

PAIN

Calliet, R. *Hand Pain and Impairment.* Philadelphia: Davis, 1964.

Calliet, R. *Neck and Arm Pain.* Philadelphia: Davis, 1964.

Hale, M. S. (Ed.). *A Practical Approach to Arm Pain.* Springfield, Ill.: Thomas, 1971.

REFLEX SYMPATHETIC DYSTROPHY

Drucker, W. R., et al. Pathogenesis of post-traumatic sympathetic dystrophy. *Am. J. Surg.* 94(4):454, 1959.
Graham, W., and Rosen, P. The shoulder-hand syndrome. *Bull. Rheum. Dis.* 12:277, 1962.
Kozin, F., et al. The reflex sympathetic dystrophy syndrome—I and II. *Am. J. Med.* 60(3):321, 1976.

WRIST

Taleisnik, J. Wrist: Anatomy, Function and Injury. In *Instructional Course Lectures,* 72. St. Louis: Mosby, 1978.

RHEUMATIC DISEASES:
Evaluation and Treatment

*Ellen Herz Silverman*

## The Rheumatic Diseases

The normal joint is composed of bone, cartilage, synovium, synovial fluid, and the joint capsule. Muscles, tendons, and ligaments are involved in the mobility and stability of the joint. There also are bursal sacs lined with synovial tissue that facilitate motion of tendons and muscles over bony prominences. Each of the rheumatic diseases discussed here affects the joints by attacking one or more of these components (Figure 4-1). The diseases can involve one joint or many, be symmetrical or asymmetrical, be inflammatory or noninflammatory, involve just the joints or other systems.

There are over 100 diseases of the joints. Only those commonly seen in rehabilitation settings are discussed in this chapter.

### OSTEOARTHRITIS

Osteoarthritis, or degenerative joint disease, is a basically noninflammatory condition resulting in degeneration of joint cartilage and formation of bony spurs. Inflammation may occasionally be seen, sometimes as a result of crystal disease (see section on crystal deposition diseases). It affects more women than men, and incidence increases with age.

Although the etiology of osteoarthritis is not known, it is currently thought that pathological changes that occur may be reactions to physical stress [6]. This in turn may result from occupation (e.g., the feet of a ballet dancer), direct

Illustrations for this chapter were drawn by Rita M. Hammond.

trauma, continually carrying heavy loads, or repeated inadequate muscle preparation before a sudden movement (e.g., stepping off a curb that is higher than expected). Genetic factors also play a role. Osteoarthritis may be secondary to other diseases that place added stress on the joints, such as the inflammation of rheumatoid arthritis.

Osteoarthritis affects weight-bearing joints of the knees, hips, spine, and feet. Although nonweight-bearing, the joints of the hands are also subject to stress, and one may see bony enlargement of the distal interphalangeal (DIP) joints—Heberden's nodes, the proximal interphalangeal (PIP) joints—Bouchard's nodes, or involvement of the thumb carpometacarpal (CMC) joint—squaring of the thumb (Figure 4-2).

Symptoms include pain with secondary muscle spasm, aching especially during cold weather, crepitation, bony enlargement with resulting decreased range of motion, and increased pain following use of the joint. Patients with osteoarthritis may experience minor difficulty moving their joints after prolonged rest; however, morning stiffness only lasts a few minutes as opposed to that of patients with rheumatoid arthritis. They tire quickly following exercise.

Therapeutic measures include medication, heat, rest to the affected joint, exercise, and patient education. Medication is usually a nonsteroidal antiinflammatory drug such as aspirin. Heat decreases pain and muscle spasm. The affected joints should be rested if there is

*111*

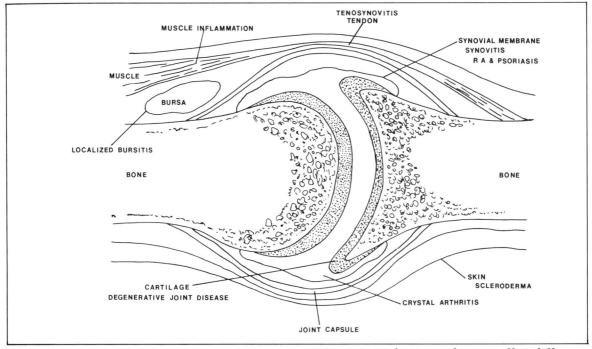

FIGURE 4-1. *Rheumatic diseases affect different parts of the joint and its surrounding structures.*

pain, as excessive use may accelerate the degenerative changes and increase pain.

Exercise, preferably isometric, is important to lessen stress on the joints by providing improved muscle support. Stress of weight-bearing can be decreased by diet or assistive devices such as a cane or walker.

Patients should be educated in joint protection, maintenance of good body alignment, work simplification, and energy conservation. Sexual counseling may be indicated for those with hip or knee involvement.

## RHEUMATOID ARTHRITIS

Rheumatoid arthritis (RA) is a systemic disease of unknown cause, characterized by chronic inflammation of the body's connective tissue—especially the synovium of the joints and tendons—and other organs. With joint involvement, granulation tissue from the proliferating synovium penetrates the joint cavity in tongue-like infiltration called pannus. Rheumatoid pannus is like a local malignancy, as it invades the cartilage giving rise to pain, swelling, joint destruction, and deformity. Inflammation often affects the small joints of the hands and feet and is usually symmetrical, but residual deformities may be asymmetrical. The disease affects more women than men, usually age 35 to 45 years. Rheumatoid arthritis is more common than previously thought, with estimates that as high as 2.5 percent of the population is afflicted [5]. The course of the disease is characterized by remissions and exacerbations.

Although RA primarily affects the joints, it may have other manifestations, including rheumatoid or subcutaneous nodules, vasculitis, lung disease, pericarditis, Sjögren's syndrome, neuropathies, myopathies, eye lesions, lymphadenopathy, and osteoporosis. It can begin with involvement of one joint or many joints. Major symptoms include prolonged morning stiffness, painful swollen

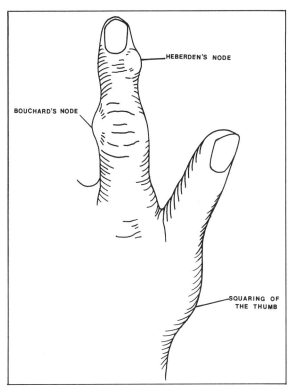

FIGURE 4-2. *Hand deformities commonly seen in osteoarthritis.*

joints with loss of motion, and muscle weakness that may be followed by atrophy. Grip strength becomes weak, and walking is difficult when there is lower extremity involvement. As inflammation increases, duration of morning stiffness lengthens. The gel phenomenon, or inability to move joints after prolonged rest such as sitting in a chair, also worsens. Fatigue may be so profound as to cause disability before joint changes occur. There may be weakness, weight loss, and low-grade fever.

The most characteristic joint changes occur in the hands and wrists. In the wrists these include synovial swelling, prominence of the ulnar styloid because of subluxation, radial or ulnar deviation, and subluxation. Tendons and ligaments no longer hold subluxed joints in their proper alignment because of inflammation, destruction of the tendons and ligaments, or muscle imbalance. One may see swelling and involvement of either the flexor or extensor tendons, and involvement of the metacarpophalangeal (MP) joints with ulnar deviation.

Ulnar drift at the MP joints results from chronic synovitis; this is often associated with radial drift of the wrist (Figure 4-3). These compensate for each other, aligning the index finger with the head of the radius, which is the normal functional position.

Characteristic changes in the finger joints include boutonnière and swan neck deformities (Figure 4-4), and the typical Z-shaped deformity of the thumb (Figure 4-5). The *swan neck deformity* is caused by contracture of the interossei and flexor muscles or tendons causing flexion at the MP joint, compensatory hyperextension at the PIP joint, and flexion at the DIP joint. A similar deformity can occur when the extensors of the thumb are displaced because of MP joint disease.

The *boutonnière deformity* is flexion of the PIP joint through the detached central slip of the extensor tendon, which serves as a "button hole" through which the joint can pop. The DIP joint is then forced into hyperextension.

Characteristic deformities of the feet include *hallux valgus* similar to ulnar drift of the hands, claw toes, hammer toes, and cock-up toes (Figure 4-6). The typical *claw toe* deformity consists of hyperextension of the metatarsophalangeal (MTP) joints and flexion of the PIP and DIP joints. *Hammer toes* differ from claw toes in that the DIP joint is hyperextended. A *cock-up deformity* results from subluxation of the MTP joint, with resulting elevation of the tip of the toe above the surface on which the foot is resting.

Therapeutic measures in RA include medication, rest, heat, splinting, range of motion (ROM) and exercise, patient education, and the use of adaptive equipment. The basic medical treatment is use of therapeutic levels of nonsteroidal antiinflammatory agents such as aspirin. If the arthritis is more severe, Plaquenil (hydroxychloroquine, an antimalarial agent), gold, or penicillamine may be used.

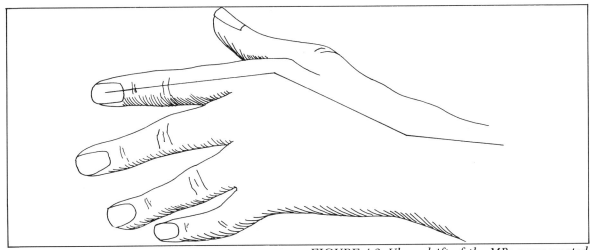

FIGURE 4-3. *Ulnar drift of the MPs compensated for by radial drift of the wrist.*

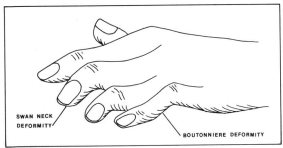

FIGURE 4-4. *Swan neck deformity and boutonnière deformity.*

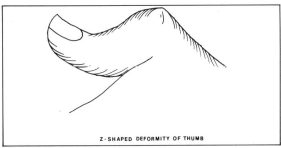

FIGURE 4-5. *Z-shaped deformity of the thumb.*

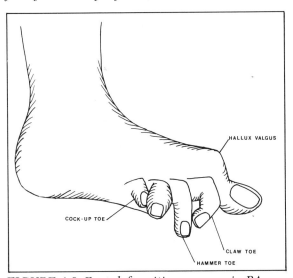

FIGURE 4-6. *Foot deformities common in RA.*

Each of these drugs has associated side effects (see Medications). Most patients will respond to one of these agents; however, less than 10 percent will have a worsening course [3].

Splinting may be used for rest, pain relief, and joint protection, and to increase function. When exercising, great care should be taken particularly during the acute stage not to overstress the joints, as this may cause further inflammation and damage. Patient education includes teaching joint protection techniques and the use and care of splints to assist in prevention of deformities. Assistive devices may be helpful in maximizing function. Sexual counseling may be indicated.

SJÖGREN'S SYNDROME
Sjögren's syndrome is a chronic inflammatory

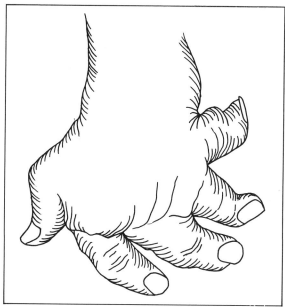

FIGURE 4-7. *Opera glass hands—arthritis mutilans.*

disease of unknown origin characterized by dry eyes and mouth, and connective tissue disease that is RA in 50 percent of the cases, but that may be systemic lupus erythematosus (SLE) or any of the other rheumatic diseases. Patients will experience decreased salivation resulting in a dry mouth, inability to eat dry foods such as crackers without drinking, and excessive dental caries. They may have difficulty chewing, swallowing, or speaking. Eye discomfort is frequent, including inability to cry and a sandy or gritty feeling. Diminished secretion of other glands also occurs, resulting in dry vaginal mucosa and bronchitis.

Therapy is symptomatic. Artificial tears may help dry eyes. Patients should have frequent sips of water while eating, and should be instructed in meticulous oral hygiene including use of a Water Pik after eating. The home environment should be humidified to decrease respiratory infections.

## PSORIATIC ARTHRITIS
Although patients with psoriasis may develop RA, there is a separate distinct disease known as psoriatic arthritis. It occurs more often in men than women, in contrast to RA. It is not a systemic disease. There are several patterns of psoriatic arthritis:

1. Asymmetrical involvement of only a few joints is present, usually as sausage-shaped digits of the fingers or toes.
2. Asymmetrical arthritis occurs as in RA, without rheumatoid factor.
3. Arthritis mutilans may be present, with bony resorption and resultant loss of phalangeal and metacarpal bone with overlying loose skin and tissue. The telescoped appearance gives it the name *opera glass hands* (Figure 4-7). Fingers feel soft and fleshy, joints are unstable and floppy. This is seen in less than five percent of patients.
4. As many as five percent of patients with psoriatic arthritis may have neck and back pain, sacroiliac involvement, or ankylosing spondylitis.

Distribution of psoriasis and arthritis does not necessarily correspond; nail-pitting, which is a psoriatic sign, does occur with joint involvement. Remissions and exacerbations of the skin disease may not necessarily correlate with those of the joint disease. When they occur, exacerbations are more sudden and remissions are more complete than in RA.

Although treatment is similar to that for RA, skin lesions require additional medications. Treatment for psoriasis includes coal tar ointments, corticosteroids, and ultraviolet light (PUVA).

Indications for splinting, ROM, and exercise are the same as in RA. Surgery is usually not attempted as there is little experience with this modality in psoriatic arthritis.

## CRYSTAL DEPOSITION DISEASES
Gout is a metabolic disease characterized by increased levels of serum uric acid resulting in characteristic recurrent attacks of acute arthritis. Attacks are usually monoarticular, but can be polyarticular. They occur in the first

metatarsophalangeal joint in 75 percent of cases. Gout may be associated with the deposition of urate crystals in and around joints (tophi), which may cause joint deformity (chronic tophaceous gout). The increased uric acid may also be deposited as kidney stones. Gout occurs mostly in men; affected women are usually postmenopausal.

Symptoms of the characteristic attack include excruciating pain in any joint but most commonly in the first metatarsophalangeal joint while the patient is at rest, which increases with touch or motion. Systemic reactions may include fever and malaise. An acute attack lasts seven to 10 days. Treatment assists in reducing the intensity of the attack. Therapeutic measures include medication, rest, splinting, and diet. Medication is particularly important, and is given to decrease acute inflammation. Some currently prescribed agents are indomethacin, phenylbutazone, and colchicine. In the chronic phase, agents such as allopurinol and probenecid directly or indirectly decrease serum uric acid.

Application of cold may relieve pain by decreasing swelling during an acute attack. Heat is contraindicated, as resulting increased blood flow may cause further deposits of crystals. Rest, possibly facilitated by splinting of the inflamed joint, can also relieve pain. Care should be taken in splinting, as the surrounding tissues may also be inflamed because of crystal deposition.

## PSEUDOGOUT

Pseudogout is so named because it demonstrates the same characteristic clinical symptoms as gout, but the inflammation is caused by a different crystal, calcium pyrophosphate. Pseudogout is not a metabolic disease. Basic treatment is the same as for acute gout.

## BURSITIS

Bursae are closed sacs lined with synovial fluid that provide a gliding surface to facilitate motion of tendons and muscles over bony prominences. There are approximately 78 bur-

sae distributed on both sides of the body. Bursitis is inflammation of one or more of them. It is caused by trauma, excessive frictional force, crystals, or infection. The most common types of bursitis include subdeltoid, olecranon, trochanteric, ischial, anserine, iliopectineal, prepatellar, Achilles, calcaneal, and bunion. Bursitis affects people of any age, and may be recurrent on the same or opposite side.

Symptoms include tenderness, pain, swelling, and inflammation. As the joint is not involved, there is no muscle spasm. Unlike arthritis, bursitis may cause motion to be limited in only one portion of the ROM, and not necessarily at its extremes.

Therapeutic measures include local injection with steroids, and protection from irritation and trauma either by modifying patients' activities, or by use of appropriate padding or heat such as ultrasound.

## ANKYLOSING SPONDYLITIS

Ankylosing spondylitis is characterized by inflammatory stiffening of the spine (spondyloarthropathy). It is not a form of rheumatoid arthritis. The major targets of this disease are the joints of the spine. These include (1) the cartilaginous joints of the intervertebral discs, (2) the synovial joints of the spine, and (3) the sacroiliac joints. It may also involve the joints of the chest wall, as well as the shoulders, hips, and knees. It is usually clinically more obvious in men than in women, appears in the 20- to 30-year-old age group, and is associated with a specific genetic determinant—an HLA antigen. Ankylosing spondylitis may also be associated with inflammation of the eye or cardiac involvement.

Symptoms include back pain and stiffness following prolonged rest, and peripheral joint involvement.

Common deformities seen initially include disappearance of normal lumbar lordosis and limited movement of the lumbar spine. Eventually, fibrosis and bony ankylosis or fusion produce the typical rigid back, resulting in the spine moving as a single unit. In advanced disease there may be marked kyphosis, fixed torti-collis, and flexion contractures of the hips and knees.

Therapeutic measures consist of medications, exercise, rest, heat, proper positioning, and patient education. Medications include nonsteroidal antiinflammatory agents. A balance of rest and exercise is crucial, as prolonged rest, although necessary in the acute phase, may lead to increased pain, stiffness, and fusion that can become permanent. Heat may be used for pain relief and prior to exercise. Exercises include ROM and strengthening of the spine, trunk, shoulders, hips, and knees in an attempt to maintain the normal extended position of the spine. Postural and breathing exercises assist in maintaining maximum vital capacity of the lungs.

The patient should be instructed in proper posture and positioning to prevent spinal fusion in a nonfunctional position. This includes sleeping on a firm mattress in a straight position and prone-lying. Prolonged flexion should be avoided whenever possible, at work and at play; for example, swimming and hiking are preferable to bicycling or bowling. Work positions can be modified to provide maximum straight body alignment. Adaptive equipment may be used to compensate for postural and mobility changes in functional tasks. Education should also include discussion of genetic implications of the disease for patients' children.

SCLERODERMA

Although scleroderma is characterized by hardening of the skin, it is often a generalized disorder also affecting blood vessels and internal organs such as the esophagus, intestine, heart, lungs, and kidneys. This generalized disorder is called progressive systemic sclerosis. Scleroderma can range from mild involvement of the fingers, hands, or face, to thickened and atrophic skin together with rapid internal involvement. Women are affected three times more than men, and symptoms may appear at any age. Prognosis is varied: patients may have periods of remission and lead full healthy lives, or they may become seriously chronically ill with multiple systemic involvement.

In about one-third of cases initial symptoms are pain, stiffness, and inflammation of the joints. The majority of patients will demonstrate arthritis at some time during the course of their illness. With skin involvement, the skin becomes puffy, swollen, and edematous, progressing to thickening and finally, atrophy. Later, the skin may show small areas of ulceration resulting from subcutaneous calcification. Tendon involvement may occur causing flexion contractures. Patients may have weakness and wasting from disuse or from myopathy, which is indistinguishable from polymyositis. About 80 to 90 percent demonstrate Raynaud's phenomenon, a disturbance of the circulation of the hands and sometimes feet, in which the patient demonstrates severe reaction to cold.

Deformities in scleroderma may result from tightening of the skin leading to decreased ROM. Skin condition should be observed to determine if it is shiny, drawn, or ulcerated.

Treatment modalities are medication, ROM, exercise, and patient education. Medications include antiinflammatory drugs for arthritis, antacids and cimetidine to inhibit gastric acid secretion, and reserpine and other vasodilatory agents for Raynaud's phenomenon. Creams and oils relieve skin dryness; paraffin treatments may also be effective. Exercise includes ROM, especially to maintain function in the hands and face; breathing for chest expansion to counteract changes in the lungs, muscle, or skin of the chest; isometric exercise to tighten muscles; and recreational exercises.

Education stresses joint protection, especially relating to maintaining good alignment for breathing and swallowing. Patient education with regard to Raynaud's phenomenon is also important.

Precautions include avoidance of household detergents because of their effect on the skin, and of exposure to cold and tobacco, which cause vasoconstriction. When patients have difficulty with regurgitation, they should have small frequent meals, not eat for two hours before bedtime, and sleep with the head of the bed at least four inches higher than the foot.

## RAYNAUD'S PHENOMENON

The majority of patients with Raynaud's phenomenon do not develop scleroderma. When they do, it may be worse because of primary hand involvement. About 20 percent of patients with systemic lupus erythematosus have Raynaud's phenomenon; there may also be mechanical causes.

In response to cold, the skin of the hands, and sometimes other body parts such as the feet or nose, turn white, then blue, then red. The skin is initially white because of vasoconstriction; this is associated with pain and paresthesias. With relaxation of the vasospasm the skin becomes a cyanotic blue. Finally, one sees the red of vasodilation.

Initial attacks resolve completely, but recurrences result in atrophy of the tissues, tapering and shortening of the fingers (bony resorption), and ulceration of the fingertips. The skin becomes smooth, atrophic, and hairless.

Treatment includes medication with vasodilating agents such as reserpine, biofeedback to assist in control of the circulatory response, and education. The patient should be instructed in methods of maintaining optimal warmth, such as mittens instead of gloves, and also be told to avoid tobacco.

## SYSTEMIC LUPUS ERYTHEMATOSUS

Systemic lupus erythematosus (SLE) is a multisystemic autoimmune disease. In an autoimmune disease the body produces antibodies that attack certain parts of the individual's cells and tissues. It affects seven times more women than men, usually between the ages of 15 and 35 years; it affects more black people than white. It is characterized by remissions and exacerbations, and prognosis is varied.

There are numerous signs and symptoms, such as arthritis; fever; decreased energy with muscle pain and weakness, often more proximally than distally; skin changes; kidney involvement; cardiac involvement; and pulmonary, gastrointestinal, and neurological problems. The last result in organic psychoses and seizures. The patient may have involvement in many systems, or proceed over a period of years with symptomatic disease first in one system, then another. During exacerbations patients may have fever, weakness, anorexia, weight loss, and malaise. During their disease, 93 percent of patients have arthritis or arthralgias. Resulting deformities are more from tendon involvement and muscle spasm than joint involvement (therefore no contractures). They may have ulcers of the mouth; skin, hair, and mucous membranes are involved in the majority; 20 percent experience Raynaud's phenomenon.

Therapeutic measures may include medication, rest, exercise for myopathies, ROM, strengthening, pain relief, and patient education in areas of energy conservation and work simplification. Medications include antiinflammatory drugs for arthritis, corticosteroids for systemic involvement, and antimalarial agents for skin lesions. Patients should be advised to avoid direct sun and use a sunscreen if necessary. If they have Raynaud's phenomenon, they should avoid exposure to the cold. Psychological counseling for body changes such as hair loss and appearance associated with taking steroids may be needed.

## Evaluation

As both patient and disease are continuously changing, so is the therapeutic regimen. Evaluation measures the disease process at a given point, and helps determine an appropriate treatment plan. It can also be used to determine effectiveness of treatment over time, and pinpoint areas in which the patient has difficulty. The regimen can then be changed as necessary.

Unfortunately, there is no standardized evaluation form on rheumatic diseases that is accurate, efficient, thorough, and reproducible, therefore each institution usually uses its own.

Some standardizations do exist for hand function. (See suggested reading.)

Evaluations may have several different formats: patient self-assessment using a questionnaire, interview, or professional assessment based on patient demonstration. A short screening or a complete evaluation may be used, or screening may pinpoint areas for more thorough follow-up. Demonstration is the most accurate.

Evaluation can be timed or untimed. The hour of the day and location must be chosen carefully, as they will affect the patient's performance. Evaluations may be objectively or functionally oriented. An objective view measures such criteria as ROM of affected joints, muscle strength, and the number of involved joints. Functional evaluation is of special interest, as deformities may exist without functional consequence.

As patients with rheumatic diseases usually have multiple joint involvement, a complete evaluation is time-consuming. It is therefore important to set priorities within the assessment so that treatment can begin within a reasonable time frame. Objective evaluation may delay therapeutic intervention, while a functional assessment may provide better guidelines. The former may, however, be used to assist in determining what is causing the functional problem.

GENERAL INFORMATION

The initial part of any evaluation must include obtaining general information about the patient and the disease. The evaluator should know the diagnosis and onset. Systemic complications such as skin ulcerations or digital vasculitis may be important in treatment planning. The presence of other illnesses is important: diabetic patients have more pain, swelling, and loss of motion than do nondiabetics; obese patients may have osteoarthritis because of the increased stress on joints; those with Parkinson's disease often cannot rest joints adequately and may have trouble with splinting.

The evaluator should ask the patient which joints are affected and examine pinpointed areas of difficulty for pain, swelling, passive and active ROM, and deformity (Figure 4-8). Deformities include subluxation, ankylosis, and contracture. Crepitation, redness, localized areas of tenderness, and instability may also be noted.

The patient should be asked about the duration of morning stiffness, the best and worst times of day, and endurance. Other important information includes age, occupation, living situation, and hand dominance. Finally, the patient should be asked to grade that day's physical well-being on a scale of one to ten. This simple numerical self-assessment can be used as a means to monitor progress and effective therapy [2].

Included here are general guidelines for evaluating ROM, muscle strength, and sensation, followed by functional evaluation.

RANGE OF MOTION

Range of motion (ROM) may vary in patients depending on the day, the time of day, or when medication for pain relief was last taken. It may be affected by deformity such as subluxation, ankylosis, and contracture. The measurement may also vary depending on the evaluator. Measurement is time-consuming, and a thorough evaluation may not always be indicated. It may be assessed more rapidly and functionally by gross measurement over multiple joints rather than by specific joints. A common screening that offers functional implications is to ask the patient to touch the top of the head and the back of the neck (as in hair care), touch the back of the waist (as in dressing and toileting), and touch the toes (as for lower extremity dressing). This technique, however, is limited, and does not give a complete picture of functional limitations. It should be used in conjunction with a hand evaluation and a more comprehensive functional evaluation to determine areas that may benefit from therapeutic modalities and adaptive equipment.

There are, however, instances in which specific joints should be measured: establishing

## EVALUATION GENERAL INFORMATION

Name                                          Age
Diagnosis                                     Onset
Other problems                                Morning stiffness
Occupation                                    Handedness
Best time of day                              Worst time of day
Living situation

| Joints | Pain | | Swelling | | Active ROM | | Passive ROM | | Deformity | |
|---|---|---|---|---|---|---|---|---|---|---|
| | R | L | R | L | R | L | R | L | R | L |
| Hands | | | | | | | | | | |
| Wrists | | | | | | | | | | |
| Elbows | | | | | | | | | | |
| Shoulders | | | | | | | | | | |
| Neck | | | | | | | | | | |
| Jaw | | | | | | | | | | |
| Hips | | | | | | | | | | |
| Knees | | | | | | | | | | |
| Ankles | | | | | | | | | | |
| Feet | | | | | | | | | | |
| Spine | | | | | | | | | | |

*Hand*

| Joints | Pain | | Swelling | | Active ROM | | Passive ROM | | Deformity | |
|---|---|---|---|---|---|---|---|---|---|---|
| | R | L | R | L | R | L | R | L | R | L |
| MCP | | | | | | | | | | |
|   Index | | | | | | | | | | |
|   Middle | | | | | | | | | | |
|   Ring | | | | | | | | | | |
|   Little | | | | | | | | | | |
| PIP | | | | | | | | | | |
|   Index | | | | | | | | | | |
|   Middle | | | | | | | | | | |
|   Ring | | | | | | | | | | |
|   Little | | | | | | | | | | |
| DIP | | | | | | | | | | |
|   Index | | | | | | | | | | |
|   Middle | | | | | | | | | | |
|   Ring | | | | | | | | | | |
|   Little | | | | | | | | | | |
| Thumb | | | | | | | | | | |
| CMC | | | | | | | | | | |
| DIP | | | | | | | | | | |

FIGURE 4-8. *Evaluation of joints.*

| Foot Joints | Pain R | Pain L | Swelling R | Swelling L | Active ROM R | Active ROM L | Passive ROM R | Passive ROM L | Deformity R | Deformity L |
|---|---|---|---|---|---|---|---|---|---|---|
| **Forefoot** | | | | | | | | | | |
| **MTP** | | | | | | | | | | |
| First | | | | | | | | | | |
| Second | | | | | | | | | | |
| Third | | | | | | | | | | |
| Fourth | | | | | | | | | | |
| Fifth | | | | | | | | | | |
| **IP** | | | | | | | | | | |
| First | | | | | | | | | | |
| Second | | | | | | | | | | |
| Third | | | | | | | | | | |
| Fourth | | | | | | | | | | |
| Fifth | | | | | | | | | | |
| **Midfoot** | | | | | | | | | | |
| **Hindfoot** | | | | | | | | | | |
| True ankle | | | | | | | | | | |
| Tibiofibular talar | | | | | | | | | | |
| Talocalcaneal | | | | | | | | | | |
| Subtalar | | | | | | | | | | |

Date _____

Therapist _____

| Self-care | I | ID | D | U | Pain |
|---|---|---|---|---|---|
| Feeding | | | | | |
| Buttering bread | | | | | |
| Cutting meat | | | | | |
| Drinking from a cup | | | | | |
| Holding utensil | | | | | |
| | | | | | |
| Personal Hygiene | | | | | |
| Brushing teeth | | | | | |
| Combing hair | | | | | |
| Washing hair | | | | | |
| Setting hair | | | | | |
| Shaving | | | | | |
| Toilet after-care | | | | | |
| Turning faucet on and off | | | | | |
| Ability to wash all areas | | | | | |

| Self-care | I | ID | D | U | Pain |
|---|---|---|---|---|---|
| Dressing | | | | | |
| UE dressing | | | | | |
| Bra | | | | | |
| Putting on shirt | | | | | |
| Coat | | | | | |
| Tying necktie | | | | | |
| LE dressing | | | | | |
| Pants | | | | | |
| Socks | | | | | |
| Stockings | | | | | |
| Shoes—laces, buckles | | | | | |
| Fine motor coordination | | | | | |
| Buttons | | | | | |
| Zippers | | | | | |
| Snaps | | | | | |
| Splints | | | | | |

FIGURE 4-9. *Functional evaluation.*

| Mobility | I | ID | D | U | Pain |
|---|---|---|---|---|---|
| Bed | | | | | |
| On/off chair | | | | | |
| On/off toilet | | | | | |
| Tub | | | | | |
| Bath | | | | | |
| Shower | | | | | |
| Car transfers | | | | | |
| Open and close door | | | | | |
| Length of time to go 50 feet | | | | | |
| Walking in home | | | | | |
|   Outside home | | | | | |
|   Level surfaces | | | | | |
|   Uneven surfaces | | | | | |
| Stairs | | | | | |
| Transportation | | | | | |
|   Driving | | | | | |
|   Public transportation | | | | | |
|   Curbs | | | | | |
| Endurance | | | | | |

| Homemaking | | | | | |
|---|---|---|---|---|---|
| Cooking | I | ID | D | U | Pain |
|   Using stove, oven | | | | | |
|   Reaching cupboards, high, low | | | | | |
|   Peeling | | | | | |
|   Cutting | | | | | |
|   Opening containers | | | | | |
|   Opening refrigerator | | | | | |
| Cleaning | | | | | |
|   Sweeping | | | | | |
|   Mopping | | | | | |
|   Stove | | | | | |
|   Oven | | | | | |
|   Laundry | | | | | |
|   Washing dishes | | | | | |
|   Cleaning bathroom | | | | | |
|   Washing windows | | | | | |
| Making bed | | | | | |
| Turning faucets on and off | | | | | |

| Outdoor activities | | | | | |
|---|---|---|---|---|---|
| Recreation | | | | | |
| Shopping | | | | | |
| Doing home repairs | | | | | |
| Yardwork, gardening | | | | | |

*I = Independent; ID = Independent with device; D = Dependent; U = Unable*

baseline ROM; pre- and postsurgery; fitting for splinting, bracing, or serial casting; determining specific changes in ROM in a given joint from the disease process; and determining changes in mobility affected by ROM.

Range of motion should be measured both actively and passively. If the limitations are equivalent it means that there is joint involvement. If passive ROM is greater than active, there is periarticular involvement. Testing may also be affected by the presence of deformity or inflammation.

A consistent evaluator should do the initial, intermediate, and final evaluations, as a change in observer may affect the tests' validity.

## MUSCLE STRENGTH

When testing for muscle strength one has some of the same difficulties found in testing ROM. Severe joint involvement can make accurate individual testing difficult because of changes in alignment resulting from subluxation, tendon involvement, and so on. Group muscle testing may therefore prove more effective and accurate, unless one is concerned with a particular muscle.

One also needs to be aware of pain and its effect on strength testing. Strength is best gauged in that part of ROM that is pain-free. Pain usually exists in extremes of ROM except with bursitis, where an intermediate area may be affected.

Because of the importance of the hand, its strength is usually measured. Two of the more common measures in arthritis are grip strength and pinch. In assessing the former one should use a dynamometer, or for the more severely involved hand, a sphygmomanometer, which provides less resistance and is more flexible.

Pinch should be measured using a pinch gauge, and should be tested in three ways: lateral pinch, tip-to-tip, and 3-jaw chuck. Lateral pinch is touching the tip of the thumb to the side of the index finger; tip-to-tip is touching the tips of the thumb and index finger to each other; 3-jaw chuck is touching the tip of the thumb to the tips of the index and middle fingers simultaneously.

## SENSATION

Sensory loss must be evaluated, particularly before splinting or using modalities such as heat. Sensation may affect hand function and the ability to manipulate objects. Sensory nerve involvement may occur in arthritis secondary to nerve compression, such as in carpal tunnel syndrome, or secondary to vasculitis.

## FUNCTIONAL EVALUATIONS

Functional evaluations can be divided into six main categories: self-care, mobility, homemaking, outdoor activities, environment, and hand function (Figures 4-9 and 4-10). Range of motion, muscle strength, and sensation testing may assist in determining the reason for problem areas.

### SELF-CARE

Self-care includes feeding, personal hygiene, and dressing.

### MOBILITY

Mobility includes posture, gait, transfers, and transportation.

#### Posture

The first step in evaluating standing posture is to observe overall balance. Body weight should be evenly supported and not shifted abnormally far forward or backward. It should be borne evenly on both feet and not shifted predominantly either to the right or left.

Lateral deviations may be evaluated by looking at a patient from the front or back. A line perpendicular to the ground should be able to divide the body into two symmetrical halves. The levels of the shoulders and hips should be equal on both sides.

Of particular note in rheumatic diseases is evaluation of the spine. There are three curves in the normal spine: concave cervical, convex thoracic, and concave lumbar. Patients with arthritis may have kyphosis, that is, increase in

| | | | | |
|---|---|---|---|---|
| Name | | Age | | |
| Diagnosis | | Date | | |
| Morning stiffness | | Time of day administered | | |
| Handedness | | Therapist | | |

| Range | Independent | Difficulty | Unable | Pain |
|---|---|---|---|---|
|   Fingers to palm | | | | |
|   Opposition | | | | |
|     Thumb touching each digit | | | | |
| Strength | | | | |
|   Power grip | | | | |
|     Dynamometer or sphygmomanometer | | | | |
|   Pinch | | | | |
|     Lateral | | | | |
|     3-jaw chuck | | | | |
|     Tip-to-tip | | | | |
|   Hook grasp | | | | |
|     Holding a purse | | | | |
| Functional tasks | | | | |
|   Applied strength | | | | |
|     Closing a snap | | | | |
|     Opening a 3-inch lidded jar | | | | |
|     Opening a door | | | | |
|     Pouring a cup of water from kettle | | | | |
|     Picking up glass and drinking | | | | |
|   Precision | | | | |
|     Opening and closing button | | | | |
|             zipper | | | | |
|             safety pin | | | | |
|     Thread and tie shoelaces | | | | |
|     Handle coins | | | | |
| Combined precision and strength | | | | |
|   Insert and turn key | | | | |
|   Dial and use a coin telephone | | | | |
|   Writing | | | | |
|   Cut with scissors | | | | |

FIGURE 4-10. *Hand function test.*

the normal thoracic curve; lordosis, an exaggerated lumbar curve; a flat back, such as a decrease of normal spinal curves; or scoliosis, a lateral curve of the spine.

Chest expansion may be measured to give an indication of thoracic flexibility. One measures the difference in chest circumference between full expiration and full inspiration at the level of the xiphoid process, using a flexible steel tape measure.

While the patient is standing, the knees, ankles, and feet should also be examined for proper alignment.

### Gait
Normal gait patterns vary widely. They may be abnormal in patients with rheumatic diseases who attempt to avoid weight-bearing on a painful joint. For example, a patient with a painful hip may demonstrate pelvic tilt because of splinting, or increased weight-bearing on the opposite side. Patients with a painful ankle or foot will attempt to splint movement while walking by rolling the foot from the lateral to the medial side, replacing the normal heel-toe gait to avoid painful joint motion.

### Transfers
Transfers include getting in and out of bed, on and off a chair or toilet, in and out of the shower or tub, and in and out of some form of transportation.

### Transportation
Accessibility to and use of transportation, either public or private automobile, are important in maintaining activities outside the home.

### HOMEMAKING
Homemaking involves such tasks as food preparation, cleaning, and laundry.

### OUTDOOR ACTIVITIES
Gardening, recreation, yard work, and shopping are examples.

### ENVIRONMENT
Environment consists of home, community, and workplace. The health professional needs to be aware of the patient's environment and continuing adaptation to it. There may be compensation for deformities and decreased ROM and strength through self-made techniques, devices, or changes in life-style.

### Home
The home may present barriers in terms of locomotion. Stairs, doorways, thresholds, or loose floor coverings such as scatter rugs may interfere with locomotion, making bathrooms or bedrooms inaccessible. Poorly organized work areas may also provide barriers. Chairs or beds, tables or counters may be too high or too low. Telephones and light switches should be conveniently located and easily operable by the patient.

It is also important to find out the patient's perception of the reaction of family and friends to the disease and its disability. The social worker may want to interview family members and friends directly to ascertain resources available.

### Community
The community may provide barriers or helpful resources. The health professional should evaluate problem areas such as the patient's ability to go grocery shopping, as well as resources the patient might currently be using such as religious organizations. This assists in determining areas that can be tapped for further contact.

### Workplace
Vocational or workplace assessment includes reviewing both the patient's job responsibilities and work setting. For the latter this includes transportation to and from work, physical barriers such as entrances and lavatories, and the patient's physical position during work. Position includes the height of the work surface, and the height and type of chair if the patient sits to perform the job.

Responsibilities should be evaluated for type of work and physical demands. The latter should be understood in terms of task and endurance required, such as walking, lifting, or bending.

Finally, if there is any doubt that the patient will be able to continue to work, possibilities for adapting the situation should be explored to ensure a useful productive existence.

### HAND FUNCTION

Because of the importance of the hand, evaluation of its function should be performed, including strength, grip and pinch, types of prehension patterns—palmar, tip, lateral, hook, spherical, and cylindrical—and application of these measurements to functional tasks (Figure 4-10).

## Treatment

### DESIGNING A TREATMENT PROGRAM

The rehabilitation team for rheumatic diseases includes several health professionals. The physician can be a rheumatologist, physiatrist, internist, orthopedist, or psychiatrist, or several of these fields may be represented. A psychologist, podiatrist, nurse, physical therapist, occupational therapist, vocational counselor, social worker, nutritionist, or recreational therapist may round out the team. Most important, however, is the patient.

The rheumatic disease is a chronic condition that cannot be cured, and that is characterized by remissions and exacerbations over which the patient may feel little control. As the patient is cognitively intact and will implement the program, it is important that he or she assist in determining the regimen. The health professional must learn the patient's perception of the illness and goals for coping with it. The patient's and the team's priorities need to agree in order to provide effective rehabilitation.

It is the responsibility of the team coordinator to be certain that all aspects of treatment are covered, for example, certain areas such as sexual counseling are not specifically the respon-

sibility of one discipline. The members will prescribe medications, rest, techniques for pain relief, splinting, adaptive equipment, exercise, and education, following appropriate evaluations to determine problem areas and set priorities. As the disease is constantly changing, it will be necessary constantly to reevaluate the regimen.

### MEDICATIONS

In general, medical therapy for patients with joint diseases can be divided into two phases. In the first, or acute phase, patients are given an antiinflammatory drug that will decrease inflammation but will not block progression of disease. One of the most common of these is aspirin (acetylsalicylic acid), which should be given in therapeutic doses (12 to 18 tablets per day). Monitored blood levels can determine if the dose is in the therapeutic range. Side effects of aspirin include ringing in the ears, gastric upset, and bleeding. Alternatives such as buffered aspirin, aspirin with antacids, or enteric-coated aspirin are available but may be absorbed less thoroughly.

If the patient does not tolerate salicylates, various other nonsteroidal antiinflammatory agents are available: Indocin, Phenylbutazone, Clinoril, Motrin, Naprosyn, Toletin, and others. These have the advantages of causing less stomach upset than aspirin, and enhancing compliance because of less frequent dosage. Increased cost and specific side effects such as headache, or psychosis with Indocin, may limit their use. As their means of action is similar to that of aspirin, there is no advantage to giving them with aspirin. In some cases, these drugs are preferred to aspirin, for example, for arthropathies such as ankylosing spondylitis and acute crystal disease such as gout and pseudogout. In acute gout, colchicine may also be given to inhibit formation of a mediator of inflammation. Aspirin and the nonsteroidals may not be effective for the systemic manifestations of RA or SLE.

In the second phase, if continued or intermittent disease persists despite aspirin or other nonsteroidal agents, other drugs capable of inducing remission are used. In RA these include gold, Plaquenil, penicillamine, and steroids. The most commonly used of these is gold. It is currently given in a series of weekly injections, although oral gold will soon be available. The patient reports each week about itching, rash, and mouth ulcers prior to injection. Other side effects include blood and kidney problems. Plaquenil appears to be as effective as gold early in RA; it may be taken as a tablet once a day. Its major side effect is eye toxicity, so eye examinations twice a year are needed. A new alternative to gold is penicillamine, which has the advantage of being given as a tablet once a day. Its toxicities are similar to those of gold, but their frequency may be increased. The efficacy of penicillamine is still being studied. All three agents have a long lag time before they begin to take effect (six weeks to three months).

The use of steroids in RA is controversial because of their serious side effects. They are indicated for local joint disease, and when used as an intraarticular injection they may suppress local inflammation. They are indicated for systemic use for management of patients with SLE.

Remission in gout is achieved by control of the metabolic disease. Special agents are used to decrease the serum uric acid, including allopurinol, which decreases uric acid synthesis, and Benemid, which increases uric acid excretion.

Unfortunately, in some patients the remission-inducing drugs do not work, and for them many experimental treatments are currently being considered.

REST
Rest decreases inflammation and stresses on the joints, and is important for the whole body as well as individual joints. Rest can be provided for individual joints using splints. (See section on splinting.)

Proper positioning is important for adequate and beneficial rest. The patient should be su-

pine with the hands and arms straight at the sides. There should be a small pillow for the head, but a pillow should never be placed under the knees. It is also important to lie prone for 10 minutes in the morning and afternoon.

It is recommended that patients with systemic diseases get 10 to 12 hours sleep per night, and a one- to two-hour nap per day. Rest should be arranged into the schedule before the point of fatigue, and patients should be taught to take five to ten minutes of rest during activities.

A balance with exercise is essential, however, as too much rest can be harmful. Prolonged, it results in muscle weakness, decreased ROM, and osteoporosis (bone loss). The amount of rest that is beneficial changes depending on the severity of the disease; in the acute stage, it plays a larger role. Some patients may respond to bedrest alone. Rest is not only physical but emotional, and hospitalization may provide emotional release from environmental pressures.

PAIN AND TECHNIQUES FOR RELIEF
Pain of arthritis may have a variety of causes. It may be articular or periarticular, or come from the bone, muscle, skin, or nerves. Articular pain may be caused by joint inflammation, or mechanical joint disturbance such as instability or surface irregularity. It is most commonly seen in rheumatoid arthritis and osteoarthritis. Periarticular pain results from bursitis, tendinitis, or tenosynovitis. Bone pain may be caused by osteoporosis or compression fractures, and muscle pain may arise with postural strain or muscle spasm. Skin pain may result from ischemia or ulcers, as in scleroderma. Nerve pain may originate with nerve root irritation or compression, as in ankylosing spondylitis or disc disease.

There are several techniques that can be used for relief, all of which are based on one or more of the following principles:

1. Increasing pain threshold

2. Introducing an external stimulus that may override the pain stimulus (gate control theory)
3. Decreasing muscle spasm
4. The placebo phenomenon; patient's expectations can decrease pain
5. Affecting the circulation

Unfortunately, quantitative measurement of the effectiveness of such techniques over time is difficult.

## HEAT OR COLD
Applications of heat or cold may be effective; heat can be superficial or deep.

### Superficial Heat
Superficial heat only penetrates into the skin a few millimeters. It is usually provided by direct contact with a warm object, for example, hydrocolator packs, moist towel, warm water, or paraffin. Contraindications include reduced sensation, impaired circulation, diabetes mellitus, marked edema, local malignancy, and ischemia.

The joint affected aids in determining the type of superficial heat that will be most efficient. Hands may benefit from paraffin, while neck or shoulder involvement would suggest hydrocolator packs.

*Paraffin* has a higher specific heat than water, which means that the heat is maintained for a longer period of time. Also, high temperatures of paraffin in oil are well tolerated because the wax transfers less heat than water.

It can be applied from a commercial unit or from a double boiler. It is mixed with mineral oil in a ratio of seven pounds paraffin for every pint of mineral oil. Precautions must be taken against fire. The temperature is checked with a candy thermometer until it reaches 130°F. The paraffin is removed from the heat and the hand immersed in it for a few seconds. The hand is removed, allowed to dry slightly and redipped in the same manner several times. The hand is then placed in a plastic bag and covered with a towel for 20 to 30 minutes. The wax is stripped off to permit exercise. The wax can be recycled.

*Moist heat* seems to provide more relief than dry heat. It should not be used for more than 20 minutes at a time, and should not be continued if it causes burning or skin irritation.

Hydrocolator packs provide moist warmth for prolonged periods. They hold heat longer than moist towels as they are made with a heat-retaining resin.

A convenient means of application at home is by wrapping a hot damp towel in a plastic bag and placing a heating pad on top of that to make a hot pack. Care should be taken to avoid wetting the heating pad. A towel should be placed between the pack and the skin to avoid burns. The number of layers of towels determines the amount of heat felt by the patient.

*Hydrotherapy* is also a form of superficial heat. The major benefit is that the buoyancy of the water facilitates exercise, particularly ROM. Although total immersion in warm water is relaxing, it causes peripheral vasodilation. As less body surface is available to dissipate heat, the water temperature must be carefully watched. Prolonged immersion of the total body at 101° to 103°F may produce transient fever and thus increase cardiac and respiratory stress. Therefore hydrotherapy is contraindicated when there is cardiopulmonary involvement.

### Deep Heat
Deep heat, or diathermy, includes use of shortwaves, microwaves, or high-frequency sound waves (ultrasound) to generate heat in deep tissues, but only ultrasound can affect deep joints such as the hip. All can be used for bursitis, and ultrasound can be used to break up adhesive capsulitis of the shoulder. There is no demonstrable advantage to deep over superficial heat for pain relief. Deep heat is contraindicated in arthritis because it may stimulate enzyme-related joint destruction [1].

Precautions include the possibility of burning patients with poor circulation, impaired sensation, or metal implants (except ultrasound, which is reflected, rather than concentrated by metal), and aggravated bleeding diatheses. Short wave and microwave diathermy are contraindicated in patients with pacemakers.

## Cold
Cold, which has long been considered displeasing, has been shown to reduce muscle spindle activity and raise the pain threshold. Abrupt application causes discomfort and potentially, cardiovascular stress. The shock can be reduced by placing a warm, damp towel on the area to be treated, and placing cold packs (ice cubes in a towel) on top of the warm towel for 20 to 30 minutes. This results in relaxation, increased ROM, and decreased pain. Contraindications include Raynaud's phenomenon and cold hypersensitivity.

Efficacy of heat and cold for pain relief has not been established. By clinical observation, however, relief for acute inflammation and traumatic states is best achieved by cold compresses. Pain of subacute to chronic inflammation is usually best relieved by superficial application of heat, but some patients may prefer cold. In inflammatory articular disease, moist heat is empirically most effective.

### TRACTION
Traction is useful for decreasing both pain and contractures of the knees and hips. Its usefulness for conditions of the cervical or lumbar spine other than for rest is under question. Stretching does, however, provide some relief when there is stiffness or tightness from cramping following exercise. It is contraindicated in acute inflammation.

### MASSAGE
The primary purpose of massage is to obtain muscle relaxation prior to stretching or strengthening exercises. Types of massage include stroking, compression, and percussion. Stroking (*effleurage*) is used superficially for its soothing effect and deep muscle relaxation. Compression (*pétrissage*) is a kneading

of tissues used to stretch adhesions, mobilize edema, and relax muscles. Percussion (*tapotement*) is a stimulating counterirritant, vibration, or vigorous percussion.

### OTHER MODALITIES
*Transcutaneous nerve stimulation* provides an electrical sensory stimulus that overrides a painful stimulus, thus making the patient less aware of pain.

*Operant conditioning* decreases the patient's focus on pain by providing a reward for non–pain-focused behavior.

*Biofeedback* teaches muscle relaxation using visual or auditory feedback. It is effective against chronic neck and shoulder pain, and may be of use in controlling the vasospasm of Raynaud's phenomenon.

*Electrical stimulation* is used to decrease muscle spasm following intermittent electrically induced contractions.

## SPLINTING
### GENERAL INFORMATION
Splints and braces relieve stress on joints by providing localized rest, pain relief, and support. They assist in maintaining proper alignment, increasing functional abilities, preventing further deformity, or maintaining a joint in a functional position if fusion occurs.

Splints may be static or dynamic. A static splint does not move. A dynamic splint has moving parts and is used to increase ROM or for exercise and strengthening, usually following surgery.

There is no evidence that splints cause reversal of deformities, with the exception of serial casting of the knee, which may assist in reducing contractures of less than 45 degrees. Splints also assist in preventing contractures in the acute phase of disease.

### Design
The design of a splint is crucial for its success. It can be used to immobilize one joint such as the wrist, or several joints such as the wrist and hand. A splint can be designed to be worn at

night or during the day. A night splint may immobilize the joint and provide total rest, while a day splint must allow functional use unless the patient is in an acute stage of disease.

Different materials provide a variety of weights, durability, rigidity, porosity (enabling the skin to breathe), and ease in contouring (molding exactly to a patient's hand). Weight for the arthritic hand is crucial. Plaster, for example, is a good material, but is often too heavy. Plastizote and the low-temperature plastics are lighter, but not as durable.

Depending on how long it will be required, it may be more useful to make a light, less durable device that will require more frequent refitting or remaking, but that will be more manageable and therefore useful.

The ability of the patient to put on and remove splints independently is also of concern, particularly if bilateral devices are required.

*Precautions*
There are many precautions to observe in fabrication:

1. One needs to be aware of the compensatory stress placed on other joints by the splint.
2. The patient should be able to put the splint on and take it off without causing stress to the opposite hand.
3. The splint should allow for distribution of pressure over the widest possible area.
4. The patient should not have pain from the splint.
5. Any redness caused by the splint should clear within one-half hour of its removal.
6. One needs to observe for rubbing, especially over inflamed areas, in splints that will be used for daily activities and in patients with sensory loss. Areas that are particularly susceptible are the ulnar styloid and the point at which the straps cross the hand.
7. The therapist must compensate for fluctuation in the size of the joint if there is swelling.

8. Splints should be used in conjunction with a program of daily ROM.
9. The purpose, design, and especially the fit of splints should be reevaluated on a regular basis to be certain that the goals are being met.

If a splint is designed to increase hand function, this should be tested both with the splint on and off.

Education is vital. The patient needs to know when and how to wear the splint, how to clean and care for it, and to contact the therapist if redness or swelling develops.

HANDS
The maximum position of function of the hand is MP, 30 to 40 degrees flexion; PIP, 35 degrees flexion; thumb MP, 20 degrees flexion; CMC, 15 degrees internal rotation and 50 degrees abduction; and thumb IP, 0 degrees.

Any hand splint should conform to and maintain the normal pattern of the hand, including the transverse and longitudinal arches of the hand and wrist, and five to ten degrees ulnar deviation of the wrist if tolerated. Where bilateral wrist splinting is indicated, one wrist should be in neutral and the other in five to ten degrees flexion for toilet hygiene. The splint should be sturdy enough to provide the desired stability for the wrist when the patient is using the hands.

The most common hand devices for arthritic patients are full-hand resting and wrist stabilization splints, those designed to counteract ulnar drift, and the thumb carpometacarpal stabilization splint.

*Full-Hand Resting Splint*
This immobilizes the wrist, thumb, and fingers (Figure 4-11). The patient with severe inflammation of both the wrist and hand, as with RA or crystal-induced arthritis, may benefit from localized rest to provide pain relief, decrease inflammation, and prevent contractures. This type of splint may also be used when there is less acute inflammation; and as a night splint to

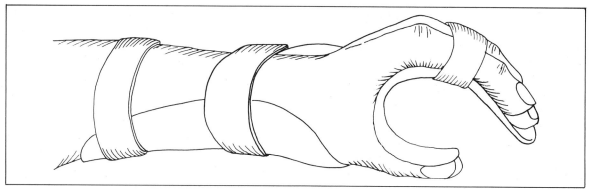

FIGURE 4-11. *Full-hand resting splint.*

provide support, optimal range and web space, and proper alignment of the joints during sleep. As it does not permit active hand function, when worn during the acute stage it must be used in conjunction with a daily ROM program.

The wrist should be in maximal pain-free extension up to 30 degrees. The thumb should be in abduction and opposition volar to the second metacarpal. Spacers may be needed between the fingers to maintain optimal alignment, or an ulnar ridge may be necessary to keep the fifth finger properly aligned.

*Wrist Stabilization Splint*
Where there is wrist involvement without finger involvement, a functional wrist splint may

FIGURE 4-12. *Wrist stabilization splint.*

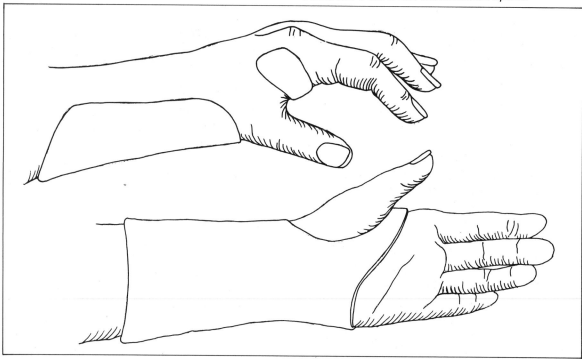

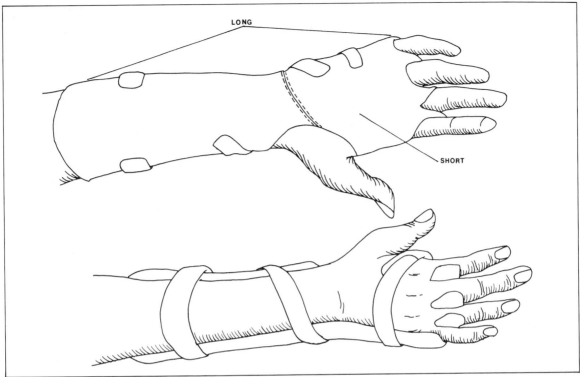

FIGURE 4-13. *Protective ulnar drift splint.*

be indicated (Figure 4-12). It partially or completely immobilizes the wrist while allowing full MP joint and thumb mobility. It is used to increase hand function and grip strength, provide localized rest to the wrist, and decrease inflammation and pain. The thenar clearance should allow full thumb opposition.

This splint may also be used in cases of carpal tunnel syndrome to relieve pressure on the median nerve. When used for this condition the wrist should be neutral in zero degrees extension. The device is contraindicated for patients with coexistent active MP synovitis, as immobilization of the wrist can cause increased stress to the MP joints, increasing the forces for subluxation and ulnar drift.

When it is prescribed to increase hand function, a careful test should be administered with the splint both on and off to determine if function is in fact improved.

### Ulnar Drift Splints

There are two basic types of splints for patients with MP synovitis that may result in ulnar drift. The protective ulnar drift splint (Figure 4-13) is used to prevent ulnar deviation and volar subluxation by maintaining the joints in normal alignment with zero to 25 degrees MP flexion. It is used where there is MP synovitis or beginning MP volar subluxation, beginning swan neck deformities, or intrinsic tightness. It can be a short unit or combined with a wrist stabilization splint. It is worn both day and night except when removed for ROM exercises. It may make hand skills awkward to perform.

The metacarpal ulnar drift splint (Figures 4-14 and 4-15) is for patients who already have severe ulnar drift or subluxation of the MP joints that interferes with function. It is designed to improve pinch and grasp, to reduce pain, and improve function by maintain-

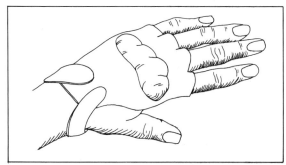

FIGURE 4-14. *MP positioning splint.*

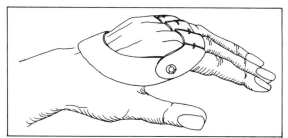

FIGURE 4-15. *Metacarpal ulnar drift splint.*

ing the MP joints in proper alignment. It is worn during activities but not at rest.

Both of these types of splints are difficult to fit, and proper effective fit is crucial. Functional hand evaluations should be administered with splints on and off.

### Thumb Carpometacarpal Stabilization Splint

The thumb CMC stabilization splint (Figure 4-16) is used primarily for patients with degenerative joint disease resulting in isolated pain with motion. When properly fitted, it relieves pain and increases hand function.

### ELBOWS

A Plastizote cylinder may be used to maintain extension when the joint is acutely inflamed. The elbow should be in 20 degrees flexion and supine. Daily ROM should be administered.

### SHOULDERS

The shoulder may be immobilized in a sling for the patient with bursitis, and daily ROM should be administered.

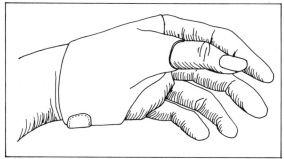

FIGURE 4-16. *Thumb carpometacarpal stabilization splint.*

### NECK AND BACK

There are many types of cervical braces, ranging from a soft foam collar to halo casting for total immobilization. The purposes of cervical bracing are to provide support to the neck, to reduce motion, and to relieve muscle tension and spasm that result from a local source of irritation in the disc or joint.

A soft collar provides general cervical pain relief in the absence of recent or progressive neurological deficit. It provides partial immobilization, and may be used as a reminder for patients not to move their heads.

The Philadelphia collar is a plastic brace with additional contact points, and can be used when more support is required.

A cervical brace or collar should be used in conjunction with isometric exercises for cervical flexion, extension, and rotator muscle groups to minimize disuse atrophy. One can also use manual resistance to assist with exercise. A special cylindrical pillow can be used to support the head.

Low back braces and corsets provide relief of pain by providing some restriction of spiral movement and abdominal compression. A corset is often most easily applied when the patient is in bed, rolling from side-lying onto the corset in a supine position, or standing and leaning with the low back against a wall for support while fastening it.

### KNEES

The knees should be kept straight or at a maxi-

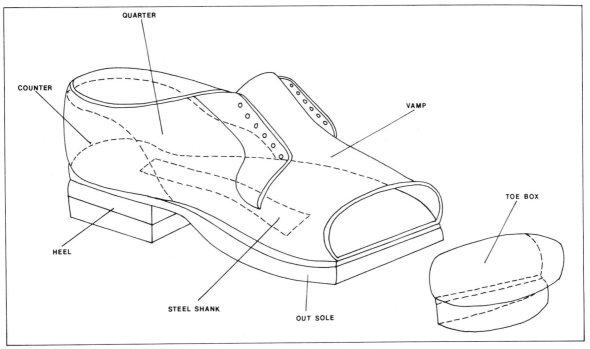

FIGURE 4-17. *Parts of the shoe.*

mum of 15 degrees flexion when inflamed. Elastic fabric splints or "cages" do provide some support and increased comfort when there is pain. Long leg braces have become more useful with the development of light-weight plastics for the patient with weakness of the knee. As with the hand, splinting the knee requires careful prescription and design. Location of hinges, straps, and bands, and ease of application must be considered.

Serial casting can be used to reduce knee contractures of less than 45 degrees. Otherwise, traction is suggested. The cast is changed every five to seven days. To facilitate maximal extension the patient lies prone prior to application of the cast.

### ANKLES

The ankles are often sources of persistent and disabling pain. When one lies in bed the ankle often goes into plantar flexion and should be positioned with a foot board. A short leg splint with a foot support, or an extension of a knee splint can also be used.

A short leg brace may aid in distributing weight-bearing over a larger surface and providing relief for the ankle. If immobilization is required, a SACH or cushioned heel with a rocker sole may compensate for ankle mobility. A below-knee weight-bearing brace may be used where subtalar pain interferes with ambulation.

### FEET

One of the most important external devices for the involved foot is the shoe (Figure 4-17). It can be modified to minimize pain and maximize position and function. The ideal shoe should provide support for the total foot including hindfoot, midfoot, and forefoot.

Hindfoot support is by a rigid steel shank extending longitudinally from the heel to the MTP line to support the midtarsal arch area, and a firm well-fitting heel counter to hold the calcaneus in optimal alignment and prevent the foot from sliding in the shoe. One single upright strut may be used for support where there is weakness. The ideal heel height is approximately one inch; a higher heel places stress on the forefoot, and a lower one stresses the ankle and heel. Crepe soles are often helpful in relieving calcaneal stress, however, if soles are too soft they may create instability and further problems. A padded heel insert designed in horseshoe fashion may take pressure off a painful calcaneus.

The shoe should have tie lacing with multiple lace holes for wide distribution of the supporting trusses over the dorsum of the midfoot. Arch supports may be used to aid weight distribution.

The toe box should have ample width, length, and depth to accommodate deformities such as splaying of the toes in RA resulting in metatarsalgia, and to mitigate any abnormal pressures on the forefoot. A crepe sole may assist during the toe-off phase of walking when there is a painful first MTP. The metatarsal pad may be helpful when there are forefoot problems.

A Plastizote insert may be molded to the painful foot and placed in the shoe to provide good equal weight distribution. It usually needs to be replaced every three months.

## JOINT PROTECTION

The structures in and around joints that have been affected by inflammation, swelling, and arthritic changes may be more easily damaged than normal joints by stresses both inside and outside the joint. Joint protection is essential to (1) decrease pain, (2) prevent deformity, and (3) maximize functional ability. This section reviews techniques that a patient can use to decrease these stresses during activities of daily life.

Respect pain; pain that lasts more than two hours after doing an activity is a danger signal that the joint has been overstressed. One needs to be aware of the activities done, and appropriate modifications should be made.

Maintain balance between activity and rest. A patient should get eight to ten hours sleep per night and one to two half-hour rest periods per day, as rest during activities is needed.

Position body properly. Proper body alignment is necessary to prevent joint stress and development of deformity, and to minimize energy expenditure. One needs to use proper body alignment in bed, sitting, standing, and moving.

### Bed

As joints tend to become deformed in a flexed position, flexion should be avoided in bed. The mattress should be firm and flat, with one small pillow under the head. Pillows should never be placed under the knees. The patient should lie prone at least 10 to 15 minutes twice a day to assist in the prevention of hip and knee contractures.

### Sitting

The arthritic patient should have at least one perfectly suited chair at home. It should have high firm seat and back, and armrests to assist in rising. It should be possible to sit with one's feet flat on the floor, and a nearby table should be at a comfortable height. If the patient is unable to flex the hips to 90 degrees, or has difficulty rising from a sitting position, a higher chair may be necessary, but the feet should still be supported.

The sitting position is determined by the task being done, but the spine should be aligned to minimize stress. Good sitting posture allows the arms to be in the best functional position and so helps to lessen fatigue. It also allows maximum lung capacity in respirations. The importance of work height to facilitate good posture should be kept in mind. The patient should not sit for long periods leaning on bent elbows, but the arms should be at the sides, in the lap, or resting on a table. Altering the height of the work surface as well as the position of illumination may allow the patient to assume a less stressful position.

Correct positioning is also of importance

when rising from sitting to standing. The patient should slide forward on the chair, bring both feet underneath the body flat on the floor, and lean forward; then with palms, or if possible, forearms, push off the chair while pushing off with the hips and knees. Twisting and pushing up on one side should be avoided. The patient should not clutch the desk or table top during pushing up, as this will put undue stress on the fingers.

### Standing

Alignment is important in maintaining good balance while standing. If the body is out of balance the muscles and joints have to work harder to keep it upright, resulting in fatigue and pain. In correct standing posture the body is erect with squared shoulders, neck, back, and hips, and with knees straight. With multiple joint involvement of RA loss of mobility in any one joint will lead to increased stress on all other joints in order to compensate for lost motion.

### Moving

Ambulation is not only a lower extremity function, so it is important to consider the upper extremities when prescribing ambulation aids. Platform crutches or walker, for example, place weight on the forearm, thus avoiding placing stress on wrists, elbows, fingers, and shoulders.

Try to avoid prolonged static positions. Maintaining a grasp or one position for a long time tires muscles so that they cannot give joints the support they need. It is best to avoid prolonged standing or sitting. When more height is needed to accomplish a job, a high sturdy stool adjusted to the working level is helpful. When standing, it is advisable to lean against a wall, counter, or desk to relieve some of the body weight from the legs. Reading materials can be supported by a bookrest. If bifocals are worn, a separate pair of glasses is useful to avoid a static neck position that can be painful. Activities involving repetitive tiring

motions or holding are especially stressful and fatiguing, and should be done for short periods of time; vacuuming, cleaning windows, and ironing are examples. Activities should be stopped before joints become tired. There are many activities involving static hand positions: writing, painting, hammering, using hand tools, and knitting. If these are to be maintained, the hands should be rested with the fingers straight at least every ten minutes. An electric typewriter can supplement writing and also provides good finger exercise. There are many other beneficial nonstatic activities including Turkish knotting, playing pool, swimming, decoupage, light gardening, and weaving, for example.

The strongest largest joint available for the job should be used. The knees, not the back, should be used when lifting heavy objects. For lifting plates, bowls, baking pans, and so on, the palms, not just the fingers, of both hands should be slipped beneath the object so that the wrists are used to lift. Oven mitts should be used for lifting anything hot. Objects should be slid whenever possible. When steadying an object, the weight of the forearm should be used instead of the fingers. A pocketbook, satchel, bookbag, or shopping bag should be carried on the forearm or shoulder rather than in the fingers. Body weight, that is, the rear end rather than the hands, should be used to move drawers, boxes, or doors. A ring-topped can should be opened with a knife instead of fingers, with the blade slipped into the ring, and the edge of the can used as a pivot. Webbing or a leather strap can be attached to the refrigerator door if it is magnetic; the arm is slipped through the strap, and when a step is taken backward the door will open.

Each joint should be used in the most stable anatomical and functional plane. The pull of gravity should be minimized, and objects should be slid and not lifted. Good body mechanics should be used. The body and hands should be positioned properly when doing a task.

Certain principles of joint protection primarily involve the upper extremities. They include:

a. Avoiding ulnar or lateral deviating pressures on the fingers
b. Avoiding positions of prolonged flexion
c. Avoiding tight grasp

## Avoiding Ulnar or Lateral Deviating Pressures

This should be done to prevent deformity. A knife should be held like a dagger, and a pulling motion used to cut. Objects should be held with their handles parallel to the knuckles. Doorknobs should be turned using wrist motion while standing sideways to the door. A doorknob helper is useful for knobs that are difficult to grip. When lifting plates, bowls, and bulky equipment or containers, the objects should be lifted with both palms under the objects, avoiding gripping the edges. When opening screwed jars, the lid should be pressed down with the palm of the hand and shoulder motion used in turning. A washcloth or piece of rubber can assist in stabilizing the jar or gripping the lid. A drinking cup with a large handle through which all fingers may be slipped should be used, or an insulated or thermal cup may be held between both palms. When wringing out washcloths and clothes, moisture should be pressed out with the palm of the hand, or the article can be stabilized around the faucet and twisted using wrist action. Clothes can also be allowed to dry in the air or in an automatic dryer.

To dial a telephone a pencil is used like an icepick and padded for easy grasp with shoulder motion used to dial; a pushbutton phone can be obtained. An electric can opener or electric scissors can be of help. Adaptive car door handles and keys can be made.

If a kettle must be filled with water, one should put in a little at a time with a small container. One should slide the kettle to the edge of stove and tip the kettle, instead of lifting it to pour.

One should avoid abnormal pressures against the pad of the thumb. The thumb should not be used to depress the latch on a car door or in sewing heavy fabric.

## Avoiding Positions of Prolonged Flexion

When resting on the hand, the fingers should be straight against the cheek. When crossing the arms, the fingers should be straightened on top of the arms.

The fingers should be kept in extension and the hand flattened as much as possible. Sponges and dust mitts should be used instead of dishcloths and dustcloths. The fingers should be kept straight when smoothing out a sheet or clothes.

One should avoid both pushing against the backs of the fingers when rising from a chair, and propping the chin on the backs of the fingers.

## Avoiding Tight Grasp

Gripping activities such as holding a purse by the handles cause harmful internal pressures. The handles of any often-used tools or utensils and pens or pencils should be enlarged by wrapping them in foam or small hand towels. Work or kitchen tools should be chosen for their light weight and larger handles. Objects should be held with both hands, palms up. Offset screwdrivers or wrenches can be used for lever action. A cutting board with spikes can hold food for cutting. Pliers and tweezers can help in securing fine grasp, and vises and clamps are good for large objects. An effort should be made to loosen the grasp on things such as steering wheels, golf clubs, work tools, writing equipment, and so on. Strong grasp combined with twisting action should especially be avoided, including such activities as unscrewing tight jars, turning door knobs, wringing clothes, and turning keys without extended handles.

Avoid activities that cannot be stopped immediately. Overambitious tasks, such as cooking a complicated meal or going downtown should not be begun if one is unsure of one's tolerance.

Use energy conservation and work simplification techniques. The effort expended to do a job should be minimized; energy conservation and work simplification techniques should be employed. The work area should be reorganized so that frequently used equipment is within easy reach and less necessary items are out of the way. Shelves should be raised or lowered for accessibility to their contents. When an activity is started everything needed from the cupboard, refrigerator, closet, or storeroom, should be obtained at one time to save steps. A tea cart or pushcart is helpful in eliminating carrying problems, and saving time, steps, and energy. The use of unnecessary tools, equipment, or dishes should be cut down to minimize cleaning up. Shopping by telephone or mail can be helpful. Simple nutritious meals should be planned, with use made of convenience foods. Lightweight equipment and tools should be used at work and at home, such as aluminum cookware, plastic utensils, Flair pens. One should sit to work whenever possible, but with regular periods of standing and stretching. The elbows should be supported on a table or washstand while combing the hair, shaving, or during facial hygiene. Adaptive devices can be used to protect joints, conserve energy, and increase function.

Activities should be planned to avoid pressure of rushing against time, as this causes one to tire quickly. All heavy activities should not be done the same day, but should be spread out over several days. Activities should be organized and done in the same manner at all times, using proper joint protection techniques. Repetition of the same methods makes one proficient and saves time and energy. The best time of day should be considered for each activity; if the morning is the most difficult time, more activities should be done the evening before, such as bathing.

The health professional needs to help the patient review regular activities and how a typical week is organized. The arthritic needs to learn to take rests during the day. Problem activities should be reviewed to consider (1) how to make them easier, such as reducing the force necessary to do the activity—screwing lids on loosely, or using energy conservation; (2) changing methods, such as sliding rather than lifting, or using two hands instead of one; (3) using adaptive equipment if necessary; or finally (4) eliminating them altogether.

ADAPTIVE EQUIPMENT

There is a multitude of ways to adapt the environment and the tools used in daily functioning. It is important to discuss the future use of any adaptive device with the patient, as there are several reasons for declining it. The patient may already have figured out a way to do the task, may be embarrassed and not wish to use the device, may not wish to be taught how to use it, may feel the cost is prohibitive, or may not think an adaptive device is needed in the first place. Following the principles of joint protection, such equipment has been developed to compensate for decreased ROM and strength. Examples include:

Reachers
Long-handled devices such as sponges and
    utensils
Toilet aids
Bathroom equipment including raised toilet
    seat and rail for the toilet and tub seat, and
    grab bar for the tub

Principles of joint protection on which such equipment is based are:

1. Respect for pain
2. Balance between rest and work
3. Proper body positioning
4. Avoidance of prolonged static positions
   a. Electric can opener
   b. Two pairs of glasses instead of bifocals
   c. Electric typewriter
   d. Electric scissors
   e. Bookrests for reading
5. Use of the strongest joint for the activity
   a. Adapting canes or crutches for upper extremity problems

b. Strap on refrigerator to open door using forearm

6. Use of joints in most stable anatomical and functional plane

7. Use of upper extremity principles
   a. Avoidance of ulnar and lateral deviation
      (1) Push-button telephone
      (2) Cup with large handle for all fingers
      (3) Thermal cup
      (4) Faucet adapters
      (5) Doorknob adapters
   b. Avoidance of prolonged flexion
      (1) Oven mitts instead of pot holders
      (2) Extended handles
   c. Avoidance of tight grasp
      (1) Pliers and tweezers
      (2) Built-up handles
      (3) Spiked cutting board

8. Elimination of activities that cannot be stopped immediately
   a. Wheeled cart to carry objects from one place to another

9. Energy conservation techniques
   a. Dycem to stabilize objects
   b. Use of bedpan, commode, urinal at night
   c. Wheeled cart

## EXERCISE

Exercise serves several purposes for the arthritic patient; principally, it maintains or increases ROM or mobility, strength, and endurance. Exercise should always be done at the patient's best time of day and following analgesia or other type of pain relief. Following exercise, pain should not last more than one to two hours; if it does, the exercise program should be decreased. Before prescribing an exercise program one must be aware of how disease has affected ROM so as not to do further damage to the joints. The ROM may be affected by ruptured tendons, swelling, subluxation, tendon constriction, and muscle impingement; exercises should be modified accordingly.

The acuteness of disease determines the objectives of the program. Different types of exercises are used to achieve different objectives, but the fewest possible movements should be done in the least stressful manner to accomplish goals.

### ACUTE STAGE

In the acute stage when there is severe inflammation, the only goal is to maintain ROM. No stretch should be placed on the joint. Passive exercises are used, and the joint moved through its range. The therapist may also do gentle active assisted ROM, which is active motion by the patient through partial range, with assistance to complete the range. Both should only be done gently to the point of pain tolerance without causing increased pain and swelling. The joint should be put through two complete exercise cycles per day to maintain range. It may take as many as two to five warmups to reach maximum range.

### SUBACUTE PHASE

In the subacute phase with moderate inflammation one needs to increase mobility and strength in addition to maintaining ROM. This can be done with active assisted ROM, isometric exercise, and simple exercise equipment. More vigorous active assisted exercise may be used, in which the external forces may be mechanical or manual. Forces include gravity assist, pulleys, water, or manual assistance provided by another person or an unaffected part of the patient's body. To increase ROM, three to ten repetitions are recommended per session one to two times per day.

For strengthening in the subacute phase, isometric exercise is suggested to achieve maximal muscle contraction without joint motion. There is less stress placed on the joint, but muscle strength can be maintained or increased. At the onset of isometric exercise the joint is positioned so that the muscles being exercised are at slightly less than maximal contraction. If this causes pain, the position with the least amount of discomfort is used. The patient contracts the muscle as tightly as possible without moving the joint, holds it for six seconds, then relaxes. In the subacute phase this should be done one or two times per day to maintain strength. Isometric exercise is especially important for the antigravity muscles such as the gluteals and quadriceps, which tend to lose strength rapidly when a patient is on bedrest, has joint swelling that causes muscle atrophy by reflex, or is not active during the acute and subacute stages.

CHRONIC PHASE

Where there is minimal or no inflammation, the goals are to maintain and increase strength and endurance. Active or active assisted exercise can be used to increase ROM. Isometric and isotonic exercise can be used to increase strength and endurance. Isotonic exercise uses joint motion to achieve a muscle contraction. This can be done graded against progressively greater resistance (progressive resistive exercise). These exercises should only be done if there is no joint pain.

## Upper Extremity ROM Exercises

I. Warmups
   A. Shrug the shoulders
   B. Wiggle the shoulders around
   C. Pendular swinging: With arms hanging at the sides, swing them side to side and back and forth
   D. Hold the arms at 90 degrees flexion with the elbows straight; reach forward and back protracting and retracting the scapulae simultaneously slowly in turn
II. Cane exercises
   A. Shoulder flexion, external rotation, and elbow flexion and extension
      1. The cane is held palms down
      2. The cane is raised overhead; elbows are straightened
      3. It is brought behind the neck
      4. The cane is raised overhead again
      5. It is brought back to starting position. If the cane cannot be raised overhead it should be raised to tolerance
   B. Elbow flexion and extension
      1. Hold the cane palms down
      2. Bring it in toward the chest

3. Straighten arms in front
4. Bring the cane back toward the chest
   C. Shoulder abduction and adduction, elbow flexion and extension, pronation and supination
      1. Hold the cane, one palm up, one palm down
      2. Move the cane on a diagonal as far as possible in the direction of the up-turned palm
      3. Return to the center
      4. Reverse hands so the other palm is facing up
      5. Move the cane on a diagonal in the direction of the upturned palm
      6. Return to center
         The therapist may give active assistance by holding the cane in the middle
III. Finger wall-climbing
   A. Stand facing the wall and walk the fingers up the wall keeping elbows straight and shoulders level
   B. Standing with one's side to the wall at arm's length, walk fingers up the wall keeping elbows straight and shoulders level
IV. Wrist extension exercises
   A. Exercise 1
      1. The hands are placed together in front of one's body with elbows straight, palms together, and thumbs toward the ceiling
      2. Keeping palms together, hands are brought in toward the chest, bending elbows out to sides. The elbows should not be kept close to sides while bringing hands in
      3. The elbows are straightened, keeping palms together
   B. Exercise 2
      1. With forearms and hands on the table palms down, the hand is picked up at the wrist, keeping fingers straight
      2. The hand is put back down on the table. The palms should not deviate ulnarly when these exercises are being done

V. Finger exercises
   A. Exercise 1
      1. The hands are placed on the table palms down
      2. Each finger is picked up one at a time
   B. Exercise 2
      1. The hands are placed on the table palms down
      2. Each finger is picked up one at a time, starting with the thumb, and moved in the direction of the thumb
      3. If there is difficulty picking up fingers, they are slid toward the thumb, but never toward the little finger
   C. Exercise 3
      1. The hands are opened and closed, spreading the fingers as the hand is opened and making as tight a fist as possible as the hand is closed
      2. The tip of the thumb is touched to the tip of each finger and pinched to make an O
   D. Exercise 4
      1. With another person present, the fingers of both people's right hands are interlocked as in thumb wrestling
      2. All MPs are extended while the PIPs and DIPs are flexed
      3. The patient should try to flex the fingers, with the fingers of the assistant giving support and assistance
      4. Ulnar deviation is avoided
      5. The same is done on the left

## Isometric Arm-Strengthening Exercises

The first two exercises are performed with the patient sitting in a chair.

1. A belt or loop of heavy elastic cord is fastened around one of the front legs of a chair; the cord is pulled up and out, using the hand opposite the cord, holding for six seconds.
2. The cord is pulled by the hand on the same side, up and across the chest, holding for six seconds.

3. The elbows are rested, flexed on the table, hands pointing towards the ceiling. The forearms are crossed; one attempts to straighten each elbow in turn for six seconds, while resisting the motion with the other arm.

## Lower Extremity ROM Exercises
   I. Hip and knee
   These exercises are done lying on the back with the legs straight
   A. Flexion and extension
      Each knee is brought to the chest in turn. The hip and knee are bent as far as they will go, keeping the other leg flat on the bed
   B. Hip abduction and adduction
      Each leg in turn is slid out as far as it will go to the side, keeping the knee straight, and then pulled in to starting position
   C. Hip rotation
      With the legs about 10 to 12 inches apart at the knees, each leg in turn is rolled inward and outward
   D. Prone-lying
      Lying prone should be done 10 to 15 minutes two times a day
   E. Combined motion
      Each heel is slid along the opposing leg toward the hip and returned to starting position in turn this exercise is done sitting erect on a hard chair with knees flexed
   F. Knee and ankle
      The knees are straightened as far as possible, with toes pointing toward the ceiling and returned to starting position;
   II. Ankle
   These exercises are done lying on the back with the legs straight
   A. The ankles are flexed with toes pointing toward the foot of the bed, and then extended so that the toes are pointing toward the ceiling
   B. The feet are turned so that the soles are facing each other and then turned so that the soles are facing away from each other

C. Circles are made with each foot in turn both clockwise and counterclockwise

III. Toes

    A. The toes are curled so that they try to touch the bottom of the foot, and then are straightened as far as possible

    B. The toes are spread out as far as possible and then brought together

## Isometric Leg-Strengthening Exercises

1. Quad setting: Lying on the back with one leg straight, the thigh muscles above the knee are tightened by pressing the knee into the bed for six seconds; after relaxing, the exercise is repeated with the other leg
2. Buttock muscle setting: While lying on the bed with the legs straight, the buttocks are tightened by trying to pinch them together
3. While sitting with a heavy elastic cord around the thighs, the knees are pulled apart as much as possible against the resistance of the cord, holding for six seconds
4. A large coffee can is squeezed between the knees for six seconds

## Arch-Strengthening Exercises

1. Sitting with the feet resting on a towel, the toes are curled to gather the towel under the arch of the foot. Rest frequently to avoid cramping
2. While patient is sitting, a marble is picked up with the toes, carried toward the other foot, and dropped into a dish, repeated with several marbles
3. Standing with the toes over the edge of a board, the toes are held flexed over the edge of the board for 6 seconds, then relaxed

## Facial Exercises

1. Open the mouth as wide as possible
2. Smile as widely as possible
3. Blow out evenly and steadily

4. Say the vowels AEIOU, exaggerating each one
5. Wrinkle the forehead and raise the eyebrows
6. Close the eyes as tightly as possible; open them as wide as possible

## Neck ROM Exercises

These exercises are done while sitting erect.

1. The chin is pulled in toward the chest, (making double chins) making sure that the back of the neck and head are straight, and relaxed
2. The head is flexed forward touching the chin to the chest, then extended backward to look up at the ceiling
3. The head is turned, bringing the chin to the left shoulder, then back to the center, and turned bringing the chin to the right shoulder and back to the center
4. While looking straight ahead the head is tilted, bringing the ear down to the shoulder, then straightened to the center and brought down to the other side (the shoulder should not be lifted)
5. The head is flexed forward and rotated in as large a circle as possible, slowly in a clockwise direction, and repeated in a counterclockwise direction

## Neck-Strengthening Exercises

Above exercises 2, 3, and 4 are done while resisting the motion with the hand, not allowing the head to move, and held for a count of six.

## Posture and Breathing Exercises

1. Ten deep breaths
2. Lying flat on the stomach on the floor with the arms at the sides, the head is lifted and the knees are bent as far as possible at the same time (the knees may be lifted, if possible)
3. Lying flat on the back on a bed with the legs straight, the heels and shoulders are pushed down into the bed simultaneously

pushed down into the bed simultaneously while the buttocks are lifted off the bed for a few seconds

4. Lying flat on the back with hands on the sides of the chest, a deep breath is taken pushing the ribs out against the hands, held a moment, the air let out, and repeated

## MOBILITY

Mobility means more than walking: it includes the ability to move into and out of bed, from lying to sitting, sitting to standing, and the reverse. Mobility occurs in the home, at work, and in the community, the last encompassing ability to use public transportation or an automobile.

When devices or techniques are prescribed to facilitate mobility, they should be designed for the individual patient and environment, taking into account how all the joints are affected by the device.

### BED

Rails can facilitate bed mobility. A wooden board under the mattress can increase firmness. A hospital bed with electric controls may help increase mobility of the patient with severe disease. These devices may be combined with teaching techniques for coming to sitting position in the most effective, efficient manner.

### TRANSFERS

Chairs should have arm rests. Blocks under chairs raise the height and facilitate transfers. Commercial chairs are available that lift the patient out by way of a seat cushion that is elevated when a button is pressed. Bathroom equipment can be used for the toilet and tub. (See Adaptive Equipment.)

### STAIRS

Rails, if not present, can be installed, and center rails may help. Some patients benefit from risers alternating every other step.

The type of floor, carpet, or linoleum can affect mobility. One may wish to modify the environment or interpose an adaptive device so that the patient can maneuver.

### WHEELCHAIRS

Chair size can be adjusted for narrow doorways or wide patients. Leg rests can be elevating or removable; arms can be removable. The back of the chair can be high.

### AMBULATORY AIDS

Ambulatory aids may assist in distributing weight off the feet, ankles, knees, or hips. Their use will be determined by weak or painful joints.

### Canes

When prescribing a cane it should be fitted in terms of length, width, and grip. The position of the hand is determined by the most comfortable elbow angle required for stability. It may be necessary to modify this for wrist or elbow contractures.

The T cane may be more appropriate for the patient with rheumatic disease, as the shape of the handle distributes weight through the entire arm, rather than placing stress on the fingers and wrist as the more common C cane does.

### Crutches

When prescribing crutches, platform models may be more beneficial for the arthritic patient. Weight is distributed to the larger joints of the elbow and the shoulder rather than the joints of the hand.

### Walkers

They may be adapted with platforms rather than having patients bear weight on their hands. Walkers may also be adapted with gliders or wheels on the front so that they do not have to be picked up, but slide across the floor. This, of course, means that they do not provide as much stability, but one must evaluate the needs of the patients to determine what is more useful and safe.

## Automobile

Extra mirrors may be added for the person who has difficulty turning the head. Steering wheels may be ordered that tilt, allowing easier access to the driver's seat.

## PSYCHOSOCIAL ASPECTS

Patients with arthritis manifest certain personality characteristics such as depression, lack of adaptability, and overconcern with bodily function. These characteristics are more likely to be consequences of the chronic disease than of a specific rheumatoid personality. A patient with chronic disease lives with the threat of constant pain, restriction of motion, weakness, loss of function, and deformity. Psychological reaction depends on:

1. The patient's personality before the illness
2. The patient's perception of the disease and its effects
3. The reactions and expectations of society, family, and friends
4. The characteristics of the patient's environment (home and workplace)
5. The patient's economic situation

### PREMORBID PERSONALITY

The patient's previous ways of handling stress may be accentuated by the disease and be of help in handling the situation, or they may be a negative influence.

### SELF-PERCEPTION

Self-esteem can be affected by pain, deformity, or drugs. The patient may be afraid of losing independence and becoming a burden on the family, or be concerned about sexual dysfunction. The patient needs to understand the disease and the limitations imposed by it. Patient education can assist in these areas.

### PERCEPTIONS OF OTHERS

The family may overprotect or expect more from the patient than is reasonable. The patient, in turn, may incur secondary gains from the attention received from family and friends while ill.

Society has its traditional expectations of people. For example, a woman is expected to take care of the house and children, and the man is expected to be the principal support. Although these stereotypes are changing, the patient of either sex may experience guilt at being unable to fulfill expected roles.

### ENVIRONMENT

Physical barriers at home may present difficulties for the arthritic patient: stairs may make him or her feel trapped; a poorly arranged kitchen may create a feeling of dependence on others. Depending on the amount of impairment, the environment can either minimize or maximize the degree of disability.

The same is true of the work environment. Levels of education and self-esteem play a role in motivation and incentive, and those in positions of responsibility tend to work longer than people in lower positions who may have the same impairment.

The patient's abilities, physical barriers at work, and possible assistive devices should be evaluated. A vocational rehabilitation counselor may offer guidance and prepare the patient for specific tasks. The counselor may educate the employer and other employees, arrange transportation, and facilitate the patient's return to work. Unfortunately, however, fewer than five percent of patients with rheumatic diseases receive assistance from vocational rehabilitation [4]. There is also a lack of incentive in the social security disabilities system, which rewards chronic persistent disease.

### ECONOMIC SITUATION

Economics may determine the patient's access to therapy, transportation, and adaptive equipment that is not available through insurance.

### SEXUAL PROBLEMS

Although sexual counseling is of concern to a patient with rheumatic disease, there is no one professional discipline generally assigned the responsibility of guidance in these problems as they relate to physical limitation. This may be because society has generally viewed people with physical limitations as sexless, or because sex is a difficult topic to discuss and no one discipline wants to be the one to handle it exclusively.

Whoever on the team assumes the role of sexual counselor should initially obtain a history, including sexual knowledge and experiences, information on contraception, the partner's history, symptoms that affect the patient's sexual functioning, and the patient's expectations. The patient with rheumatic disease may face one or several problems in areas of sexual functioning: decreased libido, deformities, impotence, contraception, and the attitude of the partner.

Libido, or sexual drive, may be decreased as a result of depression, disease, effect of medication, or diminished self-image. Deformities may affect both the patient's self-image and ability to assume customary positions. This is particularly true where there is hip or knee involvement of osteoarthritis and RA. Hand deformity or pain may interfere with foreplay. Impotence or frigidity may result from pain, fatigue, medications, or fear of failure. Scleroderma may cause erectile dysfunction.

Use of contraception may be a problem: application of a condom may be difficult with hand deformity, and birth control pills are contraindicated for patients with SLE. Methods of contraception should be discussed with the physician.

The attitude of the partner may also have an effect; for example the "joint-protecting partner" may be afraid of hurting the patient. There are, however, several ways to adapt situations to assist in maintaining normal sexual functioning, including many of the principles discussed earlier: (1) the time of day is important in minimizing pain and fatigue; (2) rest, analgesia, or a form of relaxation may be helpful prior to sexual activity; (3) heat, ROM, and muscle-strengthening exercises to the joints may be of assistance.

Positioning is a way to minimize joint stress and adapt for deformity. Often, the customary positions are not the best, and lateral or rear entry may work better. The patient may want to determine a position that is generally comfortable, and then use it in sexual activity. Also, pillows may be used to maximize comfort.

Entry may be a problem, especially in patients with Sjögren's syndrome, and KY jelly may be used for lubrication. Vaseline should not be used as it is not water-soluble and can therefore cause infection.

It is important for the patient and partner to communicate so that they can work together to achieve pleasurable sex. Such activity is also an excellent way for patients to increase self-esteem. The therapist can help the patient maximize pleasure by facilitating communication, and offering education in areas of anatomy, proper use of joint protection, and energy conservation.

PATIENT EDUCATION
Patient education gives the person with rheumatic disease a greater understanding of the disease. This reduces anxiety and increases compliance with treatment. Patients should know both the diagnosis and prognosis, and know and understand their treatment regimen including medicines and side effects, rest, exercise, use and application of splints and adaptive equipment, and permitted recreational activities. The patient should be informed about the therapeutic, psychosocial, and economic resources that are available in the community.

The information in an education program should be individualized. Patients' needs may differ according to socioeconomic levels, geographical area (i.e., urban versus rural), and living situations. Thus each patient can provide valuable input in designing the program by indicating preference for participation of family members, best time of day, duration, frequency of sessions, and method of teaching.

Patients can be taught individually or in groups, the latter in the hospital or in the community. Community groups can be formed and run by the patients themselves. Many may wish to take advantage of more than one of these resources.

A wide range of educational materials is currently available to both the patient and therapist. Local chapters of the Arthritis Foundation offer information on resources available in the community as well as patient clubs. The Arthritis Information Clearinghouse was established by the National Institutes of Health to help health professionals by screening, collecting, and organizing information on arthritis and related musculoskeletal diseases from a variety of resources. The Clearinghouse can be extremely valuable for education.

The information the therapist should review with the patient includes principles of joint protection, use of splints, assistive equipment, exercise, and purpose of the treatment regimen. The patient should be made aware of which sources can be of assistance with specific problems, for example, the therapist should be contacted if there are problems with a splint.

It is important for the therapist to be certain that the patient has assimilated the material. Useful techniques include having the patient repeat back what was heard, demonstrate techniques that were learned, and answer questions on a follow-up questionnaire.

## DIET
Diet also requires education. All patients should have a nutritionally well-balanced diet. Often, because of decreased mobility, they will make fewer trips to the grocery store, and have limited access to certain foods such as fresh fruits and vegetables.

Patients with gout should avoid foods high in purine, such as liver and sweetbreads, and avoid alcohol, as these can induce attacks. Diet is no longer as crucial with gout as in the past, however, as there are now drugs that are effective in preventing attacks.

Patients should maintain proper body weight, particularly when there is involvement of the weight-bearing joints and/or systemic involvement. Patients with gout or a systemic disease should consult a physician before making any change in diet, either for weight reduction or weight gain.

## SURGERY
Surgery does not cure arthritis, although it may result in pain relief, restored function of a joint, and improved appearance. Surgery is only indicated when there is pain despite medication, or loss of function, and should not be performed for deformity alone. It may enable the patient to be self-sufficient and earn a living, arrest further destruction of a joint, or reduce stress in related joints. It is expensive, painful, and risky, however, and may be useless if the patient does not exercise afterward. It must be noted that such exercise may be affected by involvement of joints that have not been surgically treated. Surgery is an evolving art with most experience achieved with the hip and the hand. Knee surgery is becoming more common and having increased success. The life of implanted devices is still not known, and joint replacement is therefore not usually done on young patients.

Procedures may be prophylactic, reconstructive, or reparative. Prophylaxis includes synovectomy and tenosynovectomy. The former is removal of diseased synovial tissue, and may temporarily retard disease in a given joint. Tenosynovectomy, which is removal of diseased tendons and synovial tissue, may be used to avoid tendon rupture.

The most common reconstructive surgeries are arthrodesis, arthroplasty, and total joint replacement. Arthrodesis is fusion of a diseased joint in the best position of function so that there is no motion; it is performed to relieve pain.

Arthroplasty is used to help reconstruct a damaged joint. It may replace one side of the joint, interpose a new gliding surface, or replace both joint surfaces.

Total hip replacement is a great surgical advance for patients with RA. It can reduce pain, increase ROM, and increase walking distance.

Following the surgery, patients are hospitalized two to three weeks; by three to four days they can sit for meals and can begin crutch training, ROM, and muscle strengthening. By 18 to 21 days they will be independent on crutches and ready for a home program of exercise. At the end of six weeks they only need a single crutch on the side opposite the operation, and at the end of ten weeks they begin unsupported ambulation. The most common surgery is total hip replacement (THR) using a metal ball in the femur to articulate in a polyethylene socket held in place with bone cement.

Hand surgery has also expanded, the most common reconstructive procedure being the Swanson MP arthroplasty. This is not an artificial joint, but a spacer to keep the MP joints better aligned and encapsulated by a new fibrous capsule. Its major use is for treating preexisting fusions, fixed swan neck deformities, and gross dislocation or severe ulnar deviation of the MP joints. The patient need only be hospitalized four to five days. Movement is started as soon as possible, with edema a limiting factor. Joint ROM is not restored completely, but the joint is more functional and looks better, and the operation may assist in preventing further damage. The therapeutic regimen before and after this procedure has been well worked out (see Suggested Reading).

A common form of reparative surgery is release of the median nerve in carpal tunnel syndrome. This is performed when the median nerve is trapped by constricting fibrous tissue.

*I wish to express thanks to Dr. Stuart L. Silverman, Assistant Professor of Medicine, University of Pennsylvania, and Attending Physician, Arthritis Section, Hospital of University of Pennsylvania, Philadelphia, for his advice, assistance, and patience; and acknowledge the support of Pennsylvania Home Health Services.*

# References

1. Harris, E. D., Jr., and McCroskery, P. A. The influence of temperature and fibril stability on degradation of cartilage collagen by rheumatoid synovial collagenase. *N. Engl. J. Med.* 290:1, 1974.
2. Levy, J., and Dick, W. C. Detection of change in disease activity. *Clin. Rheum. Dis.* 1(2):226, 1975.
3. Mason, M., and Currey, H. C. F. *Clinical Rheumatology.* Philadelphia: Lippincott, 1970.
4. Niederman, J. Understanding Vocational Rehabilitation as it Relates to the Total Rehabilitation of the Arthritis Victim. Presented to the American Rheumatism Association, Atlanta, 1980.
5. O'Sullivan, J. B., and Cathcart, E. S. The prevalence of rheumatoid arthritis. *Ann. Intern. Med.* 76:573, 1972.
6. Rodin, E. L. The physiology and degeneration of joints. *Semin. Arthritis Rheum.* 2:245, 1972.

# Suggested Reading

## GENERAL REFERENCES

Hart, F. D. Approach to the patient and general measures of management. *Clin. Rheum. Dis.* 1(2):217, 1975.

Hirschberg, G. G., Lewis, L., and Vaughan, P. Disabling Conditions due to Musculoskeletal Impairment. In *Rehabilitation, A Manual for the Care of the Disabled and Elderly.* Philadelphia: Lippincott, 1976. Pp. 326–347.

Katz, W. A. (Ed.). *Rheumatic Diseases, Diagnosis and Management.* Philadelphia: Lippincott, 1977.

McCarty, D. J. (Ed.). *Arthritis and Allied Conditions.* Philadelphia: Lea and Febiger, 1979.

Melvin, J. L. *Rheumatic Diseases: Occupational Therapy and Rehabilitation.* Philadelphia: Davis, 1977.

Shands, A. R., and Raney, R. B. *Handbook of Orthopedic Surgery.* St. Louis: Mosby, 1967. Pp. 141–177.

Rusk, H. A. *Rehabilitation and Medicine.* St. Louis: Mosby, 1977.

Sweezey, R. L. *Arthritis: Rational Therapy and Rehabilitation.* Philadelphia: Saunders, 1978.

## EVALUATIONS

### EXAMINATION OF THE JOINTS

Hoppenfeld, S. *Physical Examination of the Spine and Extremities.* New York: Appleton-Century-Crofts, 1976.

Polley, H. F., and Heinder, G. G. *Rheumatologic*

*Interviewing and Physical Examination of the Joints.* Philadelphia: Saunders, 1978.

FUNCTIONAL EVALUATIONS

Carroll, D. A quantitative test of UE function. *J. Chron. Dis.* 18:478, 1965.

Carthum, C. J., Clawson, D. K., and Decker, J. L. Functional assessment of the rheumatoid hand. *Am. J. Occup. Ther.* 23:122, 1969.

Jebson, R. H. An objective and standardized test of hand function. *Arch. Phys. Med. Rehabil.* 50:311, 1969.

Jette, A. M., and Deniston, O. L. Inter-observer reliability of a functional status assessment instrument. *J. Chron. Dis.* 31:573, 1978.

Kellor, M., et al. Technical manual hand strength and dexterity norms. *Am. J. Occup. Ther.* 25:77, 1971.

Loomis, B. The home visit: An integral part of occupational therapy for patients with rheumatic diseases. *Am. J. Occup. Ther.* 19:264, 1965.

McBain, K. P. Assessment of function in the rheumatoid hand. *Can. Occup. Ther. J.* 37:95, 1970.

Potvin, A. R., et al. Simulated activities of daily living examination. *Arch. Phys. Med. Rehabil.* 53:476, 1972.

Smith, H. Smith hand function evaluation. *Am. J. Occup. Ther.* 27:244, 1973.

Treuhaft, P. S., Lewis, M. R., and McCarthy, D. J. A rapid method for evaluating the structure and function of the rheumatoid hand. *Arthritis Rheum.* 14:75, 1971.


TREATMENT

REST

Mills, J. A., et al. Value of bed rest in patients with RA. *N. Engl. J. Med.* 284:453, 1971.

Smith, R. D., and Polley, H. F. Rest therapy for rheumatoid arthritis. *Mayo Clin. Proc.* 53:141, 1978.


SPLINTING

Cracchiolo, A. The use of shoes to treat foot disorders. *Orthop. Rev.* 3:8, 1979.

Malick, M. H. *Manual on Static Hand Splinting.* Pittsburgh: Harmarville Rehabilitation Center, 1973.

Malick, M. H. *Manual on Dynamic Hand Splinting.* Pittsburgh: Harmarville Rehabilitation Center, 1974.

Partridge, R. E. W., and Duthie, J. J. R. Controlled trial of the effect of complete immobilization of the joints in rheumatoid arthritis. *Ann. Rheum. Dis.* 22:91, 1973.

EXCERISE

Williams, M., and Worthington, C. *Therapeutic Exercise for Body Alignment and Function.* Philadelphia: Saunders, 1957.


JOINT PROTECTION

Cordery, J. C. Joint protection, a responsibility of the OT. *Am. J. Occup. Ther.* 19:285, 1965.

Occupational Therapy Department. *Why Joint Protection?* Philadelphia: Moss Rehabilitation Hospital.

Watkins, R. A., and Robinson, D. *Joint Preservation Techniques For Patients with Rheumatoid Arthritis.* Chicago: Rehabilitation Institute of Chicago, 1974.


ADAPTIVE EQUIPMENT

Fred Sammons Be O.K., Box 32, Brookfield, Ill. 60513.

The Independence Factory, PO Box 597, Middletown, Ohio 45042.

How-To-Make-it-Cheap Manual, The Arthritis Foundation of Southwestern Ohio, Chapter 2400, Reading Road, Cincinnati, Ohio 45202.

See Patient Education Material.


PSYCHOSOCIAL ASPECTS

Wright, V., and Owen S. Effect of rheumatoid arthritis on the social situation of housewives. *Rheumatol. Rehabil.* 15:156, 1976.


VOCATIONAL REHABILITATION

Brewerton, D. A., and Daniel, J. W. Return to work: Experiences of a rehabilitation officer. *Br. Med. J.* 2:240, 1969.


SEXUAL PROBLEMS AND COUNSELING

Ehrlich, G. E. (Ed.). Sexual Problems of the Arthritic Patient. In *Total Management of the Arthritic Patient.* Philadelphia: Lippincott, 1973.

Lachniet, D., and Onder, J. Sex and arthritis and women. *Arthritis Foundation Allied Health Professions Section Newsletter.* 7(3–4):7–9 Dec., 1973.


PATIENT EDUCATION GUIDES

*Arthritis Information Clearinghouse.* PO Box 34427, Bethesda, Md. 20034.

Arthritis Foundation (or local chapter) 3400 Peachtree Rd. N.E. Atlanta, Ga. 30326

*Arthritis Patient Education "How To" Guide About Gout, a Form of Arthritis Arthritis Quackery, a $485,000,000 Racket*

*Arthritis, the Basic Facts*

*Home Care Programs in Arthritis—A Manual for Patients*

*Living with Arthritis and Where to Turn for Help*

*New Life for Old Hands*

*Rheumatoid Arthritis, a Handbook for Patients*

*Self-Help Devices for Arthritic Patients*

*SLE*

*So You Have ... Rheumatoid Arthritis,* Patient Handbook Series

*Surgery: The New Frontier in Arthritis*

*The Truth about Diet and Arthritis*

Merck, Sharpe, and Dohme

West Point, Pa. 19486

*Living with Arthritis*

McNeil Laboratories, Inc.

Fort Washington, Pa. 19034

*Exercises for Low Back Pain*

*Home Exercise Program for Arthritis*

Purdue Frederick Co.

Norwalk, Conn.

*Arthritis Medication Information and Guide to Physical Activities*

*Coping with Arthritis*

SURGERY

Buckman, L., and Leonard, J. *Post-Operative Care in Patients With Silastic Finger Joint Implants.* Midland, Mich.: Silastic Dow Corning Corp.

Mackin, E., and Hunter, J. *Pre- and Post-Operative Hand Therapy Program With Staged Gliding Tendon Prostheses (Hunter Design).* Philadelphia: Hand Rehabilitation Foundation.

McCann, V. H., Philips, C., and Quigley, T. R. Pre-operative and postoperative management: The role of allied health professionals. *Orthop. Clin. North Am.* 6:3, 1975.

Swanson, A. B. *Flexible Implant Resection Arthroplasty in the Hand and Extremities.* St. Louis: Mosby, 1973.

# 5 BURN REHABILITATION

*Susan Koch Clark and Martha K. Logigian*

Over two million persons are burned annually in the United States. Of these, approximately 70,000 require hospitalization, and 10,000 to 12,000 die. The incidence of burns is higher in the southern states, with men and women equally affected except in the age range of nine to 15 years, when three times more boys than girls are burned [3].

Burns are generally classified as follows: scald, flame, contact, chemical, radiation, and electric. Guilfoy and associates [13] found that scalds are the most common, representing 44 percent of all reported burns, followed by flame (27 percent), contact (13 percent), chemical (five percent), radiation (three percent), and electric burns (two percent). The most frequent burn to young children is that of hot liquid. The most common scalds happen in the kitchen when hot liquids such as tea, coffee, soup, or grease are spilled. The incidence of scald burns is highest in young children and decreases after the age of eight years, at which time flame burns increase in frequency.

A flame burn inflicts the most severe injuries, with more deaths resulting from this than any other type. It usually occurs when a person contacts a single ignition source, such as a stove or match, while trying to start or use a fire. Adults are injured because they are careless, whereas children are injured because of their curiosity and fascination with fire. Chemical burns are most frequent in work-related populations, although a small percentage occur when young children touch or swallow chemicals. Radiation burns are almost always connected with misuse of sun lamps, and elec-trical burns are caused by either a household current or live wire. Electrical burns generally cause internal injury, with the greatest damage at the entry and exit sites.

A severe burn is a complicated injury that requires a specially trained medical team to provide proper care. A minor burn can be treated in a community hospital, but a major one should be referred to a specialized institution. The concept of such facilities is fairly new, with the first "burn units" established in 1947 at the Brooke Army Surgical Research Unit in Texas and the Medical College of Virginia. Burn facilities have been classified as programs, units, and centers. A hospital with a burn program has no specialized area for burn care, but follows a consistent plan conducted by a physician who is assumed to be treating at least 25 burns per year. A burn unit is a program conducted in a facility used only for burn treatment, and has at least six beds. A burn center is a larger unit with emphasis on research and teaching as well as patient care [9, 30].

## Anatomy and Physiology of the Skin

The skin is the largest organ of the body. The outer layer, or *epidermis*, consists of dead or dying cells that are compacted to form a protective covering. At the junction of the *dermis* and epidermis is a multiplying layer of basal cells that reconstitute the epidermis following partial destruction of the skin. The bulk of the skin is made up of the dermis, which is deep to the epidermis (Figure 5-1). It is composed of mature fibrous tissue and collagen, as well as

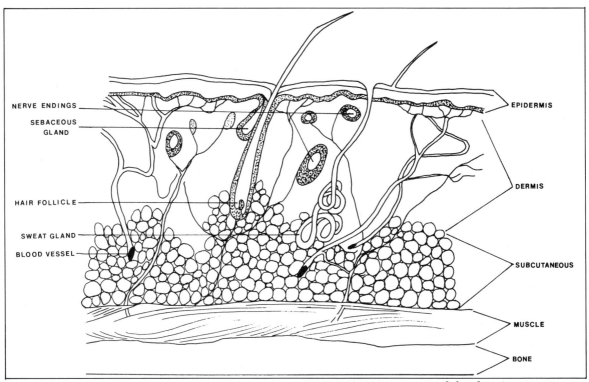

FIGURE 5-1. *Anatomy of the skin. (Artist: Rita M. Hammond)*

blood vessels, nerves, and glands of the skin. Nerve endings that provide perception of pain, temperature, and tactile sensation are found exclusively in the dermis, damage to which results in complete loss of these functions. Deep to the dermis, and with an irregular junction, is the *subcutaneous tissue,* composed primarily of fat with interspaced blood vessels.

The skin has a number of specific functions, one of the most important being prevention of invasive infection from bacteria by serving as a protective covering and physical barrier. It prevents loss of body fluids and heat, and helps maintain the delicate fluid balance required by the body. It is an extensive sensory organ that allows us to avoid damage or destruction, thus protecting us from local trauma. In addition, the skin has a gliding and stretching function to allow motion of bones and joints. Finally, the appearance or cosmetic effect of skin is important to a person's well-being.

A burn either diminishes (when it is partial-thickness) or eliminates (when it is full-thickness) these functions. The amount of skin lost and the depth of damage determine the severity of the injury.

## Classification of Burns

Severity is influenced by five main factors: depth, size, age of patient, past medical history, and part of the body injured. Burns of the head, neck, and chest are especially serious because they can lead to pulmonary problems. Burns of a joint result in increased loss of mobility, and those of the perineum are more susceptible to infection [12].

### DEPTH

There are two basic terminologies used to classify burn depth: *partial-thickness* and *full-thickness*; and *first, second,* and *third degrees.* Basically, a partial-thickness burn is either a

TABLE 5-1. *Classification of Burn Depth*

| Degree | Possible Cause | Appearance and Texture | Sensation | Course |
|---|---|---|---|---|
| *First degree* Superficial layers of epidermis destroyed; vasodilation | Ultraviolet exposure: sunburn, ultraviolet light; low-intensity flash | Redness only—will blanch with pressure and refill; no blistering; minimal or no edema; normal texture | Hyperesthesia; sensitive to temperature; slight pain; tingling | Complete recovery within 5-10 days; peeling |
| *Second degree* Superficial layer of skin destroyed; partial thickness | Contact with hot liquids; scalds; flash flame | Large, thick-walled blisters may increase in size; redness around blistered area; normal to firm texture | Painful; hyperesthesia; sensitive to heat and cold | Recovery in 16-21 days; some scarring; wound will heal by itself if nothing causes further damage |
| *Deep second degree* All but deep layers of dermis destroyed; capillary permeability | Scalds; flame | Usually no blister formation; mottled reddened base; broken epidermis; weeping surface; edema; firm texture | Very painful; may be anesthetic during first few days but sensation will return as tissues recover | Infection may convert to third degree; crust will develop and when removed tiny pigskinlike areas will be seen, and will heal very slowly; most hypertrophic scarring results from deep second degree burns |
| *Third degree* Full-thickness destruction; coagulation of protein | Flame; electrical; contact with hot objects | Usually brownish, may be white, black, or red; no blisters, or if present, thin-walled and will not increase in size; broken skin with fat exposed; edema; firm or leathery texture | Painless; insensitive to pin prick; danger of shock | Regeneration of skin not possible, cannot heal by self; eschar sloughs; grafting is necessary; scarring, loss of contour and function result; time to heal depends on whether grafts take |
| *Fourth degree* Tissue under skin destroyed; may include fascia, muscle, tendon, bone, subcutaneous tissue | Flame; electrical; prolonged contact with hot objects | Muscle, tendon, bone may be exposed; infection may soon intervene; edema | Painless | Early debridement necessary to establish adequate drainage; grafting necessary; takes months to heal |
| Char | Flame; deep electrical | Black skin; leathery texture | Painless | Should be excised early; amputation of limb probably necessary |

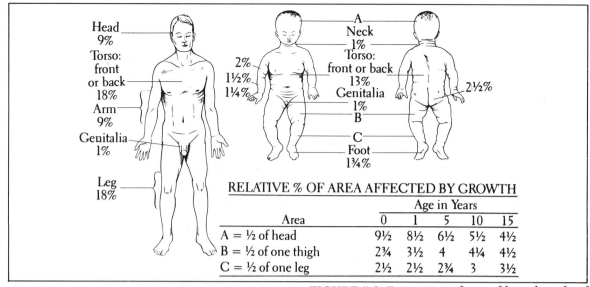

| Head 9% | Neck 1% | A |
| Torso: front or back 18% | Torso: front or back 13% | |
| Arm 9% | Genitalia 1% | B |
| Genitalia 1% | | C |
| Leg 18% | Foot 1¾% | |

2%
1½%
1¼%
2½%

**RELATIVE % OF AREA AFFECTED BY GROWTH**

| | Age in Years | | | | |
|---|---|---|---|---|---|
| Area | 0 | 1 | 5 | 10 | 15 |
| A = ½ of head | 9½ | 8½ | 6½ | 5½ | 4½ |
| B = ½ of one thigh | 2¾ | 3½ | 4 | 4¼ | 4½ |
| C = ½ of one leg | 2½ | 2½ | 2¾ | 3 | 3½ |

FIGURE 5-2. *Estimation of size of burn by rule of nines. (From C. E. Eckert,* Emergency Room Care *(4th ed.) Boston: Little, Brown, 1981. With permission.)*

first or second degree burn, and means that only part of the skin has been damaged or destroyed. A first degree burn affects only the epidermis and some portion of the dermis. In a partial-thickness burn, enough epithelial cells remain to provide new epidermis and the wound will heal by itself. It should be noted, however, that infection can change the depth of a burn causing a wound that would normally heal by itself to go to full-thickness and require skin grafting.

When the dermis is entirely destroyed, it is considered a full-thickness or third degree burn. It requires skin grafting for closure. There may also be destruction of the subcutaneous tissue, muscles, and bones, and some refer to this as *fourth degree* burn. The deeper the burn, the longer the recovery time and the more serious the problem.

Evaluation of depth is made by gross appearance, the presence or lack of sensation, and knowledge of what caused the burn (Table 5-1).

SIZE

One estimates the percentage of body burned to reach an idea of the size and extent of the injury. There are two methods used to determine this. One is the "rule of nines." The head and both upper extremities represent nine percent of the body surface area; the lower extremities are each given the value of 18 percent, and the anterior and posterior trunk are each 18 percent. With the addition of one percent for the perineum, the total is 100 percent. To determine size, the physician shades in the burned areas on an anterior and posterior diagram of the body and adds up the estimated percentage (Figure 5-2).

The other, or Berkow, method includes the factors of change in proportion by age, considering that the head is twice as large proportionately in the child than in the adult. A diagram is used for this method also, with the burned areas shaded in. One must refer to the table and summary columns to calculate the total body surface area burned (Figure 5-3).

154

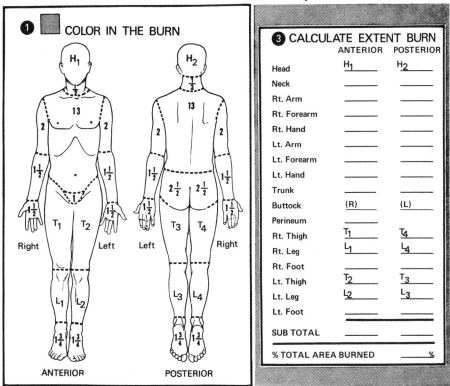

# Estimation of Size of Burn by Percent

National Burn Information Exchange

I. Feller, M.D., Director, Ann Arbor, Michigan 48104

Form Completed By: _____

Name: _____

Date: _____ Age: _____

Past Medical History: _____
_____
_____

Concurrent Injuries: _____
_____

**1** ▦ COLOR IN THE BURN

H₁

H₂

13

13

2    2        2    2

$1\frac{1}{2}$    $1\frac{1}{2}$        $1\frac{1}{2}$    $1\frac{1}{2}$

$2\frac{1}{2}$    $2\frac{1}{2}$

$1\frac{1}{2}$    $1\frac{1}{2}$        $1\frac{1}{2}$    $1\frac{1}{2}$

Right    T₁    T₂    Left        Left    T₃    T₄    Right

L₁    L₂        L₃    L₄

$1\frac{3}{4}$  $1\frac{3}{4}$        $1\frac{3}{4}$  $1\frac{3}{4}$

ANTERIOR        POSTERIOR

**3** CALCULATE EXTENT BURN

| | ANTERIOR | POSTERIOR |
|---|---|---|
| Head | H₁ | H₂ |
| Neck | | |
| Rt. Arm | | |
| Rt. Forearm | | |
| Rt. Hand | | |
| Lt. Arm | | |
| Lt. Forearm | | |
| Lt. Hand | | |
| Trunk | | |
| Buttock | (R) | (L) |
| Perineum | | |
| Rt. Thigh | T₁ | T₄ |
| Rt. Leg | L₁ | L₄ |
| Rt. Foot | | |
| Lt. Thigh | T₂ | T₃ |
| Lt. Leg | L₂ | L₃ |
| Lt. Foot | | |
| SUB TOTAL | | |
| % TOTAL AREA BURNED | | % |

**2** CIRCLE AGE FACTOR

PERCENT OF AREAS AFFECTED BY GROWTH

| | AGE | | | | | |
|---|---|---|---|---|---|---|
| | 0 | 1 | 5 | 10 | 15 | Adult |
| H(1 or 2) = ½ of the Head | 9½ | 8½ | 6½ | 5½ | 4½ | 3½ |
| T(1,2,3 or 4) = ½ of a Thigh | 2¾ | 3¼ | 4 | 4¼ | 4½ | 4¾ |
| L(1,2,3 or 4) = ½ of a Leg | 2½ | 2½ | 2¾ | 3 | 3¼ | 3½ |

(see instructions on back)

FIGURE 5-3. *Estimation of size of burn by percent-age. (Taken with permission from I. Feller and C. Archambeault,* Nursing the Burned Patient. *Ann Arbor, Mich.: Institute for Burn Medicine, 1973.)*

## PROGNOSIS

Prognosis will depend on the severity of the injury. A burn is considered critical if it includes complications with respiratory tract injury; partial-thickness burns of more than 30 percent of the body surface; full-thickness injury of more than ten percent of the body surface and involvement of the face, hands, feet, or genitalia; complications of fractures; or electrical or deep acid wounds. Moderate burns are those that include partial-thickness injury of 15 to 30 percent of the body surface, and full-thickness of less than ten percent of the body surface. Minor burns are those of partial thickness less than 15 percent of the body surface, or full thickness of less than two percent of the body surface. Mortality can be predicted based on the total area of the body surface burned and age of the victim [12]. In addition, a patient with a past medical history of heart disease or diabetes has a poorer prognosis, as do those with burns of the thorax, head and neck, or perineum because of respiratory complications and infection.

Complications are the rule rather than the exception, and are the potential cause of death. The most common complications are septicemia, pneumonia, renal failure, and heart disease. Metabolic complications occur in patients with over 40 percent burned area, or full-thickness burns over 20 percent. The stress incurred can lead to stress diabetes, Curling's ulcer, and adrenocortical insufficiency [12].

## Acute Care

Initially, the patient may be stabilized in a hospital emergency room and subsequently transferred to the burn treatment area, or may be admitted directly to a burn unit if one is available. During this time, first aid procedures are provided and the severity of the burn is determined. Medical treatment includes respiratory care, fluid therapy, and wound care [12, 24].

Respiratory care is critical, and can include the administration of moist nasal oxygen, and if necessary, a tracheostomy. The primary consideration is maintenance of a patent airway.

A burn injury causes massive fluid shift, referred to as burn shock, which is maximal by eight to ten hours. This systemic change depends on the temperature and length of time the agent contacted the skin. In a severe burn, inflammation and fluid shift are so great that they cause hypovolemic shock and death if they go untreated.

The burn trauma increases capillary permeability, allowing the capillaries to leak fluid into the interstitial spaces, thus increasing interstitial fluid. The result of this is edema. The lymphatic system normally carries away increased tissue fluid, but is unable to when the burn is large and there is a great deal of plasma leak. This shift of plasma from the blood vessels to the interstitial spaces continues for 24 to 48 hours after injury. Water and electrolytes are lost most rapidly at first, leaving the plasma with increased protein concentration. Soon after injury, the protein also leaks from the vessels. Loss of fluid from the vascular space lowers the circulating blood volume, which is termed *hypovolemia*. Fluid therapy is imperative to replace fluid volume, thus preventing hypovolemic shock. In addition, fluid input and output must be accurately monitored. A catheter is placed in the bladder to measure hourly urine output, which indicates whether the blood volume and pressure are adequate. It is also important to monitor pulse rate and blood pressure.

A patient is given tetanus protection when first seen. All other medications are given intravenously, nothing by mouth. Analgesics may be required if the burn is of partial thickness, both to sedate and relieve pain.

Initial wound care includes cleansing and removing all dead tissue that can serve as media for bacteria; preventing conversion of a partial-thickness burn to a full-thickness; preparing healthy granulation tissue for grafting by aiding separation of eschar; and providing for patient comfort. Infection control begins at the time of admission and continues until grafting is completed. The patient is autocontaminated by bacteria that survive on the hair follicles and glands under the burned tissue, and by dirt from the accident. Aseptic techniques must be used to protect the body from organisms, as the skin is no longer able to perform this function [12].

Cleansing with an antibacterial agent can be accomplished in a hydrotherapy tub. After cleansing, a topical agent and dressings may be applied. Some centers use the exposure method, with the burn exposed to the air to dry the surface. In addition, if possible the patient is placed in an antideformity position and splints are constructed as indicated.

A complication seen in burns of a circumferential nature is the constricting effect of eschar on the trunk or extremities. Edema beneath the eschar will produce enough pressure to occlude circulation, and may result in ischemic necrosis. *Escharotomy* is an incision of the dead eschar performed to reduce the pressure.

Following initial emergency care, the patient continues to be monitored for possible complications. In addition, grafting of the burn site begins. Grafting can take weeks or months to complete. During this time, the patient must be positioned properly and turned frequently to prevent skin breakdown. A Circ-O-lectric bed is often used as it facilitates position changes and provides access to the wounds.

Significant metabolic drain is produced by the burn, creating a negative nitrogen balance, loss of plasma protein, destruction of erythrocytes, and heat loss from evaporation. As a result, the patient uses up large quantities of calories and has an increased risk of infection, poor granulation tissue, and delayed healing of donor sites. Intravenous hyperalimentation is the usual course with severe burns, beginning on the third or fourth day posttrauma. If the patient can eat, supplemental foods are provided for adequate caloric intake. In general, a high-caloric, high-protein diet with supplemental vitamins and iron must be provided [10].

Among the medications required for the se-vere burn are narcotics to relieve pain and anxiety, antibiotics to control infection, antacids to alleviate gastric irritation, and laxatives to avoid constipation. Medication to correct or avoid systemic and metabolic disorders are often prescribed, as are antiinflammatory agents. Sedatives and tranquilizers may be necessary to relieve emotional stress [12].

WOUND CARE

*Debridement* is removal of eschar, the covering of dead tissue that forms after the burn. As eschar provides excellent conditions for bacterial growth, its removal is necessary in preventing infection and preparing a granulation tissue surface for grafting [27]. Two techniques of debridement are commonly used: (1) primary excision and early grafting, and (2) daily debridement. During the former the patient is taken to the operating room soon after admission and given general anesthesia, and all eschar is surgically removed and homografts or autografts are applied. Daily debridement is done at the bedside or in a Hubbard tank. There are three types: (1) natural, where the body's enzymes dissolve the eschar; (2) sharp, where the loose eschar is cut away; and (3) enzymatic, where prepared enzymes are applied to dissolve the eschar. The most common method is sharp debridement, performed daily at the time of dressing changes. If hydrotherapy or Hubbard tank is used, the patient soaks for 10 to 20 minutes and the technician then peels back the loose eschar with forceps and cuts it off. The object is to remove dead tissue without destroying viable deep dermal elements. Thus the goal of debridement is to remove all eschar as soon as possible and prepare the wound for grafting.

Hydrotherapy is used with most burn patients, whether for debridement or not. It provides cleansing of the wound by removing loose eschar and dirt, maintains range of motion, and allows relatively painless dressing changes. In addition, it provides total body cleansing and a frictionless environment in which the patient can exercise. The tub is gen-

TABLE 5-2. *Positioning to Prevent Deformity*

| Area Burned | Resulting Deformity | Position of Prevention |
|---|---|---|
| **Neck** | | |
| Anterior aspect or circumferential | Flexion contracture of neck | No pillow under head |
| **Neck** | | |
| Posterior aspect (only) | Extensor contracture of neck | Prone—pillow under upper chest to flex cervical spine; supine—small pillow under neck |
| **Axilla** | | |
| Anterior | Adduction and internal rotation | Shoulder joint in abduction (100 to 130°) and external rotation |
| Posterior | Adduction and external rotation | Shoulder in forward flexion and 100 to 130° abduction |
| Pectoral region | Shoulder protraction | No pillow; shoulders abducted and externally rotated |
| Chest or abdomen | Kyphosis | As above and hips neutral (*not* flexed) |
| Lateral trunk | Scoliosis | Supine, affected arm abducted |
| **Elbow** | | |
| Anterior surface or circumferential | Flexion and pronation | Arm extended and supinated |
| **Wrist** | | |
| Total or volar surface | Flexion | Splint in 15° extension |
| Dorsal surface | Extension | Splint in 15° flexion |
| **Hip** | | |
| Includes inguinal and perineal burns | Internal rotation, flexion, and adduction; possible joint subluxation if contracture severe | Neutral rotation and abduction and maintain extension by prone position or *pillow under buttocks* |
| **Knee** | | |
| Popliteal surface or circumferential | Flexion | Maintain extension, using posterior splints or suspend heels with plastic heel protecting boots. *No pillows* under knees while supine or under ankles while prone |
| Ankle | Plantar flexion if foot dorsiflexor muscles are weak or their tendons are divided | 90° dorsiflexion with splint if possible rather than foot board |

Source: From: I. Feller, and C. Archambeault. *Nursing the Burned Patient.* Ann Arbor, Mich.: Institute for Burn Medicine, 1973. With permission.

erally used once or twice a day until grafting begins.

Following debridement and hydrotherapy, a topical antibacterial agent is applied to the wound to help control infection and prevent loss of body fluids. Some of the agents currently in use include Sulfamylon, silver sulfadiazine creams, Betadine ointment, Furacin, Gentamicin, and saline soaks. Silver nitrate solution is used by saturating layers of gauze and applying them to the wound.

Full-thickness burns must be *autografted* (skin taken from the patient's own body) to provide complete healing. When the injury is so large that there is not enough undamaged skin, *homografts* (from cadavers) or *heterografts* (pig skin) serve as temporary cover. Fresh homografts may adhere and function as normal skin, and therefore are preferable, whereas heterografts and synthetic skin are purely temporary. These biological dressings allow healing of a partial-thickness wound and prepare the bed of a full-thickness burn for autografting.

Autografts are used to resurface full-thickness wounds, generally, around 14 to 21 days postburn. They are usually thin and are taken from the patient with a sterile dermatome. The area from which the skin is taken is called a *donor site*. The graft is placed on the burn site, rarely requiring suturing.

A mesh graft is used when the patient's intact skin is limited. Multiple incisions are made into a sheet of autograft skin with a mesh dermatome machine, allowing the skin to be stretched from three to nine times its original size. Mesh grafts are not used on the face or neck or over joints, as there is more scarring associated with these areas, and they are susceptible to trauma. Sheet grafts are used in these areas.

Most grafts "take" better if they are exposed rather than put under a dressing. In some situations, suspension of an extremity may be necessary to ensure sufficient exposure. If dressings are used they must be firm, bulky, and capable of applying even compression. The dressings should be removed after 48 hours to permit inspection. Donor sites are treated with exposure. They usually heal within 10 to 14 days, and can be used again if needed. At first after grafting, the patient should not move the area excessively, as this may cause the graft to slip and it will not take. After three to four days, the patient can usually go into a Hubbard tank and begin some movement.

## MINIMIZING CONTRACTURES

The position of comfort is often the position of deformity. There is a tendency to flex the joint nearest the burn, leading to flexion contractures. Extension, however, is the desired position that helps to prevent deformity caused by contractures, and to reduce scar formation (Table 5-2). Splinting is often indicated to assist in positioning. (See section Splints Designed to Maintain Proper Positioning.)

Range-of-motion exercises should be provided at least daily, with each joint going through its entire range. This can be most easily carried out in the hydrotherapy tub. Active range of motion is encouraged from the very beginning, but until the patient is alert and able to cooperate enough to exercise actively, assisted or if necessary, passive exercises are performed [31]. These are done gently only to the point of pain, as an aggressive approach can result in an increase in edema and a decrease in the patient's cooperation.

In addition, the team should encourage the patient to assist with self-care when possible, including feeding. Adaptive devices such as built-up utensils are available if needed.

## Rehabilitation

When a burn is reduced to less than 20 percent of the body surface, rehabilitation can begin [12]. Grafting should be completed in areas of full-thickness wounds by this time. The goals of the rehabilitation program are to return the patient to a productive place in society and to achieve functional and cosmetic reconstruction. The patient may be discharged from the program after several months, but the rehabilitation process may continue for two to five years before a maximum level of functioning is reached. In addition, many emotional problems surface during this time. (See the section on emotional adjustment for a more complete discussion.)

### HYPERTROPHIC SCARRING AND CONTRACTURE

After the burned skin has begun to heal, within three to four weeks the scar begins to hypertrophy and may cause severe deformity. In the experience of the Shriners Burns Institute [18], more than 80 percent of patients with second and third degree burns developed hypertrophic scarring.

During normal healing, granulation tissue has an increase in *fibroblasts,* the cells that synthesize mucopolysaccharides and collagen fibers needed for new connective tissue. They produce an excessive amount of collagen fibers, which adhere to each other in an irregular pattern. These bundles appear twisted and disorganized compared to normal tissue. They fuse as they come together, forming an accumulation that produces thick raised scarring at the site of the burn, and contractures [4]. *Contracture,* the result of the wound being held in a shortened position, can cause significant cosmetic disfigurement.

The burned skin and scar tissue are constantly contracting until they are opposed by a force such as that from exercise or traction. Loss of range of motion can result particularly where the burned area bridges the flexor surface of a joint. Positioning and splinting help prevent contractures, and should be continued following healing of second degree burns and grafting of third degree burns [1].

Pressure applied to the scar can greatly decrease the degree of hypertrophy and subsequent contracture [22]. Parks and colleagues [26] found that continuous pressure applied to a scar for six to 12 months reduces hypertrophy and discoloration. They have identified the required magnitude of pressure to be 25 mm Hg. Pressure also helps reduce edema, and controls both vascularity, which prevents proliferation of fibroblasts, and excessive collagen. When scar tissue is maintained under pressure, collagen is laid down in an orderly manner, becoming more compact and structured and less vascular and erythematous [25]. The result is a soft, pliable, elastic scar that allows full range of motion at the joints. Reduction in pain and itching is also a benefit of continuous pressure.

Various materials are available that provide adequate pressure, such as molded plastic splints and pressure garments. JOBST Anti-Burnscar Supports are garments measured and designed for the individual patient. They are made for all parts of the body and allow full functional range of motion while providing constant pressure. The garment is worn 24 hours a day, except when bathing, for approximately six to 12 months, or until the scar has matured. (It is recommended [21] that for patients with second degree burns that do not require grafting, the garment be worn beginning approximately one week after complete healing of the wound; for burns that require grafting it is worn beginning 10 to 14 days following surgery.) Pressure should be applied as long as the scar tissue has the appearance of an active scar, that is, while it is hyperemic and firm [1]. It is useful to have two sets so that one remains on the scar tissue, while the other is cleaned. They must be checked regularly to ensure proper fit, and new garments ordered if the individual outgrows them or they become stretched. Often after a few months, the garments require replacement.

Silastic Medical Elastomer has been used as an interface between the skin and pressure garment [23]. It has been found to be successful if the elastomer mold is applied when the scar is still red (no later than six months postburn) and worn continually under the garment until the scarred area is completely blanched white and mature. It is particularly useful on concave surfaces and soft tissue areas where direct pressure is less effective, such as the anterior surface of the trunk, neck and face, and the hands [23].

POSITIONING AND SPLINTING

Positioning a burned part of the body to maintain skin and joint integrity during recovery and rehabilitation can be accomplished through the use of pillows, blanket rolls, sand bags, and the like (see Table 5-2) during periods of rest. If the involved skin remains supple and does not restrict motion, and if the joints can actively go through a functional range, positioning may not be indicated, either nighttime or daytime. Joint stiffness may be greater than before injury, but as long as this can actively be decreased, positioning techniques are not necessary. Toward the end of the first year posttrauma, the degree of stiffness should begin to lessen. Static splints can and should be used to maintain skin length and joint range, and dynamic splints are useful in slowly and gently altering scar tissue and joint range. When serving these purposes, serial splints can be considered dynamic.

Static splints are continued for night wear up to approximately 12 months postburn. Every few weeks, the individual should not wear the splint at night. As soon as the active morning range is the same as that of evening before, its use is discontinued. If loss of range is observed at a later date, nighttime wearing may alter the change.

Serial static or dynamic splints apply constant gentle pull on scar tissue and joints. Wearing time should slowly increase from 10 to 15 minutes per hour, to two or three hours on and one or two hours off. During the off periods, the patient should attempt activity incorporating these joints. As tissues and joints accommodate the splinted position and are able to duplicate the gains actively, splint tension is increased slightly. Pressure must be applied evenly over broad areas, never restricting circulation or causing nerve compression, or edema. Fit must be assessed frequently by the therapist, and the patient should note wearing precautions and the need to have the splint altered.

Serial static splints are most appropriate when both scar tissue and joint changes are desired. If only joint range is sought, a dynamic traction splint may be used. Strict attention is directed to the line of pull, that it is perpendicular to the skeletal segment distal to the joint. Thus the distal bone will not be pushed proximally into the joint space. Both splint types should only restrict those joints necessary to assure a stable balanced fit. Warm soaks and lotion applied prior to wear can decrease discomfort. If prolonged pain is experienced when the splint is applied, the tension is too great and should be lessened. Well-fitting

splints will give the least discomfort and increase compliance with the wearing schedule.

SPLINTS DESIGNED TO MAINTAIN PROPER POSITIONING
Areas that commonly require splinting following deep second and third degree burns include the neck, anterior trunk, knees, ankles and toes, axillae, elbows, wrists, and digits. (See Table 5-2.) A topical agent is generally applied to the burned area, and the thermoplastic splint is worn over a light gauze dressing and held in place by gauze bandaging or elastic wrap. This procedure is followed in the acute stage and until major wound coverage has been attained. Subsequently, during scar maturation pressure, positioning, exercise, and splinting (when indicated) are essential in the control of hypertrophic scarring and the prevention of contractures [22].

NECK AND CHIN
To position the neck in extension, the patient is fit with a neck conformer once edema subsides. It is worn 9 to 12 months to achieve a smooth surface and adequate chin contour [32]. If it is formed while the patient is supine, it will be better tolerated at nighttime.

ANTERIOR TRUNK
Because of the complex surface with alternating areas of convexity and concavity, an orthosis for this area should provide neck and trunk extension and shoulder retraction while conforming to topography [5]. The device designed by Becker includes a two-piece plastic body jacket with a full neck and chin conformer.

LOWER EXTREMITY
A full resting leg splint may be needed if the burns cover the entire leg. A three-point splint is applied to maintain knee extension without applying pressure to the flexor surface. It has two thermoplastic cuffs, one on the thigh and one on the lower leg, riveted to lateral alumi-

num rods. A lambswool pad covers the knee anteriorly [35].

## ANKLE AND TOES
A footdrop splint or foam boot can be used to position the foot in neutral.

## AXILLA
To maintain the upper extremity in at least 90 degrees of abduction, a sling may be used or a splint constructed. This position is more easily maintained in bed; however, when ambulation begins, a shoulder abduction elevation or airplane splint is fabricated. An airplane splint may be indicated for the patient with a contracting axilla or tightening trunk skin. It must fit accurately and be made very secure to maintain the axillary angle desired and prevent skin breakdown over the iliac crest. An axilla conformer is another such splint [34].

## ELBOW
A pan, or three-point extension, splint is used to maintain the elbow in extension. The former is oval-shaped, molded directly over a light elbow dressing. The three-point extension splint keeps the elbow in extension without applying pressure on the flexor surface. It has two narrow cuffs, one on the forearm and one on the upper arm, riveted to aluminum rods. A lambswool pad covers the elbow [35].

## WRIST AND HAND
A resting hand splint is designed to position the wrist in 20 to 30 degrees of extension, MPs in 45 to 70 degrees of flexion, and the PIPs and DIPs in complete extension. The thumb is placed in abduction and extension to maintain the web space; this position helps to maintain the palmar arch as well [17, 22, 31].

"The PIP joint is the most vulnerable joint in the burned hand. If this joint is allowed to remain flexed, the middle extensor slip is caught between the overlying unyielding eschar and the underlying heads of the proximal and middle phalanges, resulting in partial destruction of the extensor slip. The lateral bands displace volarward with the hand drifting into the typical 'burned hand deformity'—that is extension of the MP joints, flexion of the PIP joints [19]." To prevent the boutonnière deformity from occurring, the hand is positioned as stated.

Internal splinting with Kirschner wires may be used as an alternative to an external thermoplastic splint. External skeletal fixation devices such as the hayraker splint may be used particularly when there are burns on both surfaces of the hand [28].

## SKIN CARE
Newly healed skin is tender and can be scaly and crusty in texture. It requires special care as it has a tendency to break down and blister on bruising and chafing. The skin around the joints is especially vulnerable to movement and bruising, and padding may be required for these areas. Splints and JOBST garments may provide protection.

Pruritus, or itching, is a common problem with scar areas because of lack of sweat glands in the new tissue and dryness of the skin. Increased blood supply may also contribute to the problem. Skin moisturizers applied to the scar tissue usually relieve this. Lotions with lanolin, cocoa butter, or mineral oil tend to be deep-penetrating and last longer than other topical agents. Application by light rubbing should be carried out three to four times a day. Antihistamines may be used for more intense itching [28].

Because of the sensitivity of new scar tissue, direct sunlight must be avoided, as direct exposure can result in a permanent change in pigmentation. Clothing and a commercial sunscreen can offer necessary protection.

Cosmesis can be a significant concern, and the therapist can be of assistance by arranging for the patient to be fit for a wig, false eyelashes, sculptured fingernails, or other prostheses. A cosmetician familiar with applying makeup to scarred skin may be helpful.

## INCREASED FUNCTION
Exercise continues on an intensive scale over

longer periods of time [31]. Primarily, active and active assistive exercise is used to attain and maintain functional joint motion. Passive ranging can be painful, cause tearing of internal tissues and consequent bleeding, which leads to the formation of additional scar tissue [33].

The goals at this stage of recovery are to increase range of motion, muscle strength, and facility in activities of daily living. Adaptive equipment may be required for independence in self-care, such as long-handled devices, built-up utensils, and the like. Home adaptation may be necessary to ensure independence.

RECONSTRUCTION

With the severely burned patient, reconstructive surgery is quite common. Separate admissions are planned for each procedure. Such surgery can be functional or cosmetic, and generally includes the releasing of scar tissue and contractures, grafting, and application of corrective splints.

## Emotional Considerations

It has been said [2] that "a person who has been burned suffers one of the most severe traumas that human beings can survive." A severe burn requires a long period of hospitalization during which the patient must face pain, helplessness, dependency, and possibly deformity and death. Health care personnel must be ready and able to deal with the patient's fear, depression, grief, loss of hope, and psychotic reactions.

MacArthur and Moore [20] have identified several predisposing factors to burning, or the burn-prone patient: alcoholism, senility, psychiatric disorders, and neurological disease, in that order. In addition, the burn itself can be frightening and uncomfortable, which can lead to further distress. The patient will normally experience emotional reactions to the trauma, and whether these have long-term effects will largely depend on the patient's care and premorbid personality.

Primary concerns include the threat to survival and the fear of permanent damage. Secondary issues result from the psychological significance of the burn and its impact on the patient's personality [7].

The patient is initially overcome with shock, which according to Andreason and co-workers [2] can take two forms. Some may enter a calm, dreamlike state in which they have little awareness of what happened or where they are. Lucid conversation with no recollection of what was said is typical. More common, however, is an acute traumatic reaction including insomnia, emotional lability, exaggerated startle response, and recurrent nightmares about the circumstances of the injury. This shock clears spontaneously, but is distressing while it lasts. During this time the patient is rarely concerned about deformity or death; these concerns materialize after the initial emotional impact has subsided.

The first concern during the acute phase is, "Will I survive?" This fear is quite intense for about one or two weeks but then subsides [15]. The patient experiences three other basic fears as noted by Jackson [16]: "Will I be disabled?" or "Will I be able to keep my job?" are first. Then eventually every patient approaches the subject of "Will I be disfigured?", "How much damage will remain?", or "Will I lose the affection of my loved ones?" The third fear concerns pain, with the patient asking, "How long will I suffer like this?" This often persists for six to eight weeks, and even longer in patients with severe burns. All these questions provoke anxiety and fear, and are complicated by the separation from family and friends at a time when their support is most needed. Their absence leads to doubts regarding the possible effects of the injury on the patient's relationships with them.

PAIN

The main characteristics of burn pain are its intensity and duration [11], and recovery demands the infliction of more with many of the treatment procedures. The amount will depend on the extent and location of the burn, together with the patient's anxiety level, pain tolerance, and age. Dressing changes and debridement can be the time of greatest pain. It is reduced with skin grafts, yet there will be some from the donor site until that heals. In the final phase of recovery there is a dull chronic pain, with small peaks caused by nerve regeneration that induces an itching and tingling sensation.

Medication can help control pain, yet often it may be inadequate. Thus painful treatment procedures must be carried out as quickly and efficiently as possible, with the team helping the patient realize that these are a necessary part of recovery. Moreover, medication must be monitored and paced so that it is provided at appropriate intervals, but is not addicting.

## EMOTIONAL REACTIONS

Burn patients lose control over their lives, and it is quite difficult for self-reliant people to accept a situation in which they are totally helpless and inadequate.

One reaction is called the *dependency-rebellion syndrome*. It often occurs two to four weeks after the trauma, during the debridement and skin grafting stages, and consists of anxiety, depression, and regression. Two personality manifestations of this syndrome are observed: one demands excessive care and attention from the staff; the other is rebellious and hostile, disguising dependency needs. The patient in the latter situation is frightened by the thought of losing control over his or her own life.

Depression is common, and is generally more severe if hospitalization exceeds one month. It starts during the middle of the hospital stay, lasting from a few days to a few weeks. Mild depression leads to a loss of interest, decreased appetite, crying spells, hopelessness about the future, and insomnia. At its deepest it may result in a loss of will to live, refusal to eat, lethargy, despondency, and inability to cry [2]. Severe depression will usually clear, but the patient requires support from the team during

this time. Mild depression may linger and require professional care.

Grief is a realistic sadness in reaction to a loss, and is to be expected for the patient following burn trauma. The patient experiences significant loss, much of it temporary, such as separation and disruption of life style. With permanent deformity, the grief reaction is quite pronounced. A major exacerbation can occur on viewing the deformity for the first time, especially facial deformity [29].

Many patients experience resentment toward healthy individuals and become frustrated and hostile. This hostility may be directed toward those providing painful treatment, or those providing the most care, and it is not uncommon to see the patient become irritable and angry with family members. It is important to understand that the hostility is directed against the situation, not any particular individual.

There is often guilt and blame associated with a burn injury, especially if others were involved. Alternatively, the patient may be resentful and vindictive toward the person responsible for the injury. Parents often blame themselves when a child is burned; they may regard the accident as punishment, or experience the need to be punished, which is manifested by depression or self-hate.

A number of patients experience delirium, exhibiting impaired orientation, fluctuating levels of consciousness, impaired cognitive function, insomnia, and worsening of symptoms after dark. Anxiety, agitation, hallucinations, and seizures can also occur. The frequency of delirium increases with age of the patient and the severity of the burn. With physical recovery comes recovery from the delirium, although the team must help the patient to remain oriented during this time [2].

Emotional difficulties occur for almost all burn patients, but major psychiatric disorders are infrequent. The most commonly observed phenomena include transient psychotic episodes immediately following injury; periods of mild to moderate depression, especially during the acute phase; episodes of anxiety; and a sullen, resentful, unappreciative attitude [15].

## COPING MECHANISMS
To cope with the emotional and physical stress of the burn, the patient develops strategies to deal with the immediate situation [14, 15]. There are numerous mechanisms to help the patient adapt.

### CONSTRICTION
The patient keeps a tight control over the recognition and expression of feelings by focusing on one part of the problem only. This may also be demonstrated as resignation to the injury.

### SUPPRESSION
The patient consciously avoids thinking of the unpleasant circumstances surrounding the trauma, and smothers emotions by mechanisms such as distraction. Suppression is generally a conscious process.

### REPRESSION
There is automatic exclusion from consciousness of the affect associated with the burn; the patient does not remember the trauma. It is basically an unconscious process, rarely found after the first week of hospitalization.

### DENIAL
The patient may deny the injury or its important consequences. The patient recognizes the fact of being burned, but will deny the severity of illness or the need for a significant amount of treatment. The problem is viewed as minor.

### REGRESSION
It is manifested by demanding, infantile, attention-seeking behavior, low frustration tolerance, complaining, dependent relationships, poor emotional control, a need for constant reassurance, and poor cooperation. A severely regressed patient cannot control anger, and thus alienates the staff with unreasonable demands and disruptive behavior. The patient should not be allowed to manipulate the staff.

### REWORKING
The patient repeatedly ruminates over the trauma in an effort to relieve associated tension.

### WITHDRAWAL
The patient withdraws from interpersonal relationships by avoiding close contact and resorting to fantasy. This is usually seen during the first two weeks following injury, and clears so that the patient does not reach a point of extreme avoidance.

### RATIONALIZATION
This mechanism is used to justify dependency, hostility, and irresponsibility [15].

### DELUSION–ILLUSION–HALLUCINATION
These mechanisms are used as forms of denial, and involve extensive, gross distortions of reality.

## DISFIGUREMENT
Our society places significant emphasis and value on physical appearance. Burn patients, particularly those with facial scarring, find themselves with disfiguring features, which, if they can be corrected at all, may require years of reconstructive surgery. Fear of rejection can cause them to become depressed, withdrawn, and isolated; it may evoke shame and even aggression [6].

Sexual attractiveness can be at issue, with the patient fearing loss of sexuality because of scarring and deformity. Sexual problems are also common among those who have burns involving the perineal area.

## RECOVERY MECHANISMS
The patient requires emotional support from the team as well as family and friends throughout the recovery process. Understanding the usual coping mechanisms can assist everyone in dealing with the patient and providing appropriate support. More severe emotional reactions may require psychiatric counseling.

Reassurance and support from others can

help in the restoration of self-esteem and mobilization of positive defenses. This can also be provided by other patients. The patient needs hope for the future as well as assurance of the interest and affection of others.

Initial coping mechanisms enable the patient to deal with the severity of the injury. Ultimately, acceptance can lead to participation in the recovery process. The patient can then be active in problem solving with regard to the injury, and learn to accept physically painful moments and the consequences of scarring. Every effort should be made to involve the patient in the treatment process and accept responsibility for what is done to aid recovery. Thus the patient has some control over the environment and feels like a person, not an object with little to say about what happens. When the patient feels respected and valued, rapid emotional recovery can occur.

## FAMILY CONCERNS

Bowden and Feller [8] have described common responses of families to the stress of the burn injury including indecision, intensification of preexisting problems, and guilt feelings. Indecision involves immobilization and inability to act in an appropriate way to manage the situation. The family does not know what to do, and therefore becomes immobilized.

If there have been prior problems, a burn injury to a family member only intensifies them. The family may attempt to control the course of the patient's hospitalization and treatment, or they may sabotage the patient's participation in the program. It is not rare for the patient to be made the scapegoat and blamed for the family's troubles [8].

The family may feel responsible for the injury. When this happens, parents often become permissive and interfere with a child's treatment, always trying to do things for the patient that the patient can accomplish independently [8]. The team must deal with these conflicts and gain the family's support in the treatment and rehabilitation of the patient.

Initial shock and grief on the part of the fami-

TABLE 5-3. *Addresses for Information on Burn Care*

P. William Curreri, M.D.
Secretary, American Burn Association
New York Hospital–Cornell Medical Center
525 East 68th Street, Room F758
New York, NY 10021

BT: Idea Exchange Bulletin for Burn Team
   Personnel
40 Signal Road
Stamford, CT 06902

National Burn Victim Foundation
439 Main Street
Orange, NJ 07050

National Institute for Burn Medicine
909 E. Ann
Ann Arbor, MI 48104

Department of Health and Human Services
Health Services Administration
Bureau of Medical Services, Division of
   Emergency Medical Services
Box 911, Rockville, MD 20852

Brooke Army Medical Center
Box 551 Beach Pkwy.
Fort Sam Houston, TX 78234

Shriners Burns Institute
610 Texas Avenue
Galveston, TX 77550

JOBST
PO Box 653
Toledo, OH 43694

ly may give way to rage, anxiety, depression, guilt, and shame. These feelings can be expressed through weeping or anger, or concealed by an appearance of detachment, control, or exaggerated attention to other things in life. The family feels helpless and frustrated as there is nothing they can do to ease the pain of the patient [8]. Often, however, with time and team support they learn to accept the injury, and assist in the recovery process, and hope emerges.

## References

1. Abston, S., et al. Techniques for decreasing scar formation and contractures in the burned patient. *J. Trauma* 11(10):807, 1971.
2. Andreason, N., et al. Management of emotional

reactions in seriously burned adults. *N. Engl. J. Med.* 286(2):65, 1972.

3. Artz, C. P., and Moncrief, J. A. *The Treatment of Burns* (2nd ed.). Philadelphia: Saunders, 1969.

4. Artz, C. P., Moncrief, J. A., and Pruitt, B. A. *Burns—A Team Approach*. Philadelphia: Saunders, 1979.

5. Becker, B. E. Hypertrophic burn scarring: Control of chest deformities with a new device. *Arch. Phys. Med. Rehabil.* 61(4):187, 1980.

6. Bernstein, N. *Emotional Care of the Facially Burned and Disfigured*. Boston: Little, Brown, 1976.

7. Blocker, R., et al. Psychological studies in burn patients. *Plast. Reconstr. Surg.* 31(4):323, 1963.

8. Bowden, M., and Feller, I. Family reaction to a severe burn. *Am. J. Nurs.* 73(2):317, 1973.

9. Crane, K., and Feller, I. Classification of burn-care facilities in the United States. *JAMA* 215(3):463, 1971.

10. Crews, E. R. *A Practical Manual for the Treatment of Burns* (2nd ed.). Springfield, Ill.: Thomas, 1967.

11. Fagerhaugh, S. Pain expression and control on a burn care unit. *Nurs. Outlook* 22(10):645, 1974.

12. Feller, I., and Archambeault, C. *Nursing the Burned Patient*. Ann Arbor, Mich.: Institute for Burn Medicine, 1973.

13. Guilfoy, V., Healer, C., and McLouglin, E. *Burn Injuries: Causes, Consequences, Knowledge, Behaviors, A Summary Report*. Boston: Massachusetts General Hospital, Shriners Burns Institute and National Fire Protection Association, 1976.

14. Hamburg, D., and Adens, J. A perspective in coping behavior. *Arch. Gen. Psychiatry* 17:277, 1967.

15. Hamburg, D., Hamburg, B., and DeGoza, S. Adaptive problems and mechanisms in severely burned patients. *Psychiatry* 16:1, 1953.

16. Jackson, D. The psychological effects of burns. *Burns* 1(1):70, 1978.

17. Kilgore, E., and Newmeyer, W. Management of the burned hand. *Phys. Ther.* 57(1):54, 1977.

18. Larson, D. *The Prevention and Correction of Burn Scar Contracture and Hypertrophy*. Galveston, Texas: Shriners Burns Institute, 1973.

19. Larson, D., et al. Repair of the boutonnière deformity of the burned hand. *J. Trauma* 10(6):481, 1970.

20. MacArthur, I. D., and Moore, F. D. Epidemiology of burns: The burn-prone patient. *JAMA* 231(3):259, 1975.

21. Making the least of burn scars. *Emergency Medicine* March, 1972.

22. Malick, M. Management of the severely burned patient. *Br. J. Occup. Ther.* 38(4):89, 1975.

23. Malick, M. H., and Carr, J. A. Flexible elastomer molds in burn scar control. *Am. J. Occup. Ther.* 34(9):603, 1980.

24. Moncrief, J. A. Burns. In S. I. Schwartz (Ed.). *Principles of Surgery* (2nd ed.). New York: McGraw-Hill, 1974.

25. Noordhoff, M. S. Control and prevention of hypertrophic scarring and contracture. *Clin. Plast. Surg.* 1:49, 1974.

26. Parks, D. H., Carvajal, H. F., and Larson, D. L. Management of burns materials. *Surg. Clin. North Am.* 57:875, 1977.

27. Peacock, E. E. J. Wound Healing and Wound Care. In S. I. Schwartz (Ed.). *Principles of Surgery* (2nd ed.). New York: McGraw-Hill, 1974.

28. Remensnyder, J. D. Management of the Burned Hand. In F. G. Wolfort (Ed.). *Acute Hand Injuries*. Boston: Little, Brown, 1980.

29. Singletary, Y. More than skin deep. *J. Psychiatr. Nurs.* 15(2):7, 1977.

30. *Specific Optimal Criteria for Hospital Resources for Care of Patients with Burn Injury*. American Burn Association, 1976.

31. Tanigawa, M. C., O'Donnell, O. K., and Graham, P. L. The burned hand: A physical therapy protocol. *Phys. Ther.* 54(9):953, 1974.

32. VonPrince, K., and Yeakel, M. *The Splinting of Burn Patients*. Springfield, Ill.: Thomas, 1974.

33. Weeks, P. M., and Wray, R. C. *Management of Acute Hand Injuries*. St. Louis: Mosby, 1973.

34. Willis, B. *Splinting the Burn Patient*. Galveston, Texas: Medical Communications Department, Shriners Burns Institute,

35. Willis, B. The use of orthoplast isoprene splints in the treatment of the acutely burned child: A preliminary report. *Am. J. Occup. Ther.* 22(1):56, 1969.

## Suggested Reading

### BOOKS

Breslau, A. *The Time of My Death*. New York: Dutton, 1977.

Garret, J., and Levine, E. *Psychological Practices with the Physically Disabled*. New York: Columbia University Press, 1962.

Jacoby, F. G. *Nursing Care of the Patient with Burns*. St. Louis: Mosby, 1972.

### PAMPHLETS AND BOOKLETS

*Burn Care Services in the United States*. American Burn Association, April, 1978.

Copeland, C., Schwartz, J., and Shehorn, P. *Mercy*

*Hospital's Burn Patient Handbook.* Pittsburgh: Mercy Hospital.

*Family Guide to Burn Care.* Ann Arbor, Mich.: Michigan Burn Center, 1977.

*Physical Therapy for the Acute Burn Patient.* Galveston, Texas: Medical Communications Department, Shriners Burns Institute, 1968.

*Protect Someone You Love.* Project Burn Prevention, U.S. Consumer Product Safety Commission, BURNS, Boston, MA 02114.

Willis, B. *Burn Scar Hypertrophy.* Galveston, Texas: Shriners Burns Institute.

## JOURNAL ARTICLES

### MEDICAL/SURGICAL

Curreri, W., and Pruitt, B. Evaluation and treatment of the burned patient. *Am. J. Occup. Ther.* 24(7):475, 1970.

Denton, B., and Shaw, S. Mouth conformer for prevention and correction of burn scar contracture. *Phys. Ther.* 56(6):683, 1976.

Halversen, R. Total care concept for burns. *AORN J.* 26:328, 1977.

Koepke, G. The role of physical medicine in the treatment of burns. *Surg. Clin. North Am.* 50(6):1385, 1970.

Peterson, P. A conformer for the reduction of facial burn contractures. *Am. J. Occup. Ther.* 31(2):101, 1977.

Schwartz, J. Splinting the burn patient. Presented at the Burn Symposium, Pittsburgh, 1974.

Wagner, M. Emergency care of the burned patient. *Am. J. Nurs.* 77(11):1788, 1977.

### PSYCHOSOCIAL

Abramson, M., and Brodland, G. Adjustment problems of the family of the burn patient. *Social Casework* 55(1):13, 1974.

Andreason, N., Hartford, C., and Norris, H. Incidence of long-term psychiatric complications in severely burned adults. *Ann. Surg.* 174(5):785, 1971.

Easing the strain in caring for the severely burned patient. *Nursing* January, 1973.

Gardner, N., Miller, W., and Mlott, S. Psychological support in the treatment of severely burned patients. *J. Trauma* 16(9):186, 1976.

Psychological adjustments of burn patients. Ann Arbor, Mich.: St. Joseph Mercy Hospital.

Young, D. Stigmatization of burn patients. *AORN J.* 20(5):802, 1974.

# 6 CARDIAC REHABILITATION

*Janice Simari*

To achieve its broadest goals comprehensive rehabilitation of a patient with cardiac disease must include complete medical evaluation and treatment, assessment of functional capacity, health and vocational counseling, modification of risk factors, and a program of graded exercise. Although cardiac rehabilitation programs have been designed primarily for patients of postinfarction status, the principles and methods used are applicable to those with angina pectoris and following coronary bypass surgery [31]. There are three phases of such a program (Figure 6-1):

Phase I: In-hospital. It involves the first two weeks postinfarction. Days one to three the patient is in the coronary care unit, and days four to 14 on the progressive care unit or ward. The phase consists of medical stabilization, a gradual increase in activity, patient education, and psychological support.

Phase II: Outpatient hospital-based or home program. It involves the third through approximately the sixth week postinfarction. The phase consists of increasing functional capacity, altering risk factors, and giving support for psychological adjustment.

Phase III: Long-term community-based or home program. This is any time from the second to the sixth month postinfarction. The program is a continuation of that in Phase II.

Some facilities designate an additional Phase IV (progressive exercise program) that is essentially the same as or a continuation of Phase III [31].

## Normal Heart Function
### HEART ANATOMY

The cardiovascular system, composed of the myocardium and blood vessels, is responsible for the distribution of blood to the cells of the body. The myocardium has four chambers, two atria that receive blood from the body, and two ventricles that eject blood from the heart. The right atrium receives the deoxygenated blood from the venous return. Blood passes from the right atrium to the right ventricle by means of the tricuspid valve. Contraction of the right ventricle forces the blood through the pulmonary valve, and the pulmonary artery delivers the blood to the lungs. At this point, carbon dioxide is released and exchanged for oxygen. The oxygenated blood returns from the lungs to the left atrium through the pulmonary vein. The blood then passes through the mitral valve into the left ventricle. The left ventricle contracts and forces blood through the aortic valve into the aorta, and oxygenated blood is distributed to the entire body (Figure 6-2).

The myocardium receives its blood supply from the coronary arteries: the left main coronary artery, which divides into the left anterior descending and circumflex branches, and the right coronary artery (Figures 6-3 and 6-4).

The heart pumps continually to maintain circulation. The two phases of this cardiac cycle are systole (contraction) and diastole (relaxation).

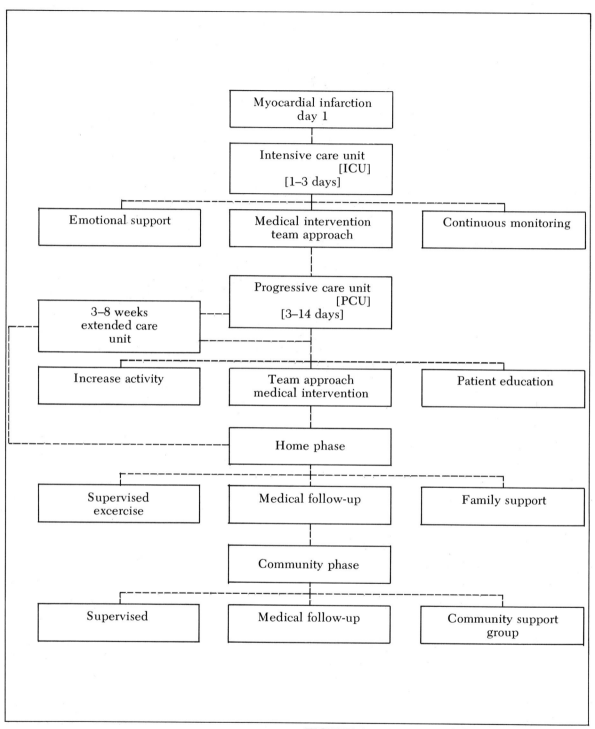

FIGURE 6-1. *Overview of the cardiac rehabilitation process.*

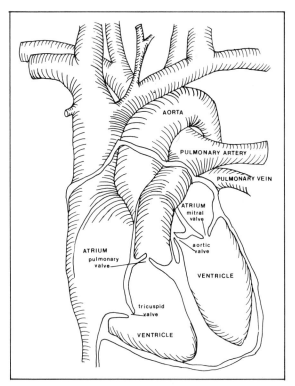

FIGURE 6-2. *Anatomy of the heart. (Artist: Rita M. Hammond)*

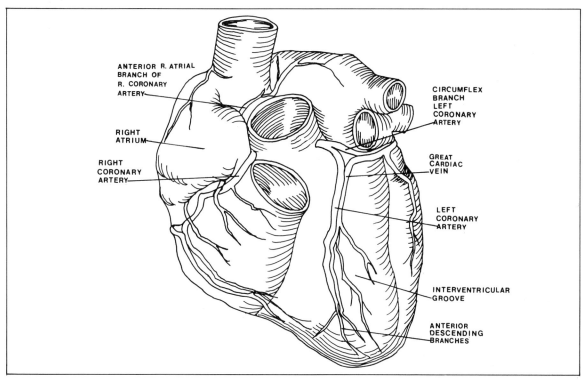

FIGURE 6-3. *Coronary arteries. (Artist: Rita M. Hammond)*

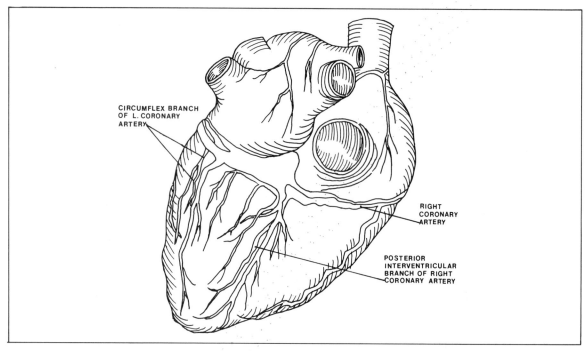

FIGURE 6-4. *Coronary arteries. (Artist: Rita M. Hammond)*

## THE CONDUCTION SYSTEM

An electrocardiogram reflects the electrical activity of the myocardium with 12 leads that allow 12 different views of the heart. This permits detection of heart rate and rhythm, axis, and chamber size, as well as evidence of myocardial infarction or ischemia.

The cardiac conduction system is innervated by the sympathetic and parasympathetic branches of the autonomic nervous system. The former increases heart rate, conduction, and contractility; the latter decreases heart rate and conduction. Although the autonomic nervous system can affect heart rate, the conduction system has its own intrinsic pacemakers that will pace the heart in the absence of the autonomic nervous system. The fastest of these is the sinoatrial (SA) node. Its impulse stimulates the atria through several pathways that end up at the atrioventricular (AV) node. From the AV node, the electrical activity spreads to the bundle of His, the left and right bundle branches, and the Purkinje fibers. Finally, the ventricles contract (Figure 6-5).

## CARDIAC ADJUSTMENT TO BODY DEMAND

During exercise, the cardiovascular system must adjust according to workload. The sympathetic nervous system is activated to increase heart rate and contractility, and thus increase cardiac output to provide increased oxygen to the skeletal muscles. Simultaneously, the rate and depth of respiration are increased mainly to expel the increased carbon dioxide formed by the skeletal muscle.

As expected, there is increased blood volume delivered to the heart with exercise, thereby increasing the end diastolic volume of the ventricles and increasing the stretch on the muscle fibers. According to *Starling's law:* the more muscle stretch, the greater the force of contraction; the myocardium responds with a more forceful contraction, and an increased volume of blood is delivered into the pulmo-

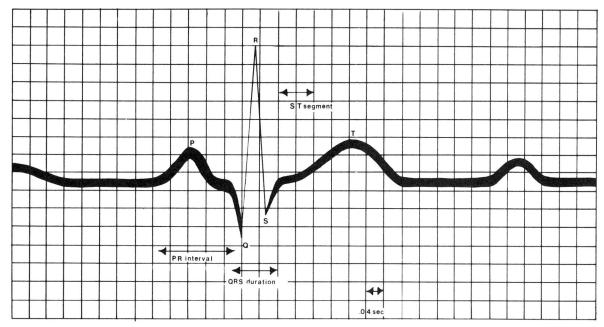

FIGURE 6-5. *The basic ECG complex. P wave indicates atrial depolarization. PR interval indicates atrioventricular conduction time. QRS duration indicates ventricular depolarization. T wave indicates repolarization of the ventricles. (Artist: Rita M. Hammond)*

nary artery from the right ventricle and into the aorta from the left ventricle. The volume of blood ejected by the ventricle into the aorta on the left (in the healthy heart, equal in amount to that ejected by the right ventricle into the pulmonary artery) is called *stroke volume.* Multiply this by the heart rate, and the result is *cardiac output*—the amount of blood per minute pumped by the ventricle. By these mechanisms exercise will increase cardiac output by increasing both heart rate (HR) and stroke volume.

Cardiac output = stroke volume × heart rate (beats per minute)
Examples:
  3.6 liters = 60 ml × 60 (HR)        cardiac
                        output at rest
19.6 liters = 140 ml × 140 (HR)        cardiac
                        output during exercise

In the healthy individual, many variables affect heart rate, one of which is cardiovascular fitness. The physically trained individual's resting heart rate and exercise heart rate will be lower than those of the untrained individual. Age is another influence. An infant may have a resting rate of 90 beats per minute, while the resting heart rate of an elderly person may be 60 beats per minute. Environmental factors such as room temperature will increase the heart rate, as will physical or emotional stress.

Blood pressure (BP) is proportional to the product of cardiac output (CO) and resistance to flow (R) in the arterial tree (BP≃ CO × R). Changes in blood pressure are blunted by the carotid baroreceptors that sense such changes and set in motion mechanisms to alter the sympathetic "tone," or outflow, to the heart and to the arterioles. Adjustments in heart rate and resistance to flow, respectively, are thereby made, tending to maintain blood pressure within certain limits. Nevertheless, emotional and physical stress increase the blood pressure. In the latter state, heart rate and stroke volume increase, but resistance decreases. The result is a slight to moderate increase in blood pressure.

## Atherosclerosis

Atherosclerosis compromises the coronary vasculature with the formation of lipid-laden focal deposits causing narrowing at or near the origins of the coronary arteries. These lesions may gradually obstruct blood flow over many years, or they may suddenly cause vascular insufficiency with ulceration, thrombosis, or embolization. This process is often referred to as coronary artery disease (CAD). Its clinical manifestations include angina, myocardial infarction (MI), congestive heart failure (CHF), and sudden death.

### ANGINA

Angina occurs when oxygen demand is greater than the oxygen supplied by narrowed coronary arteries. This condition is often manifested by chest pain of a squeezing nature, jaw pain, and pain radiating into the left arm. Although angina can occur at rest, most of the time it is precipitated by extremes in physical or emotional stress that increase oxygen demand. It typically lasts only a few minutes, until the stimulus is removed or medical treatment (nitroglycerin) is begun.

### MYOCARDIAL INFARCTION

The terms *myocardial infarction, heart attack, MI, coronary, coronary occlusion,* or *coronary thrombosis* refer to a sudden blocking of one of the coronary arteries. Onset is sudden, although it is the result of the slow development of atherosclerosis. The MI may develop as a result of a thrombus or an embolus. With the absence of blood flow to that part of the heart, the myocardium becomes necrotic.

Location and extent of MI will determine the severity of the damage, and is significant with regard to the individual's prognosis and functional ability. It has been suggested that the prognosis for an inferior wall infarction is more favorable than for an anterior wall infarction, as the anterior wall of the myocardium is larger, and is responsible for the majority of the cardiac contraction [24].

The most common site of occlusion is the left anterior descending branch of the left coronary artery. The second most common site is the right coronary artery, followed by the circumflex branch of the left coronary artery.

Its most common symptom is severe, prolonged, substernal chest pain. Pain is experienced in the left arm, neck, or jaw in 25 percent of reported cases, and frequently is associated with sweating, nausea, vomiting, weakness, shortness of breath, and anxiety. Silent MIs (without any symptoms) are not uncommon, however, particularly among diabetics and the elderly.

Laboratory tests are important to confirm the diagnosis. Electrocardiographic changes may be noted, such as ST and T wave changes, the development of Q waves, and loss of amplitude in R waves. In addition, the cardiac enzymes creatinine phosphokinase (CPK), serum glutamic-oxalacetic transaminase (SGOT), and lactic dehydrogenase (LDH) will be released into the blood, in that order, from a necrotic myocardium.

Medical treatment depends on the presence or absence of complications. At its minimum, treatment consists of admission to a coronary care unit, continuous ECG monitoring and specialized nursing, bedrest, analgesia, sedation, oxygen administration, laxatives, feedings with low sodium and caloric content, a gradual program of increasing ambulation when medically stable, and psychosocial counseling around such issues as prognosis, occupation, and sexual activity.

Although it may take up to six months for an infarct to heal by the formation of a fibrotic scar (the myocardium cannot rejuvenate), a patient with an uncomplicated MI may be discharged from the hospital after gradually increasing ambulation over seven to 14 days. On the other hand, an MI complicated by the conditions mentioned as follows may require hospitalization for months.

1. Pump failure: The loss of 40 percent or more of the myocardium, most commonly after an anterior wall infarct, may at the outset produce severe pump failure, with pulmonary edema (fluid in the lungs) and inadequate blood flow to the vital organs (i.e., brain, kidney). This condition has a high mortality (greater than 80 percent in most series), which is dependent on the functional state of the rest of the heart that is called on to compensate for the loss. This is the major cause of in-hospital mortality.

A less severe infarct leaves the patient with mild to moderate congestive heart failure (CHF), meaning that the heart lacks pump capacity to meet the metabolic demands of the body. As a result, the heart dilates and fluid accumulates—in the lung if the left ventricle "fails," in the subcutaneous tissues of the body when the right ventricle "fails", or both. Symptoms are: (1) shortness of breath on exertion or while lying flat (especially when asleep without enough pillows) in left-sided CHF, (2) edema or fluid accumulation with right-sided CHF, and (3) both.

The etiology of postinfarction CHF could be secondary to loss of myocardial tissue, or as a result of mitral regurgitation often seen in an inferior wall MI, ventricular septum rupture most common in an anterior MI, aneurysm formation, ventricular or atrial tachyarrhythmias, or bradyarrhythmias.

Treatment of cardiogenic shock is beyond the scope of this text. Treatment of mild to moderate CHF depends on its cause. In general, demands on the heart are kept to a minimum, with bedrest, treatment of infection and fever, correction of anemia, treatment of hypertension, and so on. Rupture and perhaps aneurysm require surgical intervention. Antiarrhythmics, pacemakers, or cardioversion may be necessary for the management of arrhyth-

mias compromising cardiac output. The majority of patients, however, do not fall into these categories, and are treated with digitalis glycosides to increase cardiac contractility, or diuretics to decrease lung fluid that may interfere with respiration (Table 6-1).

2. Arrhythmia: Although atrial and other supraventricular arrhythmias occur post-MI, the major cause of prehospital mortality is ventricular arrhythmia, in particular, ventricular fibrillation (VF) often preceded by ventricular tachycardia. If untreated, VF is fatal, as the myocardium cannot pump blood to the vital organs including itself. Treatment of ventricular arrhythmias may require cardioversion acutely, correction of metabolic abnormalities, and/or antiarrhythmics.

3. Conduction system: The conduction system may be interrupted anywhere from the SA node to the Purkinje cells, but the most significant is complete heart block (CHB). The most dangerous type of CHB leaves the heart with only 1 pacemaker, firing at about 40 beats per minute. This is most often caused by an anterior wall MI, and requires an emergency pacemaker to try to increase the heart rate, and thereby the blood flow to vital organs.

## Risk Factors

There is evidence that the risk of coronary artery disease is increased when associated with certain identifiable factors including cigarette smoking, hypertension, behavior or stress, physical inactivity, hyperlipidemia, diabetes, family history, male sex, and age (Table 6-2) [6, 14, 15, 26, 32, 38, 40]. The two most significant risk factors are hypertension and cigarette smoking [7, 42].

When considering the implications of these risk factors with regard to primary prevention of heart disease [7], "emphasis should be placed on the interaction of these factors with each other and with other factors." Borhani suggests that an independent change in just one of these is associated with a change in the probability of coronary heart disease.

As many risk factors are closely associated, a

TABLE 6-1. *Commonly Used Cardiac Medications*

| Generic Name | Trade Name | Therapeutic Purpose | Therapeutic Effects | Side Effects |
|---|---|---|---|---|
| Nitrates | | | | |
| Nitroglycerin | Nitroglycerin (sublingual) | Antianginal | Coronary vasodilator—increases $O_2$ supply by dilating coronary vessels; peripheral vasodilation | Bitter taste; headaches; flushing of face; occasionally produces hypotension |
| | Nitropaste (applied topically to chest) | Antianginal | Effects as above; longer-acting nitrate: 4–6 hours | Effects as above |
| Isosorbide dinitrate | Isordil (sublingual and oral) | Antianginal | Effects as above; longer-acting nitrate | Effects as above |
| Reserpine | Serpasil | Antihypertensive | Blocks storage and release of norepinephrine in CNS | Nasal stuffiness; depression; loss of appetite; weight gain; parkinsonism |
| Methyldopa | Aldomet | Antihypertensive | Inhibits formation of norepinephrine peripherally and centrally | Anemia; liver function abnormalities; drowsiness; dryness of mouth; fluid retention; fever; mood disturbance |
| Hydralazine hydrochloride | | Antihypertensive | Lowers blood pressure by dilating the peripheral blood vessels; increases cardiac output and heart rate | Tachycardia; hypotension; drug-induced lupus erythematosus |
| Furosemide | Lasix | Diuretic; antihypertensive | | Potassium loss leading to arrhythmias if not replaced |
| Hydro-chlorothiazide | HydroDiuril | Diuretic; antihypertensive | | Effects as above |
| Chlorothiazide | Diuril | Diuretic; antihypertensive | | Effects as above |
| Triamterene | | Potassium-sparing diuretic; antihypertensive | | |
| Spironolactone | | Potassium-sparing diuretic; antihypertensive | | |
| Propranolol hydrochloride | Inderal | Antiarrhythmic; antianginal; antihypertensive | Increases endurance capacity; decreases atrial and ventricular rates and ectopic activity; decreases blood pressure | Bradycardia; contraindicated for asthmatics as causes bronchial constriction; aggravates CHF in people predisposed to it; hyperkalemia |
| Quinidine sulfate | Quinidine | Antiarrhythmic | Decreases myocardial excitability | GI symptons (vomiting, diarrhea); fever; syncope; purpura |
| Procainamide hydrochloride | Pronestyl | Antiarrhythmic | Decreases myocardial excitability | Drug-induced lupus erythematosus (i.e., joint pain, arthritis, skin rash); hypotension |
| Digoxin | Lanoxin | CHF; cardiac arrhythmias (i.e., atrial flutter, atrial fibrillation, PAT) | Increases cardiac output; increases myocardial contractility; decreases AV conduction | Ventricular ectopy; nausea; vomiting; diarrhea; mental status changes |

TABLE 6-2. *Risk Factors for Atherosclerosis*

| Category | Description |
| --- | --- |
| Nonreversible | Aging<br>Male sex<br>Genetic traits—positive family history of premature atherosclerosis |
| Reversible | Cigarette smoking<br>Hypertension<br>Obesity |
| Potentially or partially reversible | Hyperlipidemia—hypercholesterolemia and hypertriglyceridemia<br>Hyperglycemia and diabetes mellitus<br>Low levels of high-density lipoproteins (HDL) |
| Other possible factors | Physical inactivity<br>Emotional stress<br>Personality type |

Source: From Thorn et al. (Eds.). *Harrison's Principles of Internal Medicine* (9th ed.). Copyright(c) 1980. Used with the permission of McGraw-Hill Book Company.

comprehensive assessment is extremely useful. In 1964, the Western Collaborative Group used a multivariate approach [38] to evaluate them. The study identified serum cholesterol, behavioral patterns, cigarette smoking, and systolic blood pressure as significantly predictive in 39 to 49 and 50 to 59 years age groups. This program, the Framingham Study, is an ongoing analysis of 1000 persons to assess the pathogenesis of cardiovascular disease.

SMOKING

Cigarette smoking has been clearly linked to coronary heart disease. Studies have demonstrated that it almost doubles the risk of developing heart disease, and that cessation will lower the risk [28, 42].

HYPERTENSION

Hypertension has been identified as the dominant contributor with regard to stroke and congestive heart failure, and is clearly associated with coronary disease [29]. It appears that systolic as well as diastolic hypertension can be potentially significant risk factors [29]. For the high-risk patient, blood pressure should be carefully monitored, as early detection and treatment decrease the chance of developing further cardiovascular disease.

BEHAVIOR AND STRESS

Specific behavioral patterns have been recognized as risk factors. Friedman and Rosenman [37, 38] have described type A behavior in association with patients who have had an MI as demonstrating a constant sense of time urgency and rapid speech. The individual is often unable to relax or use leisure time effectively, and exhibits a constant struggle to achieve [38]. It has been suggested that persons who exhibit type A behavior have an increase in coronary disease compared to type B individuals [37, 27].

As type A behavior is a lifelong pattern, it is extremely difficult to change. Relaxation exercises, time management, psychotherapy, and medication are some of the treatments recommended.

PHYSICAL INACTIVITY

Over time, a sedentary life-style can decrease the efficiency of the myocardium. Physical activity is believed to develop cardiac muscle, improve efficiency of the aerobic system, provide psychological release, and use up caloric intake. At the present time, studies have indicated that the conditioning effect of exercise produces a resting bradycardia associated with myocardial hypertrophy, improved perfusion,

Massachusetts Rehabilitation Hospital
125 Nashua Street
Boston, Massachusetts 02114
Telephone: 617-523-1818

## ACUTE MYOCARDIAL INFARCTION: CARDIAC REHABILITATION PROGRAM

Interdisciplinary Cardiovascular Program

| DAY | OT(AM) | PT (PM) | RT (PM) | ACTIVITIES |
|---|---|---|---|---|
| 2 | Turn self in bed<br>Use of commode lifted,<br>  otherwise restricted<br>  bedrest | A or AA ankle mots<br>  × 10<br>Quads—gluteus<br>  muscle contraction<br>  × 10<br>Deep breathing<br>  (exercises in bed) | Listening to music<br>Television<br>Reading<br>  (in bed) | Dangling<br>5–10,11 |
| 3 | Feed self (meat precut)<br>Partial bath; wash face<br>  and hands; electric<br>  toothbrush<br>Use of commode lifted<br>Cardiac education | Shoulder flex × 10<br>Shoulder abd. × 10 | Listening to music<br>Television<br>Reading<br>Table games<br>Light needlework<br>Light artwork<br>  (in bed) | Chair 15<br>minutes |
| 4 | Restricted bedrest<br>  feeding self<br>  (meat precut)<br>Partial bath<br>Bedside commode<br>Transfer with assist<br>Cardiac education | Complete days 1 & 2 × 2 | Listening to music<br>Television<br>Reading<br>Table games<br>Light needlework<br>Light artwork<br>  (in bed) | Chair 20<br>minutes |
| 5<br>&<br>6 | Partial bath<br>Bedside commode<br>  with assist<br>Cardiac education<br>Begin cardiac<br>  education exercises<br>  group when<br>  trendscribed | In chair<br>Active ankle mot × 10<br>Active knee ext. one leg | All stage 1 activities<br>Crafts with no<br>  isometrics | Chair 30′ TID<br>Trendscribed<br>for stage 2<br>(day 5) |

FIGURE 6-6. *Massachusetts Rehabilitation Hospital: Acute myocardial infarction cardiac rehabilitation program. (© 1979: A. 851672)*

| DAY | OT(AM) | PT (PM) | RT (PM) | ACTIVITIES |
|---|---|---|---|---|
| 7 & 8 | Partial bath; upper extremity dressing<br>Comb hair/shave at sink<br>Cardiac education<br>Cardiac exercise group | In chair<br>Active shoulder abd. × 10<br>Active shoulder flex × 10<br>Active knee ext. both legs at time 5–10 | All stage 1 activities<br>Crafts with no isometrics<br>Group diversional activity (30 minutes in wheelchair) | Chair 30' QID<br>Unassisted transfer |
| 9 & 10 | Dress self; bathroom room privileges<br>Continue personal hygiene<br>Shower self to waist<br>Cardiac education<br>Cardiac group when trenscribed stage 3 | Active hip abd. (against gravity) × 10<br>Repeat complete days 7 & 8 | All stage 1 activities<br>Crafts with no isometrics<br>Group diversional activity (30 minutes, in wheelchair) | Chair 45' QID<br>Walk in room under observation<br>Trendscriber for stage 3 (day #10) |
| 11 | Dress self<br>Unassisted transfer<br>Bathroom privileges<br>Shower self to waist<br>Cardiac education<br>Stage 3 homemaking<br>Cardiac group | Trunk twist × 10<br>Walk 100'<br>Standing arm-shoulder flex abd. × 10<br>Encourage self-monitoring | All stage 1 activities<br>Crafts with some isometrics<br>Outings outside the hospital (in wheelchair and limited good weather, 45 min. on hospital grounds)<br>Group diversional activity (30 min, in wheelchair) | Walk in hall 100' |
| 12 & 13 | Same as day 11 | Standing lateral bends × 10<br>Exercises day 7 and 11 | | Chair 10 QID<br>Walk in hall 200' day 12<br>Walk in hall 200' day 13 |
| 14 | Complete shower<br>Repeat entire program<br>Cardiac education<br>Stage 4 homemaking activities<br>Home visit if appropriate | Walking in hall<br>Begin stairs (up and down) | All stage 1 activities<br>Crafts with some isometrics<br>Outings outside the hospital (to tolerance)<br>Group diversional activity (patient may walk to activity room) | Trendscribe stage |

Accredited by the Joint Commission on Accreditation of Hospitals (JCAH)
Accredited by the Commission on Accreditation of Rehabilitation Facilities (CARF)
Accredited by the American Board of Examiners in Speech Pathology and Audiology (ABESPA)
Certified and Qualified as a Rehabilitation Facility by the Industrial Accident Rehabilitation Board.

and coronary dilation [41, 17]. Individuals who maintain an exercise schedule also tend to have lower serum triglyceride levels [39, 41].

## DIET

Desirable body weight is important to avoid undue strain on the myocardium. The Framingham Study concludes [28], "obesity seems to play an important role in the developing of coronary heart disease although no evidence has been drawn that weight reduction directly reduces the incidence of heart disease."

The American Heart Association (AHA) suggests that by lowering caloric intake, cholesterol, and saturated fats, the serum lipid concentration is reduced [20]. The AHA also suggests that dietary habits formed during the developing years may continue as lifelong patterns and influence the severity of atherosclerosis in later life. As dietary modification is still under investigation, a prudent approach should be taken in regard to eating habits.

## DIABETES

Diabetes is a significant risk factor. It is controversial, however, as to whether the degree of hyperglycemia or the medical control of blood glucose alters increased cardiac risk.

## FAMILY HISTORY

There is increased risk of developing CAD for an individual with a family history of heart disease. As this cannot be altered, consideration should be given to the cumulative effects of the reversible factors.

## MALE SEX

Coronary heart disease is the leading cause of death in men after the age of 35 years, and is responsible for nearly all premature mortality in American men [4]. In addition [4], "between the ages of 35 and 55 the death rate is five times higher in white men than in white women in the United States"

## AGING

The incidence of mortality gradually increases

TABLE 6-3. *Warning Signs of Ischemic Heart Disease*

Pain or pressure in the chest, left arm or jaw
Dizziness, light headedness, sweating, pallor, fainting, sudden weakness
Inappropriate shortness of breath
Irregular pulse
Palpitations

with age. Death rates in the United States from ischemic heart disease in 1976 are 6 per 100,000 for white men age 25 to 34 years, rising to 7954 per 100,000 for white men age 85 years and above [4].

## Cardiac Rehabilitation

Cardiac rehabilitation provides a structured program that enables the patient to regain maximum functional capacity through graded exercise and activity. Education of the patient takes place throughout to assist in the adjustment to recommended life-style modifications.

In-hospital programs are organized by stages that are designed to incorporate gradually increasing or graded activities. Within each stage there is an estimated amount of time allotted for the patient to accomplish them.

Researchers have measured the energy expended, or physiological work, of most activities that occur in a normal day. It is assessed in standard units called metabolic units, or MET. A MET refers to the energy expended per kilogram of body weight per minute of an average adult sitting quietly in a chair or at rest supine.

Based on the energy expended during activity, cardiac rehabilitation programs have been developed in which various activities of similar metabolic cost, or METs, are grouped together in specific stages, levels, or steps. Thus a program can be prescribed allowing for a gradual increase of activity by a gradual increase in MET level. The expected progression of recovery for the patient with an uncomplicated MI can be seen in Figure 6-6 (Table 6-3).

## TEAM APPROACH

Cardiac rehabilitation requires a well-integrated team approach that is essential in the management of the many areas involved. The physician provides medical care and approves the beginning and continuation of rehabilitation, such as recommendations for appropriate progression in the use of graded activity. The nurse meets the patient's immediate health needs, and often functions as the team coordinator because of close contact with all members of the team. In addition, the nurse is responsible for monitoring the patient, providing emotional support for the patient and family, and educating the patient [33] with regard to heart function and the disease process, with particular emphasis on teaching about medication.

The occupational therapist provides a program to increase the patient's ability to perform activities of daily living, reinforce specific modifications of life-style, and reduce anxiety by clarifying misconceptions that may exist regarding the medical condition. Evaluation includes assessment of self-care ability according to the patient's cardiac stage. The patient's understanding of all of these aspects is discussed. Evaluation of perception and cerebration may be indicated to determine higher cortical function.

During activity the patient's heart and respiration rates and blood pressure are carefully monitored, while observing for clinical signs of acute distress. A telemetry system or monitoring device that records heart rate and rhythm during activities is extremely valuable. Energy conservation techniques are reinforced for use while in the hospital as well as in the home. In addition to individual treatment sessions, the patient may participate in a graded exercise group to increase endurance and provide support and socialization. Closer to hospital discharge, simulated work situations are designed, including homemaking activites. A submaximal exercise test is carried out to determine an appropriate heart rate range for the patient with regard to activity. Based on these

data, the physician and other team members design a home exercise program. A home visit is carried out and a home program is provided to assist the patient in the organization of daily tasks.

The physical therapist provides an activity program to increase endurance and improve the patient's functional capacity through graded exercise and ambulation. Evaluation includes range of motion, respiratory status, and functional status. To avoid strain on the damaged myocardium, resistive muscle testing should not be performed. The patient is encouraged to use proper breathing techniques and self-monitoring of pulse while participating in the exercise program. Often a monitoring system such as a trendscriber is used to assess cardiovascular status and assign the patient to a higher activity level.

The nutritionist's primary function is to educate patient and family about appropriate diet. The patient may have problems with high cholesterol, obesity, diabetes, or hypertension, all of which require nutritional attention. In addition, existing dietary patterns and nutritional status are identified to determine a baseline for patient education. A program is designed to minimize dietary risk factors and blend with the patient's life-style [33]. Restriction of cholesterol and sodium is frequently recommended. It is essential for the nutritionist to instruct the patient and family regarding guidelines, and a written copy of any restrictions is helpful.

The recreational therapist assesses the patient's leisure interests to identify activities that may help to reduce anxiety and depression, and provide appropriate diversion within a given recovery stage. Near discharge, the therapist encourages the patient to explore available work and leisure activities. The cardiac patient may lack avocational interests; thus introduction to new activities serves as a release from daily stress when the patient is discharged home, and helps to redirect energy in a purposeful way.

The medical social worker functions as a

counselor to the patient and family by providing assistance with emotional, social, and financial concerns [33]. To clarify discharge planning and reconfirm the patient's rehabilitation program, the social worker may arrange a family-team conference early in the patient's program and again nearer to discharge.

## Psychological Adjustment

Many adjustments must be made by the patient concerning alterations in both physiological capacity and self-perception. The patient may have to adjust to a role change within the family, often from a position of dominance to one of dependence. Changes in vocational and avocational pursuits must also be considered. It is not surprising that the patient suffers from low self-esteem and is uncertain of his or her capabilities. Moreover, physiological change can affect endurance, and when this is diminished the patient's self-perception might suddenly be one of incompleteness or incompetence [5, 10, 17].

Cassem and Hackett [17, 18] have identified two major sources of such psychological stress: (1) anxiety, which occurs during the first few days after the MI, and (2) depression, commonly developing by the third hospital day. It is their impression that denial is the major coping mechanism used to adapt to this situation [16, 17].

During the first few days following an MI, continual monitoring by staff and equipment together with medication can help the patient cope; however, depression remains a serious problem. Patient education, exercise conditioning, and support groups have been strongly recommended as means of alleviating depression and anxiety [4, 18].

### PATIENT EDUCATION

The objective is to educate the patient to produce a change in behavior. This can be classified as a primary or secondary prevention strategy. Primary prevention is an educational approach to modify the individual's behavior and thus lower the risk of developing CAD.

Secondary prevention attempts to enhance the quality of life by reducing the risk of morbidity for those who have experienced heart disease. Although primary prevention in the early years would be preferable, there is evidence that secondary prevention is of value in the middle and later adult years. Intervention may be expected to have a greater short-term effect on the individual with heart disease than similar action with younger persons [1].

### PLANNING HEALTH EDUCATION

Following an MI, both the patient and family need additional health information. The patient should be involved in identifying and planning for individual needs, thus actively participating in the learning process.

Motivation and psychological readiness are crucial elements in producing effective behavioral change. When planning the educational program, one must be realistic and consider limitations that may interfere. If the patient exhibits impairment of memory or general intellectual functioning as the result of anoxia, retaining information may be difficult. Psychological adjustment to the illness—denial, anger, depression, or anxiety—may also inhibit integration of information.

### THE EDUCATION PROCESS

The program should be initiated early in cardiac rehabilitation. Before it is begun, however, the patient's general level of understanding must be assessed (Figure 6-7). The therapist should also determine the amount of knowledge specific to the situation prior to and at the completion of each meeting. The sessions are short and can be designed for individual or group instruction. Several studies [8, 10, 36] have indicated that the adult patient tends to learn more effectively in a group setting. Written materials can also reinforce teaching.

Health education helps the patient adjust to the medical condition functionally, intellectually, and emotionally. The program generally includes information on anatomy and physiology of the heart, risk factors, warning

CARDIAC QUESTIONNAIRE

Evaluation Date _____

Reevaluation Date _____

1. What does your heart do? How does it work? (Draw a picture)

2. Describe your heart problems.

3. How does your heart recover after a heart attack?

4. Are you on a special diet? Why?

5. How do you handle tension or stress? (Fill in diagram)

6. Have you taken medications before? Did you have any problems following directions? What would you do if you had forgotten to take your pills?

7. What are the three major risk factors? Can they be controlled? Can you name any other risk factors?

8. Do you smoke? How does smoking affect your heart?

9. What are the signs and symptoms of (MI, CHF, Other _____)?
(Circle appropriate diagnosis)

10. In everyday living what are some of the "do's and don'ts" for the person with heart disease?

11. What is a MET?

12. Give an example of an energy conservation technique used at home.

13. Are you interested in learning more about your heart?

14. Do you think your heart condition will improve?

15. What do you expect to gain from therapies during your stay here?

16. Do you know how to monitor your own pulse? If so, do you?

FIGURE 6-7. *Massachusetts Rehabilitation Hospital: Cardiac questionnaire.* (© 1979: A. 851672: New Edition)

MASSACHUSETTS REHABILITATION
HOSPITAL CARDIAC REHABILITATION
TEAM EDUCATION FLOW SHEET

| Responsibility | Content | Date & Teacher | Need for Further Teaching | | Person Taught | | Comments |
|---|---|---|---|---|---|---|---|
| | | | Yes | No | Pt. | Fam. | |
| Nursing | I. Orientation to MRH<br>a. Reason for admission | | | | | | |
| MD | b. Expected course of hospitalization | | | | | | |
| Nursing | c. Monitor, equipment | | | | | | |
| Nursing | d. Unit regulations (visiting, smoking, stage limitations) | | | | | | |
| Nursing | II. Cardiac rehab. program<br>a. Purpose | | | | | | |
| OT | b. Knowledge assessment, i.e., risk factors, disease process | | | | | | |
| | c. OT/RT/PT evaluations | | | | | | |
| OT/Dietary | d. Dietary education | | | | | | |
| OT | e. Formal cardiac education (refer to OT Education Flow Sheet) | | | | | | |
| MD | III. Medical referral<br>a. Implementation of cardiac rehabilitation stages | | | | | | |
| MD | b. Holter monitor | | | | | | |
| MD | c. Trendscriber | | | | | | |
| Social service | IV. Social<br>a. Family adaptations to disease, hospitalization of patient, goals (family & patient) | | | | | | |
| Social service | b. Problems (emotional, financial, etc.) | | | | | | |
| Social service | c. Patient adjustment/attitude | | | | | | |
| | V. Discharge planning<br>a. Activity | | | | | | |
| MD | 1. General | | | | | | |
| MD | 2. Restrictions | | | | | | |
| MD/OT | 3. Sexual | | | | | | |
| Team | b. Initial goal | | | | | | |
| Team | c. Final placement | | | | | | |

FIGURE 6-8. *Massachusetts Rehabilitation Hospital: Cardiac rehabilitation team education flow sheet.* (© *1979: A, 851672)*

| | Responsibility Content | Date & Teacher | Need for Further Teaching | | Person Taught | | Comments |
|---|---|---|---|---|---|---|---|
| | | | Yes | No | Pt. | Fam. | |
| OT | VI. Warning signs/precautions<br>a. CHF | | | | | | |
| | b. MI | | | | | | |
| | c. Defective pacemaker | | | | | | |
| | d. Valve infections | | | | | | |
| | e. Arrhythmias | | | | | | |
| Nursing | VII. Medications<br>a. Name | | | | | | |
| Nursing | b. Dosage | | | | | | |
| Nursing | c. Action or purpose | | | | | | |
| OT | d. Schedule | | | | | | |
| OT | e. Precautions/side effects | | | | | | |
| OT | f. When to call MD | | | | | | |
| Nursing | List medications | | | | | | |
| | 1. _____ | | | | | | |
| | 2. _____ | | | | | | |
| | 3. _____ | | | | | | |
| | 4. _____ | | | | | | |
| | 5. _____ | | | | | | |
| | 6. _____ | | | | | | |
| | 7. _____ | | | | | | |
| OT | VIII. Home visit | | | | | | |
| Nursing | IX. Posthospital<br>1. Appointments | | | | | | |
| Team | 2. Referrals<br>(i.e., VNA) | | | | | | |
| RT | 3. Community resources<br>(i.e., rec. therapy, day centers,<br>outpatient exercise prog., senior<br>citizen groups) | | | | | | |
| | 4. Phone numbers:<br>a. MD | | | | | | |
| | b. OTR | | | | | | |
| | c. RPT | | | | | | |
| | d. RT | | | | | | |
| | e. Dietary | | | | | | |
| | f. Nursing floor | | | | | | |
| | g. Social Service | | | | | | |

# MASSACHUSETTS REHABILITATION HOSPITAL
## OCCUPATIONAL THERAPY DEPARTMENT
## CARDIAC REHABILITATION EDUCATION FLOW SHEET

Name _____ Age _____ Diagnosis _____

Work History _____ Perceptual Cerebration Status _____

| Content | Date | Person Taught | | Comments |
|---|---|---|---|---|
| | | Pt. | Family | |
| Introduction to normal heart function | | | | |
| Define MI | | | | |
| Define angina | | | | |
| Define CHF | | | | |
| Define pacemakers | | | | |
| Teach self-monitoring | | | | |
| Pacing and breathing exercises (ADL) | | | | |
| Sex counseling | | | | |
| Work simplification/energy conservation | | | | |
| Risk factors: Diet | | | | |
| Smoking | | | | |
| High blood pressure | | | | |
| Obesity | | | | |
| Stress | | | | |
| Family history positive | | | | |
| Relaxation techniques | | | | |
| Warning signs | | | | |
| Precautions | | | | |

Therapist's Name _____ Date Started _____ Date Completed _____

FIGURE 6-9. *Massachusetts Rehabilitation Hospital: Occupational Therapy Department Cardiac rehabilitation education flow sheet. (© 1979: A. 851672: New Edition)*

guidelines, cardiac medications, sex counseling, energy conservation techniques, diet, stress, and time management, relaxation techniques, and family and social issues (Figures 6-8 and 6-9). Misconceptions and fears, such as of sudden death, should also be discussed, and accurate, useful information made available.

The family should be included and instructed in all appropriate areas of concern. Once knowledgeable of the patient's status and prognosis, they can deal more effectively with all necessary adjustments. If the patient exhibits significant intellectual or psychological difficulties, the family may be called on for additional support. It should be noted that family education can also be a means of primary prevention. In addition, through training in cardiopulmonary resuscitation and education as to the warning signs of an MI, they will be able to respond appropriately should an emergency arise.

## SEXUAL ADJUSTMENT

Studies have indicated that there have been significant sexual difficulties after myocardial infarction. These are seldom of organic origin, rather [30], "sexual distress arises out of a combination of misconception, anxiety, avoidance, depression, and poor self-esteem." Some fears of the cardiac patient are of sudden death or another MI with excitement and exertion; that medical advice will significantly alter or preclude sexual activities; that the MI will cause physical difficulties in sexual function; and that the MI is a warning sign of aging and therefore loss of sexual function. These concerns can be complicated by the fact that health professionals have not discussed specific recommendations with patients and their partners, which is interpreted as an unspoken prohibition [30].

Although heart rate, blood pressure, and respiratory rate do increase in healthy persons during sexual activity [30], when studying middle-aged men with heart disease and those who are susceptible, Hellerstein and Friedman [23] found that conjugal sex imposes only modest physiological cost in comparison to that of climbing a flight of stairs, walking several blocks briskly, or performing tasks of many occupations.

It has been noted [30]:

For the patient with a first heart attack and no significant medical complications (including absence of cardiac failure or arrhythmias), if exercise can be tolerated to the extent of raising the heart rate to approximately 110 to 120 beats per minute without precipitating angina or severe shortness of breath, sexual activity almost invariably can be resumed. This means that many postcoronary patients can return to sexual activity two to four weeks after discharge from the hospital.

Kolodny, Masters, and Johnson make the following recommendations for patients in this category [30]:

1. Resumption of sexual activity should occur gradually, using comfortable positions with a moderate degree of exertion, and avoiding positions that require isometric exertion. Proving anything sexually by marathon sessions or a display of athletic prowess is discouraged.
2. Sexual activity should be avoided after eating or drinking.
3. If chest pain, tightness, or dyspnea occurs during sex, the activity should be decreased or stopped, and the physician notified.
4. Partners and patients must communicate with each other about their sexual feelings. The healthy partner may decide to "protect" the patient by avoiding sex, either from misunderstanding or disbelief of the physiological facts and suggestions.

## Vocational Concerns

Difficulty in psychological adjustment to the MI may serve as a barrier to the patient's returning to work. With misconceptions regarding appropriate activity levels, both patient and family may impose unnecessary restrictions on daily tasks. They may view an occupa-

TABLE 6-4. *The Functional and Therapeutic Classifications of Patients with Diseases of the Heart with Continuous–Intermittent Permissible Work Loads*

| Functional Class | Continuous-Intermittent | Maximal | Description |
|---|---|---|---|
| I | 4.0–6.0 cal/min. | 6.5 METS | Patients with cardiac disease but without resulting limitations of physical activity; ordinary physical activity does not cause undue fatigue, palpitation, dyspnea, or anginal pain |
| II | 3.0–4.0 cal/min. | 4.5 METS | Patients with cardiac disease resulting in slight limitation of physical activity; they are comfortable at rest; ordinary physical activity results in fatigue, palpitation, dyspnea, or anginal pain |
| III | 2.0–3.0 cal/min. | 3.0 METS | Patients with cardiac disease resulting in marked limitation of physical activity; they are comfortable at rest; less than ordinary physical activity causes fatigue, palpitation, dyspnea, or anginal pain |
| IV | 1.0–2.0 cal/min. | 1.5 METS | Patients with cardiac disease resulting in inability to carry on any physical activity without discomfort; symptoms of cardiac insufficiency or of the anginal syndrome may be present even at rest; if any physical activity is undertaken, discomfort is increased |
| Therapeutic | | | |
| A | | | Patients with cardiac disease whose physical activity need not be restricted in any way |
| B | | | Patients with cardiac disease whose ordinary physical activity need not be restricted, but who should be advised against severe or competitive efforts |
| C | | | Patients with cardiac disease whose ordinary physical activity should be moderately restricted, and whose more strenuous efforts should be discontinued |
| D | | | Patients with cardiac disease whose ordinary physical activity should be markedly restricted |
| E | | | Patients with cardiac disease who should be at complete rest, confined to bed or chair |

Source: Reprinted with permission of the American Heart Association.

tion as too stressful without evaluating the work setting. The patient may consider him or herself an "invalid" and dwell on physical limitations.

Several studies have assessed the white-collar and blue-collar worker returning to work. As the latter is more often involved in work requiring physical activity, for example, laborer or machinist, it is more likely that this individual will have difficulty resuming a former job. The white-collar worker often has a more sedentary job requiring less physical stress, and would probably return to work earlier than the blue-collar worker.

Employers' attitudes, union practices, and company policies as well as physicians' recommendations may be factors preventing return to work. Naughton [34] suggests that theoretically, every stabilized patient of class II cardiovascular status or better should be employable (Table 6-4).

It has been suggested [11, 21, 34] that the most effective method of evaluating the patient for return to work is a complete physical examination including history, ECG, and an exercise tolerance test. The stress test will provide helpful information for determining functional and work capacity. Although such a test may be a viable evaluation tool as early as three weeks post-MI, a maximum stress test usually is performed eight to 12 weeks after the insult [11]. Zohman [43] suggests that the average occupational workload should not exceed one-half to one-third the maximum working capacity and intensity. A conditioning program should be prescribed to assist the patient in achieving a high functional level.

In addition to stress testing and conditioning, group programs have been used to provide support and assist return to work. During these sessions, many patients express fear of resuming their jobs, although the degree of anxiety can vary greatly [4].

A vocational assessment should be included in the cardiac rehabilitation program. Careful evaluation of the present job determines the suitability of the position itself, and physical and environmental considerations. A job description including average work hours, rest periods, and availability of emergency medical care should be obtained. The work conditions and physical requirements are assessed to determine the physical layout, for example, stairs, walking, and transportation to and from the workplace. Environmental concerns include noise level, room temperature, and stress.

## Exercise Testing

Exercise testing has recently gained popularity as an effective evaluation tool. Its two main objectives are (1) to determine the exercise capacity of an individual, and (2) to assess the cardiovascular response to an increase in myocardial oxygen demand. Exercise capacity, and therefore cardiovascular fitness, is best assessed with the maximum oxygen consumption ($VO_2$), a measure of the amount of muscle work performed [13, 40]. As the $VO_2$ is difficult to measure directly, it is estimated with the double product (heart rate multiplied by systolic blood pressure). The cardiovascular response to an increased workload depends on oxygen delivery to the myocardium. As the myocardium already extracts 70 percent of the blood oxygen content, increased cardiac oxygen delivery during work is dependent on increased coronary blood flow [13].

Other indications for an exercise test may be to establish the diagnosis of coronary heart disease, to assess effects of various therapies (medication, cardiac surgery, or physical and occupational therapy), and to detect arrhythmias. Table 6-5 presents contraindications to exercise testing according to the American Heart Association.

Appropriate candidates include people over age 35 years who plan dramatically to increase their level of physical activity, or those of any age who are symptomatic or at high risk for coronary heart disease and plan a major increase in physical exercise.

TABLE 6-5. *Contraindications to Physical Activity Including Exercise Testing*

| Level of Illness | Manifestations |
| --- | --- |
| Acute | Recent myocardial infarction; respiratory, GI, or other febrile illness; phlebitis and embolism |
| Active, chronic, systemic (uncontrolled) | Thyroid, renal, hepatic, rheumatic diseases; gout, etc. |
| Anatomical abnormalities | Uncompensated valvular heart disease; gross cardiomegaly |
| Functional abnormalities | Dysrhythmia; ventricular tachycardia; uncontrolled atrial fibrillation; second and third degree heart block |

Source: From A. A. Kattus. *Exercise Testing and Training of Individuals with Heart Disease or at High Risk for its Development: A Handbook for Physicians.* Dallas: American Heart Association, 1975. With permission.

## EXERCISE TESTS

Exercise tests may measure the maximal or submaximal levels of cardiovascular fitness. The former evaluates fitness level to maximal capacity, until the maximal oxygen uptake is reached. The submaximal test is more commonly used to assess the cardiac patient for whom a predetermined heart rate is designated the endpoint.

Capacity may be evaluated by a one-stage or a multistage test. Master's Step Test, a single-stage exercise, requires the individual to climb two consecutive steps at a predetermined rate. Although this is easily administered and economical, there appears to be individual variability in cardiovascular response, thus making it difficult to standardize. The multistage test is more commonly used for the evaluation of heart patients. Exercise workload is graded and gradually increased to the endpoint: symptoms, predetermined heart rate, or maximum VO$_2$.

These protocols may also be classified as continuous or intermittent. The former requires the individual to exercise continuously as increments increase. The intermittent test allows intervening rest periods as workload increases.

At the present time, several devices are available to assess legwork: treadmill, bicycle ergometer, and Master's Step Test. As many Americans are not accustomed to bicycle riding and develop fatigue in the thigh muscles at a relatively low working rate [12], the treadmill is more commonly used.

Arm cranking or arm ergometer is an effective tool to assess the upper extremity. It is particularly helpful to evaluate patients who are nonambulatory, and those who experience angina during upper extremity work. Some investigators report that myocardial efficiency is lower during armwork, because at peak efforts the double product is disproportionally higher than in legwork [22, 25]. It has been reported that patients with coronary artery disease are able to perform less external armwork before the onset of angina, compared to legwork. Many studies have concluded that heart rate increases more rapidly during armwork than legwork.

It appears that proper positioning is crucial to obtain accurate test results during arm cranking. Astrands [3] states that circulatory responses can fluctuate greatly, depending on the work position. When the arms are held above the shoulders, higher heart rate, blood pressure, and lactate production result.

Clearly, appropriate exercise testing and cardiovascular conditioning must be selected in conjunction with the patient's employment.

## EXERCISE PRESCRIPTION

With the clinical data gathered from an exercise tolerance test, the physician may make an exercise prescription. Haskell [19] states that it should be prescribed "so that during peak exercise, myocardial oxygen demand stays within its oxygen supply limitations while at the same time, there is a sustained increase in the oxygen delivery to the exercising skeletal muscle." The rationale of a conditioning program [39] "is to enable the individual to perform increased total body work without increasing the metabolic costs to the myocardium; that is, to enable him or her to accomplish the required physical effort with less myocardial oxygen consumption." To develop an effective exercise prescription, the type of exercise and its intensity, duration, and frequency should be defined.

Aerobic activities, such as jogging, walking, and cycling, are effective in improving cardiovascular functional capacity. These activities are characteristically isotonic, dynamic, rhythmical, low resistive exercises performed primarily by the large muscle groups [2, 9, 19, 39]. They produce far greater cardiovascular conditioning response than isometric or static exercises, which often produce a more rapid rise in heart rate and blood pressure, even though the activity itself may not be a higher-energy level task. While performing isometric exercises, the tendency to perform a Valsalva maneuver is greater, and certainly should be discouraged.

The exercise intensity may be prescribed in reference to the patient's maximum heart rate or MET level [2, 19] achieved during the test. The recommended intensity is 60 to 80 percent of the functional capacity reached, or 70 to 85 percent of the asymptomatic maximum heart rate reached [2, 19]. If the patient develops angina pectoris or inappropriate ECG changes during the test, activity should be prescribed at 70 to 85 percent of the heart rate at which the symptoms occured [19]. It appears that the conditioning effect will be reached when working at this level of intensity. Ogden and others [22, 35] state that because of individual variation in exercise, body type, room temperature, and emotional factors, MET charts should be used merely as guidelines for true energy expenditure. Maximum oxygen consumption mea-

sured by heart rate and systolic blood pressure is a more accurate way to monitor energy costs. Therefore MET costs are probably most useful in the early phase of a conditioning program, and are replaced by heart rate and blood pressure in the later phases.

To produce a conditioning effect, exercises need to be carried out for 15 to 20 minutes, three to four times weekly over a period of three to four months. Previously sedentary individuals will require more frequent low resistive exercise sessions of shorter duration than those who are more active [2, 12, 19]. For example, a patient who is unable to tolerate one half-hour of exercise would benefit from several short sessions daily to increase overall endurance.

There should always be a warmup period of five to ten minutes consisting of low-MET calisthenics to allow the cardiovascular system to adapt to the increase in physical demand. The actual session of aerobic exercises may last 15 to 40 minutes. At its completion a cooling down period of low-MET activities should continue until the resting preexercise heart rate is obtained.

EXERCISE FOLLOWING HOSPITALIZATION
Home discharge presents another phase in the recovery process. In some progressive rehabilitation programs, patients are evaluated at submaximal exercise levels to assess functional capacity at the time of discharge. During the home phase, the individual slowly resumes daily tasks (i.e., housekeeping or gardening), and is reminded to refer to a MET table as a guideline in the selection of appropriate activities (Table 6-6).

In many cases, the patient will be ready for a medically supervised exercise program eight to 12 weeks post-MI. At this time, low-level calisthenics and walking programs may be recommended. The patient should be carefully instructed in pulse-taking and signs of fatigue. The target heart rate range should be clearly understood. In conjunction with the fitness program, educational material and

TABLE 6-6. *MET Tables*

| Self-Care Activities for a 70K Man | | | Housework Activities | | |
|---|---|---|---|---|---|
| Activity | Cal/Min. | METS[a] | Task | Cal/Min. | METS |
| Rest, supine | 1.0 | 1 | Hand sewing | 1.4 | 1 |
| Sitting | 1.2 | 1 | Sweeping floor | 1.7 | 1.5 |
| Standing, relaxed | 1.4 | 1 | Machine sewing | 1.8 | 1.5 |
| Eating | 1.4 | 1 | Polishing furniture | 2.4 | 2 |
| Conversation | 1.4 | 1 | Peeling potatoes | 2.9 | 2.5 |
| Dressing, undressing | 2.3 | 2 | Scrubbing, standing | 2.9 | 2.5 |
| Washing hands, face | 2.5 | 2 | Washing small clothes | 3.0 | 2.5 |
| Bedside commode | 3.6 | 3 | Kneading dough | 3.3 | 2.5 |
| Walking, 2.5 mph | 3.6 | 3 | Scrubbing floors | 3.6 | 3 |
| Showering | 4.2 | 3.5 | Cleaning windows | 3.7 | 3 |
| Using bedpan | 4.7 | 4 | Making beds | 3.9 | 3 |
| Walking downstairs | 5.2 | 4.5 | Ironing, standing | 4.2 | 3.5 |
| Walking, 3.5 mph | 5.6 | 5.5 | Mopping | 4.2 | 3.5 |
| Propulsion, wheelchair | 2.4 | 2 | Wringing by hand | 4.4 | 3.5 |
| Ambulation, braces, | | | Hanging wash | 4.5 | 3.5 |
| crutches | 8.0 | 6.5 | Beating lcarpets | 4.9 | 4 |

[a]METS: Metabolic equivalent—approximate resting energy expenditure.
Source: Reprinted with permission from the Colorado Heart Association.

TABLE 6-6. (*Continued*)

| Industrial Activities | | | Recreational Activities | | |
|---|---|---|---|---|---|
| Task | Cal/Min. | METS | Activity | Cal/Min. | METS |
| Watch repairing | 1.6 | 1.5 | Painting, sitting | 2.0 | 1.5 |
| Armature winding | 2.2 | 2.0 | Playing piano | 2.5 | 2 |
| Radio assembly | 2.7 | 2.5 | Driving car | 2.8 | 2 |
| Sewing at machine | 2.9 | 2.5 | Canoeing, 2.5 mph | 3.0 | 2.5 |
| | | | Horseback riding, | | |
| Bricklaying | 4.0 | 3.5 | slowly | 3.0 | 2.5 |
| Plastering | 4.1 | 3.5 | Volleyball | 3.0 | 2.5 |
| Tractor ploughing | 4.2 | 3.5 | Bowling | 4.4 | 3.5 |
| Wheeling barrow | | | Cycling, 5.5 mph | 4.5 | 3.5 |
| 115 lbs., 2.5 mph | 5.0 | 4.0 | Golfing | 5.0 | 4 |
| Horse ploughing | 5.9 | 5.0 | Swimming, 20 yd./min. | 5.0 | 4 |
| Carpentry | 6.8 | 5.5 | Dancing | 5.5 | 4.5 |
| | | | Gardening | 5.6 | 4.5 |
| Mowing lawn by hand | 7.7 | 6.5 | Tennis | 7.1 | 6 |
| Felling tree | 8.0 | 6.5 | Trotting horse | 8.0 | 6.5 |
| Shoveling | 8.5 | 7.0 | Spading | 8.6 | 7 |
| Ascending stairs | | | Skiing | 9.9 | 8 |
| 17-lb. load, 27'/min. | 9.0 | 7.5 | Squash | 10.2 | 8.5 |
| Planing | 9.1 | 7.5 | Cycling, 13 mph | 11.0 | 9 |
| Tending furnace | 10.2 | 8.5 | | | |
| Ascending stairs | | | | | |
| 22-lb. load, 54'/min. | 16.2 | 13.5 | | | |

emotional support groups can be useful in helping the individual regain functional independence.

# References

1. Abramson, J.H., and Hopp, C. The control of cardiovascular risk factors in the elderly. *Prevent. Med.* 5: 32, 1976.
2. American College of Sports Medicine Subcommittee. *Guidelines for Graded Exercise Testing and Exercise Prescription.* Philadelphia: Lea and Febiger, 1976.
3. Astrands, I. Circulatory response to arm exercise in different work positions. *Scand. J. Clin. Lab. Invest.* 27: 293, 1971.
4. Bierman, E. L. Atherosclerosis and Other Forms of Arteriosclerosis. In K. J. Isselbacher, R.D. Adams, E. Braunwald, R. G. Petersdorf, et al. (Eds.). *Harrison's Principles of Internal Medicine* (9th ed.). New York: McGraw Hill, 1980.
5. Bilodeau, C. B., and Hackett, T. P. Issues raised in a group setting by patients recovering from myocardial infarction. *Am. J. Psychiatry* 128:73, 1971.
6. Blumenthal, J. A. Type A behavior pattern and coronary atherosclerosis. *Circulation* 58:634, 1978.
7. Borhani, N. O. Primary prevention of coronary heart disease: A critique. *Am. J. Cardiol.* 40:251, 1977.
8. Bracken, M. B., Bracken, M., Landry, A. B., Jr., et al. Patient education by videotape after myocardial infarction: An empirical evaluation. *Arch. Phys. Med. Rehabil.* 58:213, 1977.
9. Bruce, R. A. Methods of exercise testing. *Am. J. Cardiol.* 33:715, 1974.
10. Cassem, N. H., and Hackett, T. P. Psychological rehabilitation of myocardial infarction patients in the acute phase. *Heart Lung* 2:382, 1973.
11. Dehn, M. M., and Mullins, C. B. Physiologic effects and importance of exercise in patients with coronary artery disease. *Cardiovasc. Med.* 2:365 April 1977.
12. *Exercise Testing and Training of Individuals with Heart Disease or at High Risk for Its Development: A Handbook for Physicians.* Dallas: American Heart Association, 1975.
13. Fortuin, N. J., and Weiss, J. L. Exercise stress testing. *Circulation* 56:699, 1977.
14. Friedman, M., and Rosenman, R. H. *Type A Behavior and Your Heart.* New York: Knopf, 1978.
15. Gruen, W. A therapeutic program to change tension-producing life habits. *Pract. Cardiol.* 5(3):195, 1979.
16. Hackett, T. P. *Patient Psychology.* American Heart Association, 1975.
17. Hackett, T. P., and Cassem, N. H. Psychological Adaptation to Convalescence in Myocardial Infarction Patients. In J. Naughton and H. K. Hellerstein (Eds.). *Exercise Testing and Exercise Training in Coronary Heart Disease.* New York: Academic, 1973.
18. Hackett, T.P., and Cassem, N. H. Psychological Aspects of Rehabilitation After Myocardial Infarction. In W. K. Wenger and H. K. Hellerstein (Eds.). *Rehabilitation of the Coronary Patient.* New York: Wiley, 1978.
19. Haskell, W. L. Design and Implementation of Cardiac Conditioning Program. In N. K. Wenger and H. K. Hellerstein (Eds.). *Rehabilitation of the Coronary Patient.* New York: Wiley, 1978.
20. *Heart Facts.* New York: American Heart Association, 1979.
21. Hellerstein, H. K. Rehabilitation of the Postinfarction Patient. In *The Myocardium: Failure and Infarction.* New York: H. P., 1974.
22. Hellerstein, H. K., and Franklin, B. A. Exercise Testing and Prescription. In N. K. Wenger and H. K. Hellerstein (Eds.). *Rehabilitation of the Coronary Patient.* New York: Wiley, 1978.
23. Hellerstein, H. K. and Friedman, E. H. Sexual activity and the postcoronary patient. *Arch. Intern. Med.* 125:987, 1970.
24. Hellerstein, H. K., and Wenger, N. K. (Eds.). *Rehabilitation of the Coronary Patient.* New York: Wiley, 1978.
25. Hjeltnes, N. Oxygen uptake and cardiac output in graded arm exercise in paraplegics with low-level spinal lesion. *Scand. J. Rehabil. Med.* 9:107, 1977.
26. Jenkins, C. D. Recent evidence supporting psychologic and social risk factors for coronary disease, part 2. *Engl. J. Med.* 294:1033, 1976.
27. Jenkins, C. D. Coronary-prone behavior: One pattern or several? *Psychosom. Med.* 40:25, 1978.
28. Kannel, W. B. Some lessons in cardiovascular epidemiology from Framingham. *Am. J. Cardiol.* 37:269, 1976.
29. Kannel, W. B. Recent findings of the Framingham study—I. *Med. Times* 106(4):23, 1978.
30. Kolodny, R. C., Masters, W. H., and Johnson, V. E. *Textbook of Sexual Medicine.* Boston: Little, Brown, 1979.
31. Leach, C. N., and Scoppetta, D. J. Cardiac

rehabilitation: The New Britain program. *Conn. Med.* 41:270, 1977.

32. Mann, J. V. Current concepts, diet–heart: End of an era. *N. Engl. J. Med.* 297(12):644, 1977.

33. Matheson, L. N., Selvester, R. H., Rice, H. E. The interdisciplinary team in cardiac rehabilitation. *Rehabil. Lit.* 12:366, 1975.

34. Naughton, J. Vocational Aspects of Rehabilitation After Myocardial Infarction. In N. K. Wenger and H. K. Hellerstein (Eds.). *Rehabilitation of the Coronary Patient.* New York: Wiley, 1978.

35. Ogden, L. D. Activity guidelines for early subacute and high-risk cardiac patients. *Am. J. Occup. Ther.* 33: 291, 1979.

36. Owens, J. F., McCann, C. S., Hutelmyer, C. M. Cardiac rehabilitation: A patient education program. *Nurs. Res.* 27(3): 148, 1978

37. Rosenman, R. H., and Friedman, M. Neurogenic factors in pathogenesis of coronary heart disease. *Med. Clin. North Am.* 58:269, 1974.

38. Rosenman, R. H., Brand, R. J., Sholtz, R. I., et al. Epidemiology: Multivariate prediction of coronary heart disease during 8.5 year follow-up in the Western Collaborative Group study. *Am. J. Cardiol.* 37:903, 1976.

39. Scheuer, J., et al. *Modern Concepts of Cardiovascular Disease.* Dallas: American Heart Association, 1978.

40. Shaper, A. G. Prevention of coronary heart disease. *Lancet* 2(7996):1203, 1976.

41. Simonelli, C., and Eaton, R. P. Cardiovascular and metabolic effects of exercise. *Postgrad. Med.* 63(2):71, 1978.

42. Stamler, J. *Lifestyles, Major Risk Factors, Proof and Public Policy.* Chicago: Department of Community Health and Preventive Medicine, Northwestern University Medical School, 1978.

43. Zohman, L. R. *Beyond Diet . . . Exercise Your Way to Fitness.* Dallas: American Heart Association, 1974.

# Appendix

*Lecture Series for Cardiac Education. Designed to educate the cardiac patient and family regarding the heart and heart disease, risk factors, diet management, energy conservation, and stress management. Lectures are presented by the team members once weekly, each session lasting approximately one and one-half hours.*

I. The heart and heart disease

A. Basic anatomy and physiology of the heart including the concept of the heart as a pump, size and rate, the circulatory system, normal blood pressure, and the coronary arteries

B. Heart disease, including CAD, angina, MI, CHF, and how the heart recovers from MI

C. Warning signs such as chest pain, shortness of breath, dizziness or fainting, sudden change in heart rate, swelling in the lower extremities, sudden weight gain, and general weakness

D. Cardiac medications emphasizing common side effects, contraindications, and medication schedule

*Educational Materials*

Film: Heart Attack—Recognition and Response. Produced by KCET-TV in conjunction with the Los Angeles County Heart Association, 1971 (28 minutes).

Handouts: *The Heart and Blood Vessels.* New York: American Heart Association, 1973.

*Your Heart and How It Works.* American Heart Association.

Hollander, L. *Take Heart.* Boston: Massachusetts Rehabilitation Hospital, 1976.

Additional resources:

From the American Heart Association

*About Your Heart and Your Blood Stream,*

*After A Coronary,*

*Facts About Congestive Heart Failure,*

*Facts About Your Heart and Blood Vessel Disease,*

*Fears, Fables and Facts About Heart Disease,*

*Heart Attack,*

*If You Have Angina,*

*The Heart and Blood Vessels,*

*You and Your Heart.*

Further reading:

*Back in Circulation.* North Carolina Myocardial Infarction Rehabilitation Program. North Carolina Heart Association, 1975.

Jenkins, D. *Coronary Artery Disease.* North Carolina Heart Association, 1976.

Lee, E., et al. *Heart*. Maryland: Robert J. Brady Corporation, 1973.

II. Risk factors

A. Review of risk factors with emphasis on those that can be modified

B. Hypertension and the damage it causes if untreated; control of hypertension through medication, diet, avoiding stress and smoking

C. Explanation of use of a blood pressure cuff and demonstration of how to use it

D. Smoking and its impact on heart disease with information on community "quit smoking" programs and common sense approaches to giving up smoking, such as substitutes, e.g., exercise, activity

E. Discussion of the risk of a sedentary lifestyle and the benefits of moderate exercise

F. Precautions such as avoiding extremes in environmental temperature when exercising, including avoiding exercise in polluted areas; allowing enough time when walking to incorporate rest time; not pushing

G. Discussion of the necessity to control diabetes through diet and weight adjustment and use of insulin

*Educational Materials*

Film: Our Way of Life. Produced by the American Heart Association, 1974(27 minutes).

Handout: *Reduce Your Risk of Heart Attack*. Dallas: American Heart Association, 1974.

Additional resources:

From the American Heart Association

*Heart Quiz,*

*Why Risk Heart Attack.*

Hypertension

Film: What Goes Up. Produced by the American Heart Association

Booklets: *High Blood Pressure and How to Control It*. American Heart Association.

*Hypertension: High Blood Pressure*. DHEW Publication No. NIH 1714.

*Let's Talk About Hypertension*. New York: Bristol Laboratory, Division of Bristol-Myers Company, 1975.

*Understanding High Blood Pressure*. San Juan, Puerto Rico: 1976.

*Watch Your Blood Pressure!* The High Blood Pressure Information Center. Bethesda: National Institutes of Health.

Smoking

Films: Bill Talman. Trigger Films, American Cancer Society.

Ashes to Ashes. Produced by the Searle Educational Systems.

Quit, Quit Again. Produced by the National Clearing House for Smoking and Health, U.S. Public Health Service.

The Embattled Cell. Produced by the American Heart Association.

Booklets: *How to Stop Smoking*. American Heart Association.

*If You Want to Give Up Cigarettes*. American Cancer Society.

*Staying Alive*. DHEW Publication No. HSM 73-8705.

*Unless You Decide to Quit*. National Clearing House for Smoking and Health.

*When a Woman Smokes*. American Cancer Society.

*Yes, There Are a Lot of Good Reasons for Women to Quit Smoking*. DHEW Publication No. HSM 73–8713.

Physical Activity

Book: *Exercise Your Way to Fitness and Heart Health*. Englewood Cliffs, N.J.: Best Foods Division, CPC International.

Diabetes

Booklets: *Understanding Diabetes*. New York: Pfizer Lab Division, Pfizer Inc., 1972.

*You and Diabetes*. Upjohn Company, July, 1971.

III. Diet

A. Review of importance of dietary management with regard to heart disease

B. American Heart Association Prudent Diet

C. Explanation of terms such as: cholesterol, lipids, polyunsaturated, monounsaturated and saturated fats

D. Principles of modifying eating behavior and weight reduction

E. Discussion of sodium restricted diets

F. Information on careful grocery shopping, such as reading labels of products to determine the ingredients and nutrition content, thus enabling dietary management

G. Suggestions for dietary management when eating in restaurants

*Educational Materials*

Film: Eat to Your Heart's Content. Produced by the American Heart Association, 1968 (12½ minutes).

Handout: *The Heart Saver Eating Style.* Chicago Heart Association, Nutrition Education Project, American Heart Association, 1975.

Additional resources:

From the American Heart Association

*A Guide for Weight Reduction,*

*Eat Well but Eat Wisely,*

*Planning Fat-Controlled Meals for 1200–1800 Calories,*

*Planning Fat-Controlled Meals for 2000–2600 Calories,*

*Recipes for Fat-Controlled, Low Cholesterol Meals,*

*Save Food, Money and Help Your Heart.*

*The American Heart Association Cookbook.* New York: David McKay.

*The Way to a Man's Heart*

Mueller, J. F. Plain talk about a confusing matter. *Nutrition Today.* May/June, 1974.

*Sensible Eating Can Be Delicious.* Elm City, N.C.: Fleischmann's.

Additional films:

Eat Right to Your Heart's Delight. Produced by the International Producers Services.

Food, Energy and You. Produced by the Wexler Film Productions.

One Way of Life. Produced by the American Heart Association.

Three Times a Day. Produced by MEDCOM.

IV. Energy conservation

A. Reinforcement of principles of energy conservation and work simplification during activities of daily living

B. Energy conservation techniques: sit whenever possible, use both hands in opposite and symmetrical motions, slide objects and avoid lifting, eliminate unnecessary motions, use gravity, pre-position tools

C. Work simplification techniques: establish work centers; locate switches, appliances, etc., within easy reach; use modern conveniences and appliances; eliminate unnecessary work, e.g., no-iron sheets, clothing; use trays, push carts, etc., to carry several items

D. Alternatives to heavy work activities, i.e., let another family member do it, hire assistance

E. Reinforcement of the need for rest periods throughout the day

F. MET charts for assistance with recognizing appropriate activity levels

*Educational Materials*

Slide show: Energy Conservation. Produced by Aim for Health, Boston.

Handout: *Easy Does It.* Michigan Heart Association, 1969.

Additional resources:

May, E. E., et al. *Homemaking for the Handicapped.* New York: Dodd, Mead, 1966.

V. Stress management

A. Review of the effects of daily stress and suggest alternative behavior

B. Discussion of the body's physiological response to stress

C. Ways to reduce tension and stress in our lives: avocational activities, proper amount of sleep at night, physical exercise, pacing activities, established time for relaxation, time management techniques such as setting priorities, developing a daily agenda that includes leisure activities,

rest periods, and job-related tasks, flexibility in scheduling
D.Relaxation techniques
*Educational Materials*
Film: Gotta Lotta Livin' to Do. Produced by the New Jersey Heart Association (14 minutes).
Handout: *Stress.* Metropolitan Life Insurance Co., 1967.
Additional resources:
Bensen, H. *The Relaxation Response.* New York: Avon, 1975.
*Stress Management.* New England Memorial Hospital, Stoneham, Mass.

## Addresses

American Cancer Society
219 East 42nd Street
New York, NY 10017

American Heart Association
7320 Greenville Avenue
Dallas, TX 75231

Best Foods Division, CPC International
International Plaza
Englewood Cliffs, NJ 07632

Fleischmann's
Box 1180
Elm City, NC 27822

International Producers Services
3518 Cahuenga Blvd.
West Hollywood, CA

MEDCOM
2 Hammarskjold Plaza
New York, NY 10017

National Clearing House for Smoking and Health
5401 Westlund Avenue
Bethesda, MD 20016

Superintendent of Documents
U.S. Government Printing Office
Washington, D.C. 20402

Searle Educational Systems
G. D. Searle Company
Box 5110
Chicago, IL 60680

Wexler Film Productions
Los Angeles, CA 90038

# 7 PULMONARY REHABILITATION

*Judith Falconer*

Pulmonary rehabilitation represents perhaps the newest of the rehabilitation medicine specialties. In recent years, more attention has been paid to this field because of massive and increasing incidence of pulmonary disease, and the failure of medical care alone to provide effective treatment. In addition, the rising cost of pulmonary disease to the economy in terms of unemployment, hospitalization, and medical care has stimulated interest in finding more effective, cost-efficient methods of treatment.

By nature of the problems inherent in the disease it is frustrating and difficult to treat. The insidious onset often prevents early diagnosis and intervention. Late stages of medical management are characteristically symptomatic rather than curative. Pulmonary disease effectively remains an irreversible, progressive condition.

Rehabilitation has not been documented as causing improvement in respiratory function, yet the functional gains reported by patients postrehabilitation cannot be overlooked. Although the disease appears to remain essentially unaltered and the incidence of mortality unaffected, it has been demonstrated that patients can improve in functional abilities, endurance, comfort, and general well-being through rehabilitation. They reportedly breathe more easily, experience less anxiety, and retain a higher level of functional independence for a longer time. Patients who have completed rehabilitation programs describe themselves as more hopeful, optimistic, and active. Some evidence also exists that suggests

that they may require less hospitalization than patients who have not had such a program [6, 7].

Exactly why they improve remains unclear. It has been said that perhaps it is a result of the supportive, encouraging atmosphere provided by an interested team of professionals. It may be that limitations in understanding respiratory physiology preclude analysis of the true effect of rehabilitation on function. For these reasons, the approach to the patient with pulmonary disease should be positive, dynamic, multidisciplinary, and progressive. The general aims should be (1) to improve the quality and comfort of life, (2) to increase functional independence, and (3) to decrease the need for costly hospitalization.

Although acute respiratory care will be occasionally mentioned, it is not the function or intent of this chapter to discuss it. The minimal inclusion is only to foster a general understanding of the types of medical treatment administered, and their possible effects or complications on rehabilitation. The purpose is rather to describe a practical approach to the evaluation and treatment of pulmonary dysfunction, and to encourage a positive investigatory attitude in therapists involved in the care of these patients.

## Respiration and Respiratory Disorders

*Respiration* is the process by which oxygen is transferred from the atmosphere into the blood, and the waste product of metabolism,

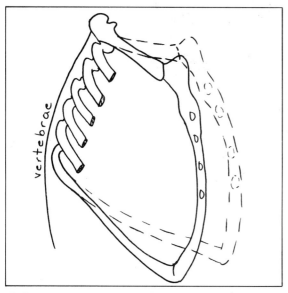

FIGURE 7-1. *Movement of the ribs during inspiration (dotted line) and expiration (solid line).*

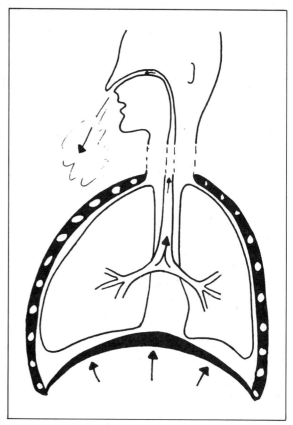

FIGURE 7-3. *Elevation of the diaphragm and deflation of the lungs on expiration.*

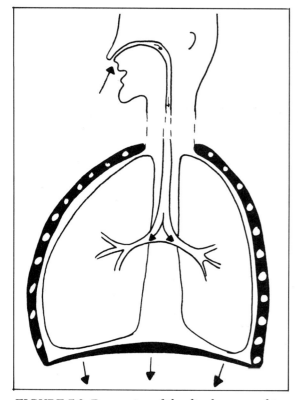

FIGURE 7-2. *Depression of the diaphragm and inflation of the lungs on inspiration.*

carbon dioxide, is removed from the body. Although it can be voluntarily controlled to some extent, it is essentially a subconscious procedure. Difficult breathing is the body's attempt to compensate for ineffectual respiration.

On inspiration, thoracic volume is increased by (1) contraction of the intercostal muscles which elevates the ribs (Figure 7-1), and (2) contraction of the diaphragm that depresses the floor of the thoracic cavity (Figure 7-2). This volume change allows the elastic lungs to expand, thereby drawing air in from the upper air passages. On expiration the reverse occurs (Figure 7-3). Relaxation of the diaphragm and intercostal muscles decreases total thoracic volume. The lungs recoil and air is forced out through the upper air passages. This is the basis of the complex process of *ventilation.*

Mechanical air filtering and mucociliary clearance action in the airways protect the lungs from microbial invasion. Small hairs in the nose act as the mechanical filters that help purify inspired air. Foreign particles also adhere to the mucous linings of the bronchus and are then brought up for expulsion by ciliary action. Irritants such as cigarette smoke depress ciliary action and alter mucous viscosity, thereby damaging the pulmonary defense mechanisms.

Within the lungs *diffusion* occurs. Oxygen diffuses or is transferred across the alveolar walls into the pulmonary capillaries, and carbon dioxide is transferred from the capillaries back into the alveoli for expiration. From the pulmonary capillaries oxygen can then be circulated in the blood to the tissues. *Perfusion* refers to passage of gases to and from the tissues.

The respiratory center in the medulla oblongata regulates the rate and depth of ventilation. When carbon dioxide and oxygen tensions in the blood are altered as with exercise, the center signals the respiratory muscles to adjust the ventilation rate, thereby restoring normal gas tensions.

For clarity, it is convenient to categorize pulmonary disorders into two descriptive groups. In the most prevalent are the *airflow obstructive disorders,* most commonly occurring as chronic bronchitis, emphysema, asthma, bronchiectasis, and cystic fibrosis. These disorders resemble each other in that they all obstruct or in some way increase resistance to the normal flow of air into the lungs. They differ, however, in pathology, etiology, and prognosis.

Chronic bronchitis, for example, is a condition of increased mucus production along the bronchial walls. The excess secretions clog the air passageways. On normal inspiration insufficient air would be delivered to the lungs. In asthma, bronchoconstrictions, or spasms, narrow the bronchi, increasing the resistance to air flow particularly on expiration. Chronic bronchitis is thought to be induced by cigarette smoking and exposure to atmospheric pollution, while asthma appears to be an allergic reaction of unclear etiology. Nevertheless, they both result in obstruction of normal air flow, and for the purpose of rehabilitation can be discussed together.

The term *chronic obstructive pulmonary disease* (COPD) usually refers to chronic bronchitis, emphysema, and asthma. By far the greatest majority of obstructive disorders are COPD. The rehabilitation modalities for all are similar, and most of this chapter will focus on these disorders.

In the second category of pulmonary dysfunction are *restrictive disorders.* Air flow may be normal, but gas exchange is insufficient because of a reduction in interthoracic spaces or small lung volume. Restrictive disorders occur with some neuromuscular diseases such as poliomyelitis and spinal cord injury. In these conditions, paralysis of the external muscles of respiration prevents normal chest expansion on inspiration, thus reducing the available space for ventilation and diffusion. Severe skeletal disorders such as kyphoscoliosis may also cause a restrictive defect in respiration as a result of the physical derangement of respiratory structures (Figure 7-4). Following thoracic surgery, ventilation may be impaired due to

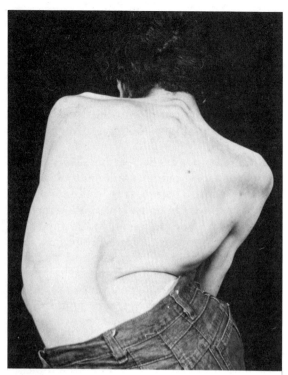

FIGURE 7-4. *Severe spinal deformity that causes a restrictive defect.*

trauma to the intercostals, pain, suturing of the respiratory accessory muscles, or removal of lung tissue.

In restrictive disorders, pulmonary dysfunction is frequently secondary to the patient's overall functional disability. In addition, treatment regimens are well-defined medically accepted practices, and do not for the most part require a comprehensive rehabilitation team approach. The procedures for restrictive disease management are therefore given less attention in this chapter. The reader is referred to the sources in Suggested Reading for more detailed information regarding treatment of restrictive disorders.

## Problems Associated with Pulmonary Disease

The most apparent dysfunction of obstructive pulmonary disease is *dyspnea*, difficult breathing. Its degree and frequency are not reliable indexes of the severity of disease, but it is the most distressing symptom in these disorders. Dyspnea occurs whenever respiration is insufficient to supply the body's oxygen requirements. On normal exertion, the demand for oxygen is greater and the rate of respiration increases to supply the need. In the diseased state, when the capacity to increase oxygen consumption and carbon dioxide expulsion is impaired, the medulla still signals for greater ventilation. The result is rapid but shallow, ineffectual airway exchange. Compensatory measures increase the effort and rate of breathing, but not efficiency. The patient begins to gasp for air or inhale in excess of proportional exhalation. This further disturbs the gas exchange balance and the net result is the frightening, painful sensation of dyspnea.

Dyspnea may be induced by emotional upset or exposure to lung irritants and polluted atmospheric conditions, but usually occurs on physical activity when the body's energy demands increase. It varies depending on the disease state from minimal, occurring only with strenuous activities; to severe, occurring at rest. The patient consequently attempts to reduce physical activity to avoid dyspneic attacks until gradually a more sedentary lifestyle results. The insufficient gas exchange compounded by a progressive reduction in physical activity eventually creates a generalized debilitated state characterized by low endurance and weakness. At the time they experience waning energies patients withdraw from social, vocational, and leisure activities that exceed their activity tolerance. As the disease worsens greater physical restrictions are imposed. It is not uncommon for patients with severe COPD to be physically limited to life within the confines of their homes.

Anxiety, depression, and preoccupation with somatic concerns frequently accompany obstructive pulmonary disease. Characteristic decreasing physical abilities, fear of dyspnea, and social withdrawal contribute to the creation of the respiratory cripple. An excessive concern with breathing and failing health further exacerbates the symptoms of pulmonary dysfunction. Ironically, efforts to avoid respiratory distress often result in unnecessary restrictions in patients' daily lives, and greater losses in functional independence and physical health.

Obstructive pulmonary disease is a vicious cycle of inefficient respiration that results in discomfort and neuromuscular deconditioning, which reduce physical and mental capabilities and lead to even less efficient respiration. A well-coordinated, intensive multidisciplinary approach can reduce the degree of disability and provide effective rehabilitation by intervening in these closely related aspects of dysfunction.

## Evaluating the Patient

In evaluating the patient with pulmonary disease, two important aspects must be explored: medically, the type and extent of disease; and therapeutically, the resultant degree of dysfunction.

Physical examination, chest radiography, pulmonary function testing (PFT), auscultation, and blood gas analysis are performed. Although these are a physician's functions, proper assessment and implementation of all therapeutic modalities require an understanding of these measures by every member of the team. Measures of strength, range of motion (ROM), activity tolerance, activities of daily living (ADL), independence, social adaptation, vocational potential, perception and cerebration, and mental status are the foundations for determining functional deficits.

### PHYSICAL EXAMINATION

In addition to a careful examination of the patient's upper and lower respiratory tracts, temperature, rate and character of respiration, volume and description of sputum, frequency and quality of cough, electrocardiogram, and medical history are noted. Posture, general appear-ance, and vocal quality are also observed and recorded.

### RADIOGRAPHS

Chest radiographs are commonly ordered whenever respiratory dysfunction is suspected. Posteroanterior (PA) views of the chest on maximum inspiration are usually taken. A normal appearance does not necessarily indicate absence of early pulmonary disease; in general, however, radiographs are of greater benefit in diagnosing later stages.

### PULMONARY FUNCTION TESTS

Spirometry is the simplest yet most valuable tool to measure ventilation. It uses the measures of forced expiratory volume in 1 second ($FEV_1$) and forced vital capacity (FVC) to differentiate obstructive from restrictive disease, and to quantitate the extent of lung damage. Briefly, $FEV_1$ is the maximum volume of air a patient can forcibly expire in one second, and FVC is the volume of air that can be forcibly expired after maximum inspiration. The former measures air flow, and the latter measures lung volume. The results are calculated against normal values for the height, age, and sex of the patient.

In restrictive defects, both $FEV_1$ and FVC are reduced indicating small lung volumes. In obstructive defects FVC may be normal, but $FEV_1$ is decreased indicating an air flow obstruction within normal volumes.

A simple spirometer measures these volumes. The patient breathes into the machine (Figure 7-5) and the information is returned on a graph of volume over time (Figure 7-6). A simpler device, the peak flowmeter, may also be used to measure expiratory volume (Figure 7-7).

Spirometry with helium dilution measures static lung volumes (Figure 7-8). Helium gas is not absorbed in the lungs and can be used to measure air flow volumes. This procedure quantitates the total lung capacity (TLC), which is the vital capacity (VC—amount of expired air following one maximum inspiration)

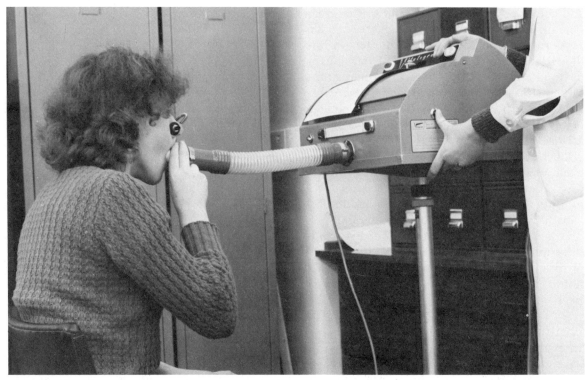

FIGURE 7-5. *Simple spirometry measuring FEV₁ and FVC. (Lung Function Laboratory, The London Hospital, Whitechapel)*

plus the residual volume (RV—amount of air remaining in the lungs after maximum expiration):

$$TLC = VC + RV.$$

The VC and FVC are the same with normal lungs, but may be different in COPD because of "air trapping." Air is trapped in the alveoli because of bronchiole collapse, thus reducing expiratory volume.

In restrictive disorders TLC, VC, and RV are all reduced indicating lung volumes smaller than normal. In obstructive disorders, TLC (air space) may be normal, but VC (air flow) is reduced and RV (residual static air) is increased, indicating resistance to air flow.

Transfer factor (diffusion capacity) is a slightly more complex measurement of gas exchange across the alveolar membranes. Reduced transfer factor usually indicates a restrictive defect.

AUSCULTATION

Auscultation, the use of a stethoscope to detect chest sounds, gives valuable information as to the nature of the obstructive or restrictive disorder. Crepitations, or fine crackly sounds on inspiration are characteristic of alveolar congestion, as in pulmonary edema or lung fibrosis. Rhonchi, lower-pitched longer wheezing sounds, signify airway obstruction, or "clogs," usually in the bronchioles. The physician must identify the particulars of the many breath sounds, but the chest therapist should know the most common ones and understand their origins and implications for treatment. Chest sounds before and after therapy should be

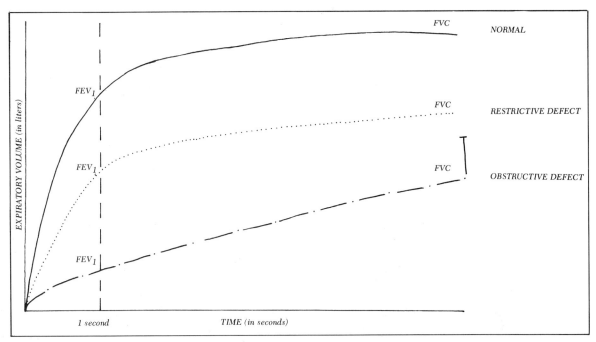

FIGURE 7-6. *Results of simple spirometry demon-strating the differences among restrictive, obstruc-tive and normal air flow, and lung volumes on expi-ration.*

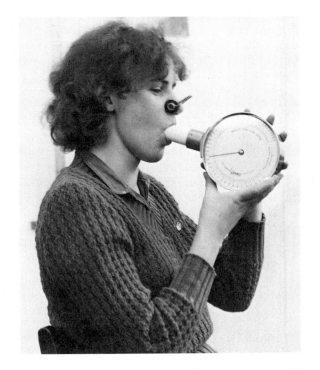

FIGURE 7-7. *Use of the peak flowmeter. (Lung Function Laboratory, The London Hospital, White-chapel)*

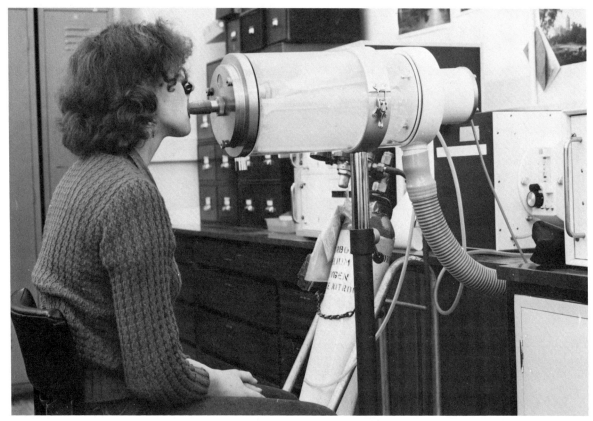

FIGURE 7-8. *Measuring TLC, VC, and RV, static lung volumes. (Lung Function Laboratory, The London Hospital, Whitechapel)*

studied to determine the value of the treatment.

## BLOOD GAS STUDIES

Blood gas studies evaluate perfusion, arterial tensions of oxygen, and carbon dioxide. The partial pressure of oxygen ($PaO_2$), partial pressure of carbon dioxide ($PaCO_2$), hemoglobin saturation of oxygen, carbon dioxide content, and acidity (pH) of arterial blood are measured. Abnormalities indicate insufficient alveolar/capillary gas exchange and lung ventilation, although these are not exclusively caused by pulmonary disease. Anemias, hysterical hyperventilation, and cardiac disease, to name a few, also result in abnormal blood gas studies.

In a healthy person, $PaCO_2$ remains constant at about 40 mm Hg, whereas $PaO_2$ falls slightly throughout adult life from about 104 mm Hg in the newborn to about 72 mm Hg in the 72-year-old. Oxygen hemoglobin saturation, however, is sufficient until the $PaO_2$ drops below around 60 mm Hg.*

The regulatory mechanisms of respiration in the medulla are sensitive to changes in arterial gas tensions. Increased $PaCO_2$ acts as a respiratory stimulant. The patient breathes harder to expire the excess carbon dioxide and restore gas balance. A fixed increase in $PaCO_2$ indicates severe lung disease. At very low levels

*These numerical values apply only to measurements taken from patients who live at sea level.

206

mental status changes such as memory deficits, confusion, irritability, and restlessness may occur.

## FUNCTIONAL ASSESSMENT

A good evaluation of functional abilities not only defines the dysfunction, but helps to establish goals of rehabilitation. It also delineates the specific areas requiring intervention, provides a means to measure improvement or change, and gives valuable assistance in recognizing the limits of rehabilitation. Improving function is undoubtedly the most important aspect of pulmonary rehabilitation, therefore great care should be taken in proper assessment. The time required to do so is justified when it results in more realistic, goal-oriented, time- and cost-efficient programs.

## STRENGTH AND RANGE OF MOTION

Strength and range of motion can be measured using standard practices of goniometry and manual muscle testing. As this is unlikely to be an area of major deficit, a quick estimation of the percentage of full range of motion at the large joints is usually adequate. Gross motor muscle strength can be similarly recorded as within normal limits, or minimally, moderately, or severely impaired.

## ACTIVITY TOLERANCE

Timed repetitive activity best measures activity tolerance. Pulse and respiratory rates taken before and after activity give some indication of the effort involved. The quantity of work produced and the time required to do it indicate activity tolerance. Walking, stair climbing, stationary bicycling, and so forth can all be used effectively to measure tolerance. In some instances, it may be appropriate to evaluate the patient sitting and performing upper extremity repetitive activity using reciprocal pulleys or nonresistive range-of-motion exercises.

As these are intended to be measures of activity tolerance and not maximum work capacity, evaluation should be discontinued when dyspnea obviously impairs performance or when the patient is no longer able to continue. Endurance, not strength, is the important feature, therefore the use of resistive activities is discouraged.

## ADL

Ability to perform each activity of daily living (ADL) is less important to evaluate than the ability to perform a series of activities comfortably in a reasonable amount of time.

Dyspnea on exertion and early fatigue are likely to be the major limiting factors to self-care. A task such as dressing should be assessed in terms of the length of time needed to complete it, the degree and intervals at which dyspnea occurs, and the effort it requires. The patient who can independently bathe and dress, but finishes totally exhausted and dyspenic is functionally and practically not independent.

Mobility requires similar assessment, but it is slightly easier to document the distances walked or number of stairs climbed in a given amount of time. Equally important as time or distance is the energy an activity requires and the degree of discomfort it causes. As with any other aspect of ADL, mobility must be evaluated in terms of functional independence and not of individual tasks. Again, a patient who can climb a flight of stairs by stopping after each step and resting a minute is not functionally independent.

Home and work responsibilities should also be given consideration. The patient's energy needs must be individually determined as there is obviously no standard of performance against which life-styles can be measured. If exertional dyspnea prevents a patient from fulfilling daily tasks at work, home, or socially, functional independence is impaired and should be so assessed. For these reasons, evaluation should first be done by interview and then through observation of the patient performing a normal routine.

An interview will provide information regarding the home and work situation. A

TABLE 7-1. *Correlation of Dyspnea Classification with ADL Performance*

| Classification | ADL Key |
|---|---|
| I    No significant restriction in normal activity; employable; dyspnea occurs only on more than normal or strenuous exertion | 4–No breathlessness, normal |
| II    Independent in essential ADL, but restricted in some other activities; employable only where job is sedentary or under special circumstances; dyspneic on climbing stairs or incline, but not level walking | 3–Satisfactory, mild breathlessness; complete performance possible without pause or assistance, but not entirely normal |
| III    Dyspnea usually occurs during usual activities such as showering or dressing; not dyspneic at rest, can walk several blocks at own pace, but cannot keep up with others of own age; does not require physical assistance; is probably not employable in any occupation | 2–Fair, moderate breathlessness; *must* stop during activity; complete performance possible without assistance; performance may be too debilitating or time-consuming |
| IV    Dependent on some help in essential ADL; dyspneic on minimal exertion and must pause on climbing 1 flight, walking over 100 yards, or dressing; often restricted to home if on own | 1–Poor, marked breathlessness; incomplete performance; assistance necessary |
| V    Entirely restricted to home and often limited to bed or chair; dyspneic at rest; dependent on help for most needs | 0–Not indicated; too difficult |

Source: Reprinted with the permission of the American Occupational Therapy Association, Inc. Copyright 1977 ©, *The American Journal of Occupational Therapy*, vol. 31, p. 436, Figure 2; and copyright 1970 ©, *The American Journal of Occupational Therapy*, vol. 24, p. 183.

description of the physical environment including such things as number of stairs, general layout of rooms, availability of toilet and laundry facilities, accessibility to shops, transportation, and so forth should be recorded. It is important to know if the patient lives alone or with others, and respective roles if the latter. The presence of an able-bodied partner, for example, may decrease the need for outside services such as domestic help and meals provision. Details of the work environment should include location, accessibility, usual work position, plus the type of responsibility and its physical demands.

In some instances a visit to the home or workplace may be indicated. In addition to the physical features mentioned, room ventilation and humidification, exposure to lung irritants, storage space and facility for oxygen or intermittent positive-pressure breathing

(IPPB) machines, and temperature regulation in the area require attention. Next, the individual should be observed in the daily routine, and dyspnea (frequency and severity) and time and effort required to perform the job evaluated.

Any set evaluation that describes the patient's limitations can be used to evaluate ADL dysfunction and provide changes or improvements. There are several such systems. One used at Moss Rehabilitation Hospital in Philadelphia defines five broad categories of functional disability with dyspnea as the evaluation criterion (Table 7-1).

Another method may be to assign numerical values to selected tasks using observable shortness of breath, time requirements, and ability to complete the task in scoring. The following point system could be used to describe performance:

2—Independent in the task within a reasonable amount of time without significant shortness of breath

1—Independent, but impractical; may be too exhausting, cause severe dyspnea or distress, or take too much time

0—Unable to complete the task for any reason

A net score for several activities such as grooming and dressing, household chores, meal preparation, shopping, and transportation can then be totaled.

## SOCIAL CONSIDERATIONS

Some knowledge of the social factors influencing the patient's life assists the therapist in realistically planning the rehabilitation program. The type and extent of support and encouragement received at home and from peers can markedly affect the outcome of rehabilitation. It is essential that friends and family understand and support the plan to obtain the patient's maximum cooperation. Leisure interests and opportunities are also important considerations in assessing function.

## VOCATION

The single most significant factor of vocational potential is whether the individual is employed at the time rehabilitation is initiated. Once the disease state has progressed to the point where the patient has lost a job, it becomes considerably more difficult to reinstate him or her in the work force. If the patient is still employed, even with great difficulty, the possibility of maintaining employment, either by adapting the work environment or changing to a less strenuous position is greater.

Some attempts have been made to correlate vocational rehabilitation potential with intelligence quotients (IQ) [1] and personality traits [2]. One study found that following hospitalization patients who were able to work longer than 6 months tended to be more gregarious and deny symptoms more than others who worked for shorter periods of time. Patients who could not be employed after hospitaliza-

tion were characteristically more anxious and less self-confident. Others have shown that IQ could, with surprising accuracy, be used to predict vocational rehabilitation success. Previous to these studies the value of $FEV_1$ had been used to correlate with vocational potential. Further investigation is needed to determine the most accurate measures of assessing vocational rehabilitation potential.

Counseling is a complex process in which the psychosocial, financial, and medical aspects of disability are integrated. As early as possible, a patient's needs should be explored. Initially, attempts are made to adapt the present employment and prevent relocation. A change to more sedentary or part-time work may be a necessity, and in some instances, further retraining is indicated. For the more severely disabled, sheltered workshops are given consideration. If it is clearly impossible to return to gainful employment, counseling in leisure interests becomes even more appropriate.

## CEREBRATION AND PERCEPTION

Hypoxemia and chronic respiratory failure may cause alterations in cognitive and perceptual skills. Evaluations of cerebration (orientation, memory, abstract reasoning, judgment and problem solving, attention span, comprehension, intelligence) and perception (space, form, depth, praxis, figure–ground, body scheme, part–whole integration) as in neurological testing can be used to identify problem areas that may have relevance to rehabilitation.

## MENTAL STATUS

Careful observation of the patient's general mental status assists in setting goals, assessment, and planning the rehabilitation program. Both how a patient appears to others and self-perception provide valuable clues to overall functional abilities and well-being. The apparent degree of anxiety, depression, denial, or passivity should be subjectively noted on initial evaluation, and periodically reviewed throughout rehabilitation and follow-up.

TABLE 7-2. *Comprehensive Evaluation Used at Massachusetts Rehabilitation Hospital, Boston*

| Measurement | | First Week | Last Week | Measurement | | First Week | Last Week |
|---|---|---|---|---|---|---|---|
| Arterial blood gases (ABG) | $p0_2 < 40$ | 1 | 1 | | $pCO_2 > 65$ | 1 | 1 |
| | $p0_2$ 40–54 | 2 | 2 | | $pCO_2$ 56–65 | 2 | 2 |
| | $p0_2$ 53–70 | 3 | 3 | | $pCO_2$ 46–55 | 3 | 3 |
| | $p0_2 > 70$ | 4 | 4 | | $pCO_2 < 45$ | 4 | 4 |
| Pulmonary function tests (PFT) | % predicted VC < 40% | 1 | 1 | % predicted $FEV_1$ | < 40 | 1 | 1 |
| | 40–60% | 2 | 2 | | 40–49 | 2 | 2 |
| | 60–80% | 3 | 3 | | 50–59 | 3 | 3 |
| | > 80% | 4 | 4 | | > 60 | 4 | 4 |
| Oxygen use per day | 24 hrs./day | 1 | 1 | Mechanical respiratory therapy use per day | > 4 hrs. | 1 | 1 |
| | 12–23 hrs. | 2 | 2 | | 2–4 hrs. | 2 | 2 |
| | 3–12 hrs. | 3 | 3 | | ½–2 hrs. | 3 | 3 |
| | 0–3 hrs. | 4 | 4 | | < ½ hr. | 4 | 4 |
| Perception and cerebration evaluation | < 100 | 1 | 1 | Nutrition | Normal weight ± | 1 | 1 |
| | 100–110 | 2 | 2 | | 31–50 | 2 | 2 |
| | 111–118 | 3 | 3 | | Normal weight ± | 3 | 3 |
| | 119–124 | 4 | 4 | | 11–30 | 4 | 4 |
| | | | | | Normal weight ± 10 | | |
| | | | | | Normal weight | | |
| Bicycle no resistance at 10 MPH | 3–5 min. | 1 | 1 | Completed exercises in group | < 90 | 1 | 1 |
| | 6–8 min. | 2 | 2 | | 91–100 | 2 | 2 |
| | 9–12 min. | 3 | 3 | | 101–110 | 3 | 3 |
| | > 12 min. | 4 | 4 | | 111–120 | 4 | 4 |
| Relaxation group | Pulse decrease 0–2 | 1 | 1 | Relaxation group | Respiratory rate decrease 0–2 | 1 | 1 |
| | 2–5 | 2 | 2 | | 3–6 | 2 | 2 |
| | 6–8 | 3 | 3 | | 7–9 | 3 | 3 |
| | 9–10 | 4 | 4 | | 10–12 | 4 | 4 |
| ADL score | < 16 | 1 | 1 | Chest physical therapy | > 1 hr. | 1 | 1 |
| | 16–21.9 | 2 | 2 | | ½–1 hr. | 2 | 2 |
| | 22–25.9 | 3 | 3 | | ¼–½ hr. | 3 | 3 |
| | 26–28 | 4 | 4 | | < ¼ hr. | 4 | 4 |
| Ambulation | 10 or </min. | 1 | 1 | Stairs climbed per minute | < 5/min. | 1 | 1 |
| | 11–50/min. | 2 | 2 | | 6–10/min. | 2 | 2 |
| | 51–99/min. | 3 | 3 | | 11–20/min. | 3 | 3 |
| | 100 or >/min. | 4 | 4 | | >20/min. | 4 | 4 |

| Measurement | | Pre | Post | Measurement | | Pre | Post |
|---|---|---|---|---|---|---|---|
| Pulmonary education 16 questions | < 4 | 1 | 1 | Medication education 12 questions | < 3 | 1 | 1 |
| | 5–8 | 2 | 2 | | 4–6 | 2 | 2 |
| | 9–12 | 3 | 3 | | 7–9 | 3 | 3 |
| | 13–16 | 4 | 4 | | 10–12 | 4 | 4 |

Each item is given a value of 1, 2, 3, or 4. All values are totaled for the score.

Source: From Massachusetts Rehabilitation Hospital, Boston, MA. Reproduced with permission.

Attention to this area, although a continuous process, should not be a focus of therapy; formal testing is usually not necessary, but should be considered in cases of severe emotional distress.

EXAMPLE OF EVALUATION

The demand from within health professions and from third party payers more objectively to document functional improvements has led to the establishment of evaluations that quantitate rehabilitation. Table 7-2 is an example of a good comprehensive evaluation used at Massachusetts Rehabilitation Hospital in Boston. Scoring criteria for arterial blood gases (ABG), pulmonary function testing (PFT), oxygen use, perception and cerebration, work tolerance, ADL, nutrition, relaxation, chest therapy, and pulmonary education have been set to assess facets of pulmonary dysfunction. The overall score is sensitive to changes, and can be used to indicate the effectiveness of a program when compared to the patient's status at the time of hospital discharge.

Although the form shows to some degree what has changed, it does not indicate how or which modalities were effective. Further, it does not indicate improvements in mental or vocational status, or adaptive functioning within the environment. Nevertheless, its value as an indicator of dysfunction and change should not be overlooked.

The use of evaluations of this nature is encouraged to prescribe and assess pulmonary rehabilitation programs less subjectively and more accurately.

## Treatment

To alleviate some of the anxiety associated with pulmonary disease, the patient must be approached with optimism and enthusiasm. A confident, positive attitude helps discourage the tendency toward preoccupation with disability so common among the chronically ill. Treatments need to be presented clearly and concisely to minimize apprehension and create an environment conducive to learning. Effective rehabilitation implies that the patient ultimately accepts full responsibility for his or her health and well-being. It is the rehabilitation team's responsibility to provide the means to such ends within a supportive and encouraging atmosphere.

The following are descriptions of treatment modalities available. The need for postural drainage, percussion and vibration, coughing exercises, oxygen therapy, and mechanically assisted ventilation must be individually determined; the numerous medical contraindications to these treatment modalities will not be discussed. Virtually all patients with COPD would benefit from physical reconditioning, breathing retraining, relaxation exercises, instruction in energy conservation, vocational counseling, and educational programs.

POSTURAL DRAINAGE

Normally, airway secretions are mobilized through bronchociliary action and the cough reflex. In the disease state, such as bronchiectasis, secretions are not only excessive and of altered viscosity, but the normal mechanisms for removal are either damaged or insufficient to maintain clear airways. In addition to causing ventilatory obstruction, excessive mucus accumulation may lead to infection.

Postural drainage is one method of removing excess lung secretions. The patient is positioned so that gravity will assist the flow of mucus from the lungs up toward the trachea, where it can be expelled by coughing or suctioning. There are approximately ten basic positions for postural drainage, each of which facilitates clearance of a particular lung segment. A bronchodilator inhaled before postural drainage may also assist in mobilizing secretions.

Patients and their families should be taught this procedure, however, it may be necessary to improvise the means by which effective drainage can be achieved at home. Figures 7-9, 7-10, and 7-11 illustrate applied positions that can be assumed in a home regimen. In some instances the patient's bed may need to be tipped with large blocks under the legs at one

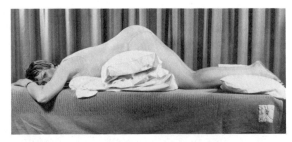

FIGURE 7-9. *Postural drainage of bronchi.*

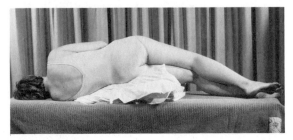

FIGURE 7-10. *Postural drainage of the lower lobes.*

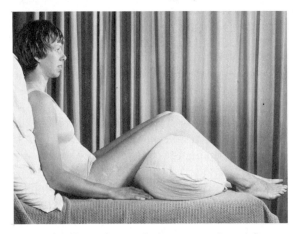

FIGURE 7-11. *Postural drainage of apical segments of the right upper lobe.*

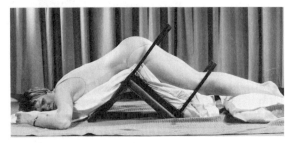

FIGURE 7-12. *Adapted position for postural drainage of the lower lobes.*

end. Cushions that collapse can be replaced by a thick wad of newspaper with two pillows covering it for correct positioning. Alternatively, an upturned chair may also achieve the desired position (Figure 7-12).

A good understanding of lung anatomy is essential in using this technique, as improper positioning may force the secretions deeper into the lungs where they will be more difficult to expel.

PERCUSSION AND VIBRATION

Percussion and vibration are manual techniques used in conjunction with postural drainage to facilitate the expectoration of excess lung secretions when postural drainage alone is ineffective. Percussion is a light rhythmical tapping with cupped hands over the external surface of lung segment being drained. Vibration is a rapid in and out motion also performed over the lung segment being drained. As vibration is less vigorous than percussion, it is recommended postsurgically or for any patient unable to tolerate percussion comfortably. When possible, the patient or a family member should be taught both techniques. In some instances the use of an electric vibrator may also be indicated.

There are three possible explanations for the effect of percussion and vibration: (1) the rhythmical jarring may mechanically loosen secretions, (2) the motions may have an internal vibratory effect that mobilizes the mucus, or (3) each blow of the cupped hands may cause a brief suction effect that releases secretions from the bronchial walls. In any case, correct administration of the techniques is essential to their success.

The patient is usually positioned for postural drainage for approximately five to ten minutes, and simultaneously percussed or vibrated approximately three to five minutes. This, however, is extremely variable. During acute exacerbations of respiratory infections drainage may be needed every two hours, whereas in chronic obstructive pulmonary disease once daily may be adequate.

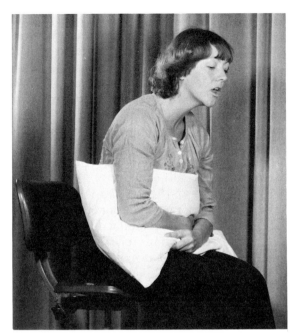

FIGURE 7-13. *Position for correct coughing.*

breath, flex the trunk slightly forward, and gently perform a series of small coughs (Figure 7-13). If no sputum is raised the procedure should not be forced.

### BREATHING EXERCISES

Patients with obstructive pulmonary disease should learn diaphragmatic (abdominal) breathing to improve endurance and reduce dyspnea. In the diseased state, the lungs' elastic recoil is lost, impairing normal diaphragmatic contraction and relaxation. The diaphragm tends to flatten, the lungs remain hyperinflated, and normal gas exchange is impaired. To compensate, the patient substitutes at higher energy costs the accessory muscles of respiration—the pectorals, sternomastoid, upper trapezius, scalene, and arm adductors. Diaphragmatic breathing reduces the effort and facilitates easier breathing by using the lower costal and abdominal muscles to assist diaphragmatic excursion, rather than these less efficient neck and accessory muscles. It further increases tidal volume and ensures more even distribution of ventilation, thereby facilitating gas transfer.

During dyspnea when the patient seems to be choking for air, the tendency is rapidly and shallowly to inhale more air. This further increases lung hyperinflation and interferes with gas exchange. Properly performed during an attack, abdominal breathing should help to reduce dyspnea. Anxiety, which worsens dyspnea, should also be lessened if the patient feels able to control breathing.

Breathing exercises should first be taught in a supine position, with pillows to support the head and knees for comfort. The patient is instructed to place one hand over the abdomen and the other over the chest for kinesthetic awareness and feedback. The patient is told to inhale gently and feel only the abdomen expand, and is then encouraged to relax and exhale slowly while gently depressing the abdomen. Slow, relaxed expiration is of greatest importance in preventing lung hyperinflation and in retraining ventilatory musculature. Ex-

The long-term value of these techniques is not yet known, but immediate gains in expectoration with productive coughing and in patient comfort can be easily shown.

### COUGHING

Coughing is one of the primary mechanical defenses of the respiratory system. It protects by expelling foreign or bacterial matter trapped by the mucous linings in the respiratory passageways. It further aids in removal of excess secretions that may lead to infection or alveolar hypoventilation.

Unproductive coughing where no sputum is produced irritates membranous linings, causes discomfort, and may induce dyspnea. The patient must therefore learn how to cough correctly. Productive coughing must also follow all postural drainage and percussion treatments.

Sitting with a pillow supporting the abdominal region, the patient should relax the neck and shoulders, then inhale a deep abdominal

piration should be longer than inspiration. It is more important to establish control of breathing than any "preferred" or "normal" rate of breathing.

Some patients automatically purse their lips during expiration. This is an effective technique that reduces the rate of expiration and decreases air trapping by helping to prevent bronchiole collapse, and should be taught if it does not occur spontaneously.

Gentle, rhythmical abdominal breathing should be encouraged. As the patient begins to feel comfortable, inspiratory volume should gradually increase. The slow, deep breathing should then be progressively practiced in sitting, standing, and finally in functional activities such as walking, climbing stairs, or dressing.

In applying correct breathing techniques to activities, it is important to understand that the stressful part of any activity is performed on expiration, the relaxed phase of respiration. Simple repetitive tasks are useful in teaching the patient to control breathing and establish a comfortable pace. Motions of reaching and bending lend themselves to the instruction and reinforcement of efficient breathing patterns. In sitting, for example, a patient can be instructed to inhale gently while allowing an overhead pulley to raise the arms bilaterally. (This also increases thoracic volume and ventilatory space, which facilitates inspiration.) This should then be followed by gentle expiration as the patient pulls against resistance. These motions rhythmically repeated also reinforce the efficiency of paced activity in increasing tolerance.

Nonrepetitive activities should be practiced last. Although the application of breathing techniques is designed to improve function in these tasks, if the patterns are not learned and understood first, a patient may find it confusing and frustrating to apply them to ADL. Indeed, any application of breathing exercises to ADL has been criticized as confusing and difficult to learn.

Abdominal breathing can also be illustrated with a task such as dressing. The patient should dress the lower extremities first, as this is the more stressful part of the activity. It is helpful to practice in sitting, bending down toward the feet on inspiration, and on slow prolonged expiration, returning to upright to put on trousers, socks, and so forth.

It must also be reinforced that ventilation is to be maintained throughout all parts of the activity, and the tendency to hold the breath on exertion must be eliminated.

Figures 7-14, 7-15, and 7-16 demonstrate some of the proper positions for efficient application of abdominal breathing during an attack of dyspnea. All positions relax head and shoulder muscles, reduce overall skeletal muscle tension, and promote diaphragmatic elevation by slightly flexing the trunk.

Often, dyspnea appears to occur suddenly without warning, so the patient must be taught to recognize the symptoms of its approach. In some instances, it is recommended to challenge the patient with a stressful task to demonstrate the signs preceding an attack, and to illustrate the efficiency of modifying activity, relaxed posturing, and abdominal breathing in preventing respiratory distress.

Deep breathing before postural drainage is also recommended to help relax the patient and prevent atelectasis. After drainage, deep breathing may help to inflate cleared alveoli and promote gas exchange.

RECONDITIONING EXERCISES

The debilitation secondary to impaired ventilation, lessened activity, and fear of dyspnea on exertion can be significantly reduced with a program of neuromuscular and cardiorespiratory exercises. It is well accepted that physical training improves endurance; some evidence also exists that it increases work capacity, improves strength, and enhances confidence and feelings of well-being. Physical training appears to reduce the distressing symptoms of respiratory disease and thereby increase functional capabilities in ADL. It is the one aspect of rehabilitation in which dramatic and

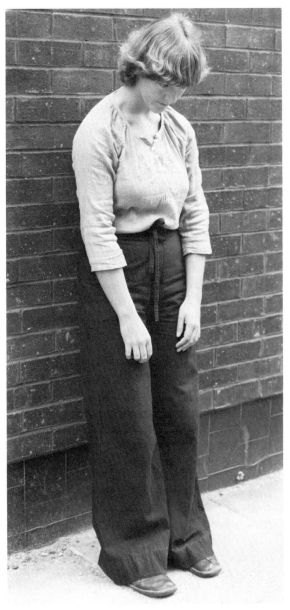

FIGURE 7-14. *Relaxed standing with trunk slightly flexed, head and shoulders relaxed, and feet approximately 12 inches from the wall.*

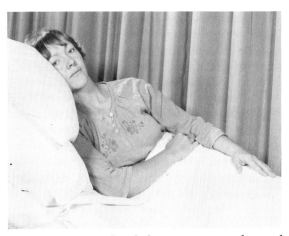

FIGURE 7-15. *High side-lying position to be used during acute respiratory distress. A pillow placed slightly forward for the left arm to rest upon may increase comfort.*

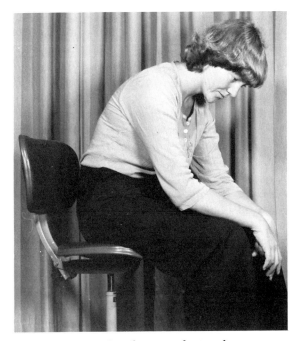

FIGURE 7-16. *Relaxed sitting during dyspnea.*

measurable improvements can be made in relatively short periods of time.

The underlying mechanisms for observable improvements are less clear. Significant improvements in lung function as measured by pulmonary function tests (PFT) have not been demonstrated. To some extent, training improves physical performance in the patient with COPD much as it does in the healthy individual. Perhaps more important for the patient is that it interrupts the destructive pattern of dyspnea, reduced activity, and deconditioning that results in greater dyspnea.

Progressive ambulation, climbing stairs, treadmill and stationary bicycle exercises, and progressive resistive exercises are most commonly prescribed. Any activity, however carefully selected and graded to meet the needs of the individual patient, can and should be used. In eliciting cooperation, it is imperative that the chosen activity or exercise be relevant to the patient's life-style and interests. It is advisable to train with an activity or exercise not only that the patient accepts, but that can be continued at home.

The degree of physical improvement depends on many variables such as severity of the disease, motivation, extent and duration of the program, and the combination of training with other treatment modalities. The length of time a reconditioning program should be administered varies with each patient. Neuromuscular reconditioning must be continued throughout the patient's life to maintain the gains and improve on them. Short-term benefits of a reconditioning program are quickly lost if the patient returns to a previous habitual sedentary life-style after discharge from the program.

Asthma presents some particular problems in regard to training. Bronchospasms often increase with exercise and frequently occur following activity. Postexertional respiratory distress may be at its worst several minutes after the physical activity ceases. It follows that asthmatic patients particularly fear the dyspnea associated with exercise, and unnecessarily restrict their activities. It is not well established to what degree asthmatic patients suffer from diminished physical fitness. Nevertheless, it is generally believed that they should also be encouraged to increase their activity, and that they would most likely feel better if they did [8]. It is advisable to begin a session with a short warmup period of light cardiorespiratory and ROM exercises, and complete similar tapering off activity postexertion. If exercise tolerance is significantly limited, more frequent rest periods are advocated.

BIOFEEDBACK
Biofeedback training techniques can be used to increase control over physiological processes by providing visual or auditory cues of autonomic body functions. They may be applicable to the pulmonary patient suffering from anxiety and dyspnea. Although some investigative work has been done in this area [4], no particular conclusions can be drawn at this time.

RELAXATION EXERCISES
Persistent anxiety, frequently occurring in the patient with chest disease, encourages a chronic state of increased muscular tension, particularly in the neck and upper trunk. In addition, the compensatory posture often adopted aggravates this condition and increases the body's oxygen requirements to maintain the inefficient position. Relaxation exercises teach the patient voluntarily to relax the skeletal muscles, increasing efficient use of oxygen and reducing associated discomfort. Decreasing muscular tension further facilitates overall feelings of well-being.

Voluntary relaxation is at first quite difficult to achieve. To be effective, it requires much patience, perseverance, and practice. Although emphasis is not on breathing patterns, mastery of relaxation will result in slower, deeper, more evenly distributed ventilation. Many techniques exist; Jacobson's description of progressive relaxation exercises is perhaps the most well known [5]. Relaxation is first learned in a supine position in a quiet environment. Pillows supporting the head and under the knees increase comfort and reduce tension. The patient is instructed to contract maximally and then relax individual body segments in a controlled rhythmical, nonstressful manner. As each body part relaxes, the patient proceeds to the next until total relaxation is achieved.

Although the patient initially learns to relax following contraction, eventually, relaxation without contraction should be mastered. Ideally, through repetition and increased kinesthetic awareness of tension and posture, a habitual pattern of relaxation should follow.

Other types of active exercise such as stretching, bending, and swinging may also be effective in reducing muscular tension if they are performed correctly and consistently.

### PRESURGICAL CARE

It is recommended that the therapist meet with and evaluate the patient presurgically and begin instruction of the program, as postsurgically the patient may be drowsy or confused. A good rapport with the therapist and some knowledge of what is to come elicits cooperation and helps reassure the anxious patient.

### POSTSURGICAL CARE

Following thoracic surgery, vigorous prophylactic therapy is required to prevent secondary pulmonary disease. Rapid shallow breathing often occurs because of trauma to the respiratory muscles and pain. The derangement of the chest muscles results in diminished chest expansion (decreased ventilatory space) and impaired cough mechanisms. The patient may be hypoventilating and unable adequately to expel excessive respiratory secretions.

Postural drainage, percussion or vibration, coughing, and deep breathing exercises are routinely employed postsurgically to improve ventilation and maintain clear airways, thus preventing the development of secondary lung disease. Deep breathing exercises in particular should begin as soon as the patient is conscious, and continue at regular intervals until normal ventilation and activity are reestab-

lished. Postural drainage positions frequently require modification, as the patient may be unable to tolerate standard ones.

General debilitation secondary to postoperative inactivity can be reduced by reconditioning exercises. A program consisting of passive, active assistive, and later resistive exercise is usually indicated. Light range-of-motion, initially done in bed, is begun as soon as possible. The programs are progressively increased in duration and intensity as medically feasible.

In effect, deep breathing and range-of-motion exercises should be regularly taught to all inactive patients as prophylactic measures against neuromuscular deconditioning and hypoventilation.

### RESTRICTIVE DISORDERS

Deep breathing and postural exercises should be emphasized in restrictive disease secondary to neuromuscular and skeletal disorders. Increased ventilatory space can best be achieved through postural improvement, and an emphasis on maximum ventilation per inspiration as in deep breathing training. In some cases of respiratory muscle paralysis, such as quadriplegia, resistive exercising of the respiratory musculature improves ventilatory endurance.

In severe cases of neuromuscular disease or mechanical derangement of the thoracic cage (restrictive disorders), body respirators, iron lungs, or other devices may be needed to assist ventilation and maintain arterial gas balance. These machines encase the patient to produce negative pressures to the external chest wall to depress the diaphragm, elevate the rib cage, and induce the negative pressure that draws atmospheric air into the lungs. The patient may need to spend the night in such a device to restore arterial oxygenation that is depleted by the day's activity.

The patient with paralysis of the respiratory musculature may be helped by periods in a rocker bed. This facilitates diaphragmatic excursion by mechanically rotating the supine patient horizontally 40 degrees toward the

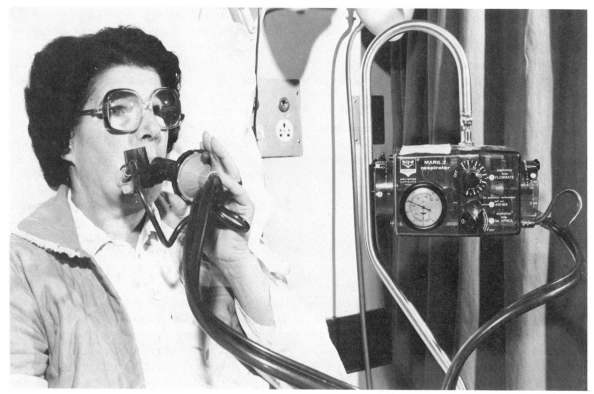

FIGURE 7-17. *Intermittent positive-pressure breathing (IPPB) machine in use.*

head, and then 40 degrees toward the feet throughout the night.

Although rarely used, these ventilation machines still have some application.

## INTERMITTENT POSITIVE-PRESSURE BREATHING

This technique (IPPB) can be used in conjunction with other forms of chest therapy to facilitate removal of excess secretions, and to assist in administration of oxygen or inhaled drugs through a nebulizer. It is most effective in treating cases of severe respiratory insufficiency such as acute episodes of chronic bronchitis or asthma. Particularly in the instance of acute respiratory failure, IPPB may be valuable in the aggressive treatment for secretion removal and reestablishment of arterial gas balance through improved ventilation. In restrictive

disease such as obesity, quadriplegia, and kyphoscoliosis, IPPB may be indicated periodically to hyperinflate the lungs to prevent atelectasis or alveolar collapse in the hypoventilated lung (Figure 7-17).

Machines can act as mechanical aids to respiration. A slight inspiratory effort begins the delivery of a preset gas flow through the mouth to the lungs. When the required ventilatory pressure is reached, the machine cycles into expiration by sealing the inspiratory flow valve and releasing built-up expiratory pressure. Either oxygen or compressed air may be used for inspiratory flow. Treatment is discontinued when the patient can adequately expectorate secretions, or when arterial gas balance is reestablished. For greater efficiency, IPPB can be combined with postural drainage.

For the few patients unable to clear their

excess secretions without mechanical aids, IPPB may be needed at home. Proper instruction in its use and care is essential, as improperly cleaned equipment may be sources of infection [3].

## OXYGEN THERAPY AND RECONDITIONING

In chronic obstructive pulmonary disease associated with low blood/oxygen tensions, oxygen therapy may increase exercise capacity, and improve general cardiorespiratory status, cognitive functions, and mental well-being.

Arterial blood gas analysis determines the need for oxygen therapy. When the patient's resting $PaO_2$ is significantly low, supplemental oxygen may be required during physical activity, when short of breath, or at night for restlessness and irritability. If the $PaO_2$ drops markedly during exercise, or if the patient is severely limited by exertional dyspnea, oxygen may also be indicated during exercise. Only when the $PaO_2$ is consistently below 60 mm Hg is continuous low-flow oxygen therapy necessary.

In a patient with impaired sensitivity to carbon dioxide supplemental oxygen must be administered with care to avoid increasing carbon dioxide retention. Reduced levels of blood oxygen act as respiratory stimulants. If the oxygen is increased, the stimulant is diminished, and carbon dioxide concentrations may continue to rise, eventually contributing to respiratory failure.

If carbon dioxide retention is not a problem, performance may be improved by oxygen-supported exercise. If the vicious cycle of inactivity resulting in deconditioning and further inactivity is interrupted by such a program, significant neuromuscular reconditioning, and consequently improved ventilation, may occur.

## OXYGEN THERAPY AND RESPIRATORY FAILURE

At $PaO_2$ tensions of less than 60 mm Hg the patient is said to be in respiratory failure. Respiratory infections usually precipitate acute

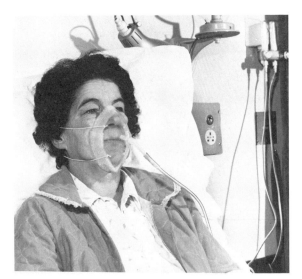

FIGURE 7-18. *Oxygen therapy.*

respiratory failure, whereas chronic respiratory failure is a constant state secondary to the pathology of pulmonary disease. Both are commonly treated with carefully controlled oxygen therapy (Figure 7-18). In chronic respiratory failure, administration of oxygen may be a regular or constant necessity.

In acute respiratory failure, oxygen is administered continuously until the underlying cause can be identified and treated. When controlled oxygen therapy combined with chemical ventilatory stimulants is inadequate to restore more normal gas balance, mechanical ventilation must be employed.

## HUMIDIFIERS

Dehydration contributes to viscous bronchial secretions and airway obstruction. Patients should be encouraged to increase fluid intake to maintain adequate hydration. In some instances, inhalation of a warm moist mist or humidified air assists in mobilizing tenacious secretions. Several types of humidifiers exist for this purpose. Whenever continuous low-flow oxygen is employed, supplemental humidifi-

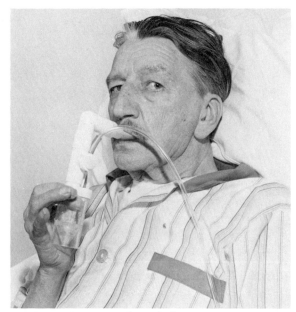

FIGURE 7-19. *Use of a nebulizer.*

cation is indicated to prevent drying of the airways, and to assist in mobilizing secretions.

### NEBULIZERS AND AEROSOLS

Nebulizers and aerosols can be used to administer drugs that are more effective when inhaled (Figure 7-19). Nebulizers disperse the drug in a gas before inhalation, whereas aerosols deliver the drug as a mist by simple pressure. To relieve bronchospasms as in asthma, bronchodilating drugs are commonly administered by either method. Both are occasionally used with antibiotics and mucolytic drugs.

Correct nebulizer and aerosol techniques need to be learned to achieve even distribution of medication throughout the lungs. Excessive or improper use, as with any medication, can lead to serious side effects.

### WORK SIMPLIFICATION

All patients with pulmonary disease can learn to maximize productivity by incorporating into their daily lives the principles of work simplification and energy conservation. Regardless of their respiratory status, functional ability can

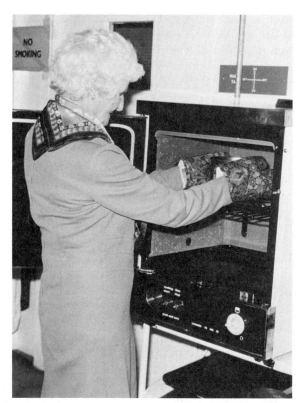

FIGURE 7-20. *Correct height of oven to reduce lifting and bending to conserve energy.*

be improved through more efficient movement and reduction in unnecessary activity. Efficient use of limited energies results in an increased capacity to perform what is necessary or interesting. The principles that apply to any disability resulting in weakness and low endurance apply to patients with diminished pulmonary capacity.

The extent to which energy conservation can be employed is endless. The function of instruction is to demonstrate how the patient can be more efficient and increase awareness of the efficiency of motion. It is ultimately the patient's responsibility to devise the many ways in which to economize on movement in all aspects of life.

Following are the basic principles on which to build energy-efficient patterns. The goals are to increase activity by establishing habits that require less effort, yet accomplish the same ends.

1. Organize work and leisure space to minimize lifting, bending, and walking (Figure 7-20). Arrange storage space so that only the items seldom used are placed above or below the level of comfortable reach.
2. Sit rather than stand whenever possible.
3. Avoid pushing, pulling, and carrying by using push carts, wheeled baskets, etc., wherever possible.
4. Eliminate tasks that do not have to be done. This particularly applies to the homemaker whose standards of cleanliness tend to be higher than necessary.
5. Use labor-saving devices and electric appliances when available.
6. Preplan activities with adequate allowance for rest periods to avoid unnecessary haste and stress.
7. Perform at a moderate pace, methodically.

## PATIENT AND FAMILY EDUCATION

Patient and family education regarding pulmonary disease should be a continuous process provided throughout all phases of rehabilitation. In some instances it may be more effective to provide additional information in a structured setting. Lectures, visual aids, written instructional materials, and discussion groups all can be used to help patients and their families understand the disease. It is essential that formal instruction be kept simple and concise. Materials such as booklets and audio-visual aids should focus on the most relevant issues, but be as brief as possible. Care must also be taken continually to reinforce the positive effects of therapy and minimize the attention given to irreversible facets of pulmonary disease.

In addition to careful clear explanations of the goals of rehabilitation, information concerning the following topics assists in motivating the patient and improving cooperation.

## NATURE OF THE DISEASE

Descriptive information concerning the disease process and its functional effects should be provided. Although it has not been proved, it is reasonable to assume that a patient who understands the disease is more likely to cooperate with a proposed treatment program.

## NUTRITION

Severe weight loss and anorexia frequently accompany COPD. Conversely, obesity adds stress to the cardiorespiratory system, and in the extreme form may cause respiratory insufficiency. Good instruction in proper nutrition improves health and function.

## COMMUNITY RESOURCES

Various community resources exist to meet the patient's medical and social needs. Information concerning their function and availability should be offered.

## PREVENTION

Some guidance concerning preventive measures may be invaluable in maintaining functional status. Patients should be taught to recognize the signs of early infection such as increased shortness of breath or cough; changes in sputum volume, color, or consistency; and low-grade fevers. Early medical attention may prevent more severe respiratory distress and possibly hospital admission. The need to avoid further exposure to lung irritants, particularly smoke and vapors, gases, and dusts should also be stressed. Patients should be made aware of the many conditions that exacerbate respiratory disease symptoms (extreme hot, cold, humid, or dry environments; excessive fatigue, emotional stress, etc.) and be taught how to avoid them. A timely change from an occupation that contributes to respiratory disease may prevent later disabling symptoms.

## MEDICATIONS

Medications most commonly associated with pulmonary disease include bronchodilators and steroids for relief of bronchospasms, diuretics in cases of pulmonary edema or ventricular failure, and antibiotics to combat respiratory infections. Oxygen should also be considered a medication.

Education on their function, application, and possible side effects should be included as a part of any rehabilitation program. The importance of adhering to recommended dosages must be stressed. Particularly in regard to bronchodilators administered by aerosol, the dangers of excessive use must be emphasized, and alternatives (e.g., mastery of breathing or relaxation) suggested. Patients frequently find it difficult to continue with prophylactic drugs in the absence of respiratory distress or disease symptoms. Clarification of purpose that reinforces the physician's instructions helps elicit cooperation with drug therapies.

GROUP COUNSELING
Opportunities for peer interaction often provide emotional support and encouragement to those with respiratory illness. Sharing experiences and feelings among patients of similar disability can for some be an invaluable aid in combating depression. Group leaders should strive for a constructive, relaxed atmosphere that encourages participation of all members. Psychotherapy is rarely indicated, and should not be attempted unless the patient clearly develops a psychological problem [14].

## Conclusion
As in any chronic disease, the emphasis of therapy should always be on function rather than dysfunction. Particularly in regard to the obstructive lung diseases, anxiety and preoccupation with dyspnea may play a major role in debilitating the patient, and focusing on disabling symptoms may actually create more fear and anxiety, and result in greater functional losses. The therapist must avoid further encouraging this state with intricate, prolonged programs and instructions.

At best, medical care retards or halts the disease process. At best, rehabilitation improves

physical performance and increases comfort. Neither treatment, however, can repair the damage or reverse the process of destruction of lung function. The problems of patients with pulmonary disease are far from being solved with presently available treatment.

Perhaps future hopes lie in preventive rather than curative or adaptive aspects of management. Although genetic factors, infectious agents, and allergies appear to play a role in pathogenesis, environmental pollutants and tobacco exceed them in importance as causative agents. Eliminating these two causative factors alone would probably dramatically reduce the incidence of these conditions. Preventing pollution and getting people to stop smoking are difficult to achieve. Attempts to alter habits, particularly in early stages of disease when a person is asymptomatic, meet enormous resistance; the ability to stop smoking requires tremendous effort and motivation.

While eliminating the disease remains the ultimate goal, its increasing incidence demands improved methods of treatment. In addition to the modalities of rehabilitation, application and distribution of comprehensive programs require further development and investigative study. More efficient application of rehabilitation principles in ambulatory care may also offer promise for future improvements in care. Better public education on prevention would probably decrease the incidence of COPD and eliminate much of the need for comprehensive rehabilitation. Thus the goals are not limited to improving on known treatments, but include making what is known more available.

In view of supporting scientific evidence, it is easy to be critical of the value of rehabilitation for pulmonary disease. It is equally easy to be unrealistically optimistic about its future role. Neither approach is fair or acceptable. What is needed is a reasonable balance of optimism—to motivate the patient and maintain professional interest—and criticism—to promote growth and encourage investigative study—to prevent the disease and develop improved methods of treatment. Although no easy task, the field of pulmonary rehabilitation offers enormous challenges and opportunities to improve the quality of life for a great number of people.

## References

1. Daughton, D. M., et al. Physiological-intellectual components of rehabilitation success in patients with chronic obstructive pulmonary disease (COPD). *J. Chron. Dis.* 32:405, 1979.
2. Fix, A. J., et al. Personality traits affecting vocational rehabilitation success in patients with chronic obstructive pulmonary disease. *Psychol. Rep.* 43:939, 1978.
3. Gaskell, D. V., and Webber, B. A. Physiotherapy for Patients Receiving Mechanical Assistance. In D. V. Gaskell and B. A. Webber (Eds.). *The Brompton Hospital Guide to Chest Physiotherapy* (3rd ed.). Oxford: Blackwell, 1977.
4. Hodgkin, J. E., et al. Chronic obstructive airway disease. *JAMA* 232:1243, 1975.
5. Jacobson, E. *Progressive Relaxation* (2nd ed.). Chicago: University of Chicago Press, 1938.
6. Lertzman, M. M., and Cherniack, R. M. Rehabilitation of patients with chronic obstructive pulmonary disease. *Am. Rev. Respir. Dis.* 114:1145, 1976.
7. Petty, T. L. Pulmonary rehabilitation. *RC* 1:68, 1977.
8. Shephard, R. J. Exercise for the asthmatic patient: A brief historical review. *J. Sports Med. Phys. Fitness* 18:301, 1978.

## Suggested Reading

Cotes, J. E. *Lung Function: Assessment and Application in Medicine* (4th ed.). Oxford: Blackwell, 1979.

Gaskell, D. V., and Webber, B. A. (Eds.). *The Brompton Guide to Chest Physiotherapy* (3rd ed.). Oxford: Blackwell, 1977.

Lane, D. J. Interpretation of blood-gas measurements and respiratory function tests. *Medicine* 22:1136, 1979.

Rusk, H. A. *Rehabilitation Medicine* (4th ed.). St. Louis: Mosby, 1977.

# 8 STROKE REHABILITATION

*Nancy Wall*

Stroke is the third leading cause of death and disability in the United States, and one of the most common conditions necessitating referral to physical rehabilitation. Approximately 500,000 adults a year suffer strokes, and an estimated two million adults are living following an episode at any one time [34]. A stroke affects an individual's medical, physical, emotional, social, intellectual, financial, vocational, and recreational life. Rehabilitation must deal with these aspects and their interrelationships.

This chapter follows the stroke and rehabilitation processes chronologically from onset to discharge. The primary objective is to provide as many treatment options as space will allow. References provide additional information on particular theories or procedures.

## Etiology of Stroke

Cerebrovascular accident (CVA) or more appropriately, cerebrovascular disease (CVD) involves a pathological process in one or more blood vessels of the brain. This may be caused by an abnormality of the vessel wall, rupture or occlusion of the vessel, lack of blood flow from a fall in blood pressure, alterations in the vessel lumen, and other less common conditions. There are two basic situations that can lead to CVD: ischemia and hemorrhage. Ischemia results from occlusion of the nutrient-supplying vessel because of thrombosis or embolus. A thrombus is a clot that develops in place; an embolus is a clot formed in another part of the circulatory system, usually the heart, that breaks off and becomes lodged in a narrower

cerebral vessel. When ischemia occurs, the brain tissue that does not receive the essential blood and oxygen suffers anoxic damage and subsequent necrosis or infarction. Hemorrhage is a rupture of the vessel causing extra blood to leak into the brain tissue (intercerebral), the subarachnoid space, or both, resulting in physical disruption of the area and increased pressure on the surrounding tissue. If disruption is severe and prolonged, anoxic damage and eventual necrosis can occur [29].

The final consequence of CVD is stroke. Clinical signs and deficits depend on the particular vessel or vessels involved. A lesion is generally isolated in one side of the brain, which results in the most common syndrome of stroke—hemiplegia or hemiparesis of the opposite side of the body. In addition, depending on the location of the lesion, there may be sensory deficit, dysphasia, visual and perceptual impairment, and changes in mental and cognitive states. Space does not allow a closer look at specific damage and symptoms of change [29, 31].

Prognosis for functional recovery depends on several factors, one of which is location of the lesion. Studies have shown that disease in the area of the carotid distribution has a poorer prognosis than does disease in the vertebral basilar distribution, and that a bilateral stroke has a poorer prognosis than unilateral insult [31]. Another factor is etiology, mainly the pathological process and its severity. A patient

Illustrations for this chapter were drawn by Nancy Wall.

with a cerebral hemorrhage may have more severe initial illness and prolonged recovery than one with thrombosis or embolus. A patient with hemorrhagic stroke may make the most significant gains between six and 12 months as opposed to gains made in the first three months following thrombotic or embolic insult. Diabetes, rheumatic heart disease, arteriosclerotic heart disease, elevated serum lipids, and especially hypertension are medical conditions that have been found to predispose to stroke [31] and influence prognosis. In one study, 23 percent of patients had associated heart disease [27]. Age at onset is also significant, as Mossmann [31] says, related to the "changes in the vascular, especially cardiac and other organic systems." Also, 44 percent of victims survive the first months, and of these patients who receive rehabilitation, (again from Mossmann [31]) 60 to 80 percent "eventually become relatively independent and 40-65% eventually return home."

## Acute Phase

In the acute phase of illness the patient's medical condition may be progressing or evolving from comatose to consciousness, with stabilization of accompanying neurological symptoms. During these critical days the patient will be totally dependent, immobile, and probably confused and frightened. Diagnostic tests at this time include computerized tomographic scan, angiography, brain scan, complete neurological workup, and blood tests. Problems such as bowel and bladder incontinence, respiratory complications, immobility, nutrition and fluid intake, and emotional factors are the primary foci of nursing and medical care.

Procedures to maintain survival are coupled with preventive measures to maintain passive range of motion (ROM), skin integrity, and proper body positions and alignment. Depending on diagnosis and etiology, limited activity may be necessary. If no other complications exist, a patient with thrombotic stroke may be mobilized in two to three days, whereas it may

be 10 to 14 days before one with subarachnoid hemorrhage can be mobilized [41]. Activity of a patient with stroke and associated myocardial infraction (MI) is a controversial issue, and depends on clinical signs such as arrhythmias, and cardiological assessment [41]. Thrombophlebitis could be a serious complication, and preventive steps including elastic stocking, foot board, active foot exercises of the sound leg, and early mobilization as appropriate may be necessary [41].

Preventive and supportive treatment would be passive and active ROM, positioning, swallowing activities, early mobilization, immediate functional tasks, and emotional support. Many of these problems are not restricted to the acute phase, however, and will need to be dealt with in a variety of ways throughout rehabilitation. It is the responsibility of the therapist to identify high-priority needs and deal with them promptly. A general screening format would gather the necessary information to allow immediate assessment of the acute needs and establishment of priorities for treatment goals. Treatment implies a sense of urgency and need for efficient use of time and skills.

A passive ROM program should begin within 24 hours following onset. When the patient is unable to actively move the joints because of paralysis or changes in conscious condition, it is necessary to move them passively. The ROM sessions provide an opportunity to evaluate the patient, offer additional sensory input—tactile, verbal, visual, and proprioceptive—and to develop a therapeutic relationship. The program can be shared by all team members, including the family when appropriate.

Positioning the patient begins immediately and is essential for maintaining body posture, joint alignment, functional range of motion, and skin integrity. In addition, from the beginning this may assist in preventing contractures, lessen the effect of abnormal tone, and assist in promoting a realistic body image. Positioning does not imply a static condition, but rather a

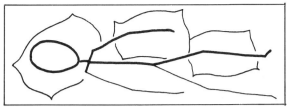

FIGURE 8-1. *Supine position. When patient is totally dependent, position with pillows under head and under shoulder for protraction; under extended arm and hand, with hand elevated if edematous; under calf with some knee flexion and no pressure on heel. Trunk should be aligned.*

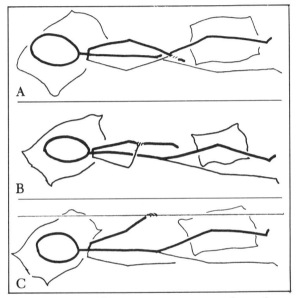

FIGURE 8-2. *When patient is more independent, use fewer pillows with A. Arms extended, hands clasped together, resting on abdomen. B. Involved arm extended by side, in supination if possible, with sound hand keeping involved elbow extended. C. Involved hand on side rail, legs extended, pillow under calf with some knee flexion, and no pressure on heel.*

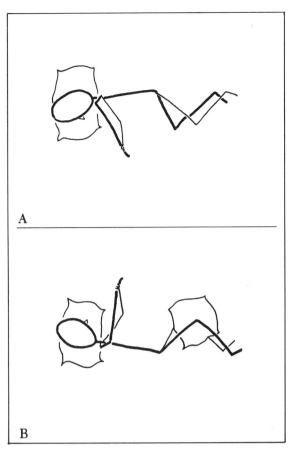

FIGURE 8-3. *Side-lying. When patient lies on either side (A and B), position with scapula protracted, arms extended with hands clasped together, or sound hand holding involved wrist; or knees and hips flexed, pillow between legs if necessary to keep bony prominences apart. Elevate hand on pillow if it is edematous (not shown).*

constant process, as the patient's position in bed must be changed frequently—every two hours or less—to be effective.

Not only the position itself, but how the patient is assisted into it, is part of the process. Initially, the patient may require maximum assistance, and may need to be "packed in pillows" to maintain a position (Figures 8-1, 8-2,

and 8-3). The goal is for the patient to assume responsibility for positioning; thus the method of assistance can set a precedent for the way it is accomplished independently. This opportunity to teach independence and safety may be one of the first steps in rehabilitation. Basic guidelines should be followed: (1) pressure off bony prominences and keeping skin dry to prevent decubitus ulcers, (2) good trunk alignment to protect internal organs, and (3) elevation of edematous extremities to reduce swelling. In addition, each position change will require moving the call bell, bed control, urinal, and so on depending on the patient's needs.

Swallowing or deglutition is a coordinated combination of oral, pharyngeal, and esophageal sensorimotor activities and reflex reactions [13]. Inability to swallow, or dysphagia, may result with stroke. Impairment of jaw and tongue motion, function of the soft palate and esophagus, and the presence of primitive reflexes, spasticity, or weakness can make deglutition difficult or even dangerous.

If swallowing problems are severe a nasogastric tube or a gastric tube may be placed as the means of ensuring sufficient fluid and food intake, and this may require periodic suctioning. Mouth and dental care are provided by nursing personnel to prevent dehydration, facilitate salivation, keep the oral cavity clean and free of infection, and provide sensory input.

Careful evaluation must be made and a treatment program developed according to the needs of the patient with dysphagia. In acute illness, limited time and other priorities may preclude all but a basic screening to assess the primary components of swallowing to determine if a feeding program would be appropriate [35]. These components include the status of gag and cough reflexes, sensation, and motor control of the face and tongue, and oral and neck muscles. It is important to assess if swallowing is possible on command, as a reflex, or both. (See section on problems in speech and languages.)

The major indications for safe initiation of oral feeding are the presence of gag and cough reflexes and mental alertness. For oral intake the patient must be supported in an upright sitting position with the neck slightly flexed and knees and hips flexed. The best first introduction of food might be a lemon-glycerine swab, followed by foods with a texture such as applesauce or Jell-O. Liquids are introduced later, as they are more difficult to handle and are easily aspirated.

If swallowing problems continue during rehabilitation, facilitation techniques should be

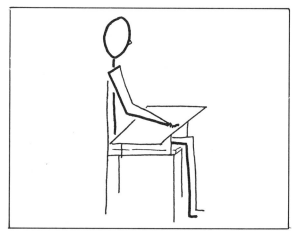

FIGURE 8-4. *When sitting in wheelchair or standard chair, patient is positioned with: head in midline (may need head support), trunk aligned with pillows or side supports, buttocks with special cushion to protect skin and provide comfort, thighs parellel to floor, weight evenly distributed along thighs, knees with 90° flexion, if possible. Feet are flat, with weight evenly distributed on both feet, foot rests, or floor, seat belt is used as indicated. Arms are extended in front and supported on a pillow, rolled-up blanket, lapboard, arm board or table. If legs are elevated, put cushion under calves, heels free and ankles dorsiflexed.*

part of the program. Use of these techniques assumes a firm understanding of the normal swallowing process, a complete and careful evaluation, and requires coordination among the rehabilitation team members [13, 35].

When the medical condition allows, careful mobilization of the patient is important to prevent loss of strength and endurance, sensory deprivation, and mental and psychological deterioration. This, in addition to passive range of motion, may take the form of active assistive or active range-of-motion exercises to all four extremities. Routine sitting up in bed with support or in a high-back chair or wheelchair may be appropriate. If balance allows, assisted and supervised sitting on the bed edge with feet well supported on the floor or a stool can follow (Figure 8-4).

The acute phase is the time of greatest dependency for the patient. What was once second nature will now be impossible. The desire to carry out an activity may exist, yet the physical ability to accomplish it will be difficult if not impossible. At this point any activity the patient can do unassisted will be a positive step toward independence and will provide a feeling of control. The call bell should always be accessible and adapted, if necessary, for the patient's use. Eye glasses, urinal, and water glass should be within the patient's reach and visual field, with other environmental controls, television and radio available. The bed or chair should be in positions that allow the patient to see and hear what is going on in the immediate area. When the medical condition stabilizes, a rehabilitation program with well-defined goals and vigorous methods may be prescribed.

## Rehabilitation Phase
### FUNCTIONAL MOBILITY
Functional mobility is the physical ability to move into, maintain, and use a variety of basic body positions. It provides the foundation on which functional independence and safety are built. It depends on normal status of reflexes, motor control, muscle tone, and sensation. These physical components interact with perception, cognition, praxia, and social and emotional components to allow an individual to develop and sustain independence.

When a stroke occurs, mobility is impaired because of abnormal reflexes and sensation, and changes in muscle tone and motor control. These abnormalities are manifested as primitive reflex behavior, flaccidity or weakness, spasticity, synergies, lack of motor control, and impaired sensation. Treatment techniques of facilitation and inhibition have been developed on the basis of neurophysiological sensorimotor theories (Table 8-1) [14, 21]. These techniques share the following general principles:

1. Sensation and motion are intimately related and rely on each other for normal behavior.
2. The sequence of normal motor development is important, and provides the

basis for a treatment program to establish return of motor functions.
3. Reflexes are used to influence motion.
4. Repetition of activity, frequency of stimulation, and sensory cues are concepts of learning common to everybody.
5. The whole body is considered as a working unit; the individual parts are not seen in isolation.
6. Personal interaction between the patient and the therapist is an important ingredient for success.

### SENSATION
Thorough evaluation of sensation is essential for every patient with stroke, as normal movements and responses rely on normal sensation. Research supports the close relationship among sensation, perception, and movement, and acknowledges the considerable influence sensory loss can have on motor performance and self-care [37, 43].

Sensation, defined by Mossmann [31] as "appreciation of stimuli" involves the organs for vision, hearing, smell, and taste, the skin or peripheral cutaneous system for sensations of temperature, touch, pressure, and location, and the deep receptors of the muscles, joints, and viscera. Clinical studies of sensory deficits in patients with hemiplegia found the average hospital stay was significantly increased for those who never recovered the sensation of pain, vibration, and two-point discrimination. It is also suggested that rehabilitation prognosis may be poorer if two-point discrimination is impaired [31].

Initial assessment provides a comparison to the norm and a baseline on which all future assessments can be made. Evaluation of the hemiplegic patient must follow a standard format, yet allow for variations of verbal comprehension and expression, perceptual impairments, cultural differences, and additional medical complications. The areas evaluated include light touch, deep pressure, pain, localization of stimuli, kinesthesia, proprioception, two-point discrimination, temperature

TABLE 8-1. *Procedures Used in Therapeutic Exercise*

| Procedure | Effect Desired | Purpose | Patient Status |
|---|---|---|---|
| Electrical stimulation of nerve or muscle; electromyograph (EMG) recording and feedback to patient | Facilitative | Maintain tissue elasticity, prevent muscle atrophy, and demonstrate to patient potential for recovery in terms of artificially induced overt muscle contraction and electrically recorded manifestations or residual motor unit activity | Flaccidity or near 0 muscle response |
| Recruitment of contraction of weak muscles into synergistic action patterns (associated reactions and reflex responses) through overflow or irradiation | Facilitative | To bring weak muscles into play under conditions of maximal voluntary effort with the residually functioning musculature against resistance; for breaking up spasticity | Extreme weakness of important prime movers (elbow extensors, knee flexors) |
| Superficial skin massage, deep muscle vibration, passive manipulation through the range of motion; guiding weak or erratic voluntary movements through the correct track, providing enhanced sensory feedback, verbal feedback, and cueing the patient's attention to sensations in the process | Facilitative | To focus attention on affected body parts while they are static, and help patient attend to kinesthetic input while body parts are in motion | Apraxic (i.e., capable of movement but inattentive to the affected extremities); easily fatigued because of extreme weakness |
| Placement in reflex-inhibiting positions (involves using vestibular stimulation to produce widespread modification of muscle tone) and/or slow, prolonged stretch of tight muscles | Inhibitive | To free patient from the restrictions that spasticity places on range of movement; for altering tone to allow more normal resting postures | Prime movers moderately strong, but resting position and phasic movement limited by spasticity |
| Prolonged application of cold compresses; immersion of limbs in ice bath | Inhibitive | For localized, discrete reduction of spasticity limiting range of motion and hampering functional use of extremity | Capable of movement and moderately strong in its execution, but range limited and coordination poor |

TABLE 8-1. *(Continued)*

| Procedure | Effect Desired | Purpose | Patient Status |
|---|---|---|---|
| Movement of head and body so as to elicit tonic labyrinthine and neck reflexes, and equilibrium reactions of limbs and trunk | Mixed | For modifying the resting distribution of muscle tone; to give patient wider range of postural and movement experiences | Muscles strong in isolated contraction, but muscle imbalance or lack of reciprocal relaxation influences posture and limits certain movements |
| Quick stretch (or, slow stretch of antagonists followed by quick stretch of agonist); repetitive tapping or vibration applied to muscle belly | Facilitative | Applied locally before and during call for voluntary movement | Prime movers still relatively weak but delivering increasingly more contractile tension under volitional effort |
| Cutaneous stimulation (brushing and icing) | Facilitative | For discrete facilitation of contraction of individual muscles, used as a refinement to maximize effectiveness of proprioceptive stimulation | Same as above |
| Application of any facilitation procedures listed above to antagonists of tight muscles | Inhibitive | To relax tight muscles through reciprocal innervation. Applies both to cutaneous and proprioceptive stimulation, as gamma efferent activation and spinal reflexes directly involving alpha motoneurons follow same reciprocal innervation principle | Muscle tone requires local adjustment to normalize muscle balance and thus permit patient to assume more normal postures and perform smoother phasic movements |
| Kinesthetic sensory enhancement or substitution (i.e., use of artificial electronic sense organs to provide position feedback and reinforce patient for improved postural stability and control of phasic movements based on this information) | Mixed | For refining motor skills | Muscle tone within normal range when patient is relaxed, but fluctuates erratically when voluntary movements of any degree of complexity are attempted, as in athetoid cerebral palsy |
| Successive induction; rhythmic stabilization; joint compression | Facilitative | To promote co-contraction of agonist and antagonist for proximal postural stability | Generalized hypotonicity, ataxia, and athetosis |

Source: From P. A. Harris. Facilitation Techniques in Therapeutic Exercise. In J. V. Basmajian (Ed.). *Therapeutic Exercise* (3rd ed.). Baltimore: Williams and Wilkins, 1978. With permission.

discrimination, stereognosis, and graphesthesia. It is important for the therapist to assess the patient's ability to feel and perceive these sensations so that lack of understanding or cooperation or short attention span is not misinterpreted as sensory loss. Careful observation of the patient's verbal and nonverbal reactions and spontaneous motor performance during activities of daily living (ADL) and functional tasks can provide additional valuable information.

Before beginning testing the patient should be informed about the procedure and its reasons, and then reinstructed and given a trial on the uninvolved side before each subtest. All testing is done with the patient's vision occluded, preferably with a screen. The stimuli are applied in an unpredictable fashion, the sequence of which may be indicated on the test form. Responses are usually recorded as follows:

Intact: Patient is consistently correct
Impaired: Patient responds inconsistently or incorrectly
Absent: Patient is unable to identify stimuli, motion, etc.
Unable to test: Patient is unable to participate in testing because of lack of cooperation or severe communication impairment

The rate of response should also be considered.

Treatment consists first of providing for safety and maximum independence. This includes educating the patient and family about the nature of the loss or change, and the role the patient must now take for self-protection and independent function. Use of compensatory techniques and devices that provide visual and auditory information about the limbs and body can be taught and reinforced by the team and family. Watching the affected limbs during ADL, gross motor, and ambulation activities; wearing bright colored bands or bracelets with bells; use of a mirror during some activities (e.g., facial exercises); developing routines for checking affected limbs (e.g., clasping hands) and wiping face during meals and going through a verbal or written inventory of steps of bilateral activities are some techniques.

Sensory education may be another approach, although there is little scientific evidence to support its effectiveness. It consists of providing more stimuli in increased intensity to the affected body parts. Specific activities of gentle rubbing with a towel; touching and identifying various textures and objects; ROM, mobility, and mat programs using facilitation techniques; ADL, and bilateral exercises all involve use of sensory stimulation.

PRIMITIVE REFLEX BEHAVIOR
Trombly and Scott [42] note that "a reflex is an involuntary, stereotyped response to a particular stimulus." Reflexes develop in the fetus and dominate movement in infancy. They provide the foundation on which less primitive, more selective motions and skills are developed. The primitive reflexes never completely disappear, but newer, more sophisticated cortical control develops and dominates in adult life [26]. When a stroke occurs this highly developed cortical control of movement can be lost, and as a result, more primitive reflexes may prevail in motor performance. These are manifested by a variety of abnormal motor behaviors that are influenced by changes in muscle tone, sensory loss, and perceptual impairment.

Just as normal human development follows a pattern from primitive to sophisticated and from mass patterns to selective movement, so recovery from a stroke follows these same patterns [43]. The primitive patterns and reflexes are inhibited as more isolated, voluntary sensorimotor control develops. Recovery of motor control reflects the sequence of normal human development and forms the basis of most treatment procedures.

It is useful and important to assess reflex behavior as part of hemiplegic evaluation. Determination of primitive responses will estab-

TABLE 8-2. *Primitive Reflexes and Their Influence on Motor Behavior*

| Reflex | Influence |
|---|---|
| Symmetrical tonic neck reflex (STNR) Head flexes, arms flex, legs extend Head extends, arms extend, legs flex | Reinforces flexion synergies of extremities Difficulty maintaining 4-point kneeling, interferes with reciprocal motions |
| Asymmetrical tonic neck reflex (ATNR) Head turns to one side, limbs on face side extend, limbs on skull side flex | Interferes with rolling to side as arm extends Influences loss of sitting balance to one side Difficulty maintain 4-point kneeling or standing balance when head turns If very strong, arm movements only possible by turning head May reinforce contracture, scoliosis |
| Crossed extension Stimulus to medial aspect of leg, opposite leg adducts, extends internally, rotates, plantar flexes (scissor pattern) | Interferes with reciprocal leg movements, e.g., walking, stairs |
| Tonic labyrinth reflex (TLR) Prone position stimulates flexion of extremities Supine position stimulates extension of extremities | Interferes with head extension when prone and head flexion when supine Contributes to poor sitting balance, e.g., if head extended may fall backward Back hyperextension interferes with rolling Supine position limits flexion of limbs |
| Positive supporting reaction Pressure on sole of foot stimulates lower extremity extension with ankle in plantar flexion | Limits reciprocal flexion of lower extremities Limits proper heel strike in gait Reinforces extension synergy of lower extremity When seated with lower extremities flexed, unable to support weight to stand |
| Flexor withdrawal Quick stimulus to sole of foot results in total flexion of lower extremity | Reinforces total mass pattern of lower extremity |
| Associated reactions Effort of one limb results in increased flexion tone of another limb (normally present in adult but under control, more evident after stroke) | Any effort will elicit increased flexion tone in upper extremities and increased extension tone in lower extremities, and thus interfere with ambulation and hand use |
| Grasp reflex Pressure on palm of hand results in persistent gross grasp | Inability to let go of objects Reduces functional safe use of hand |

lish the patient's "developmental level" and allow proper treatment to begin from that point. Specific reflex testing formats, although developed for children, can be adapted for use with the adult stroke patient [7, 16]. For example, the basis of Bobath's evaluation [7] is the presence of abnormal primitive reflex behavior and its influence on body posture, mobility, and performance.

Clinically, primitive reflex behavior is mani-fested by the presence of synergies with spas-ticity, a dominance of involuntary responses to stimuli, and lack of coordination or loss of skilled selective performance. (See section on spasticity.) The ones that most commonly in-fluence motor performance in the adult hemi-plegic are shown in Table 8-2. They generally involve the proximal body parts and are seen as total flexion or extension [16, 22, 39, 42]. These reflexes are seldom seen separately, but gener-

TABLE 8-3. *Normal Reflexes and Their Influence on Motor Behavior*

| Reflex | Influence |
|---|---|
| Protective extension<br>Arms and fingers extend when person is pushed toward side or with sudden threat to head or face | May bring about active motion of arm on involuntary basis |
| Equilibrium reactions (in developmental sequence)<br>Change in center of gravity brings about increased tone and protective extension of exemities on lower side with abduction and extension of opposite limbs in attempt to regain balance | Allows development of balance, proximal control, and distal skill sequentially through prone, supine, four-point kneeling, sitting, kneel-stand, standing, and walking<br>Allows fine adjustments of body posture in all functional positions |

ally, are present in a variety of combinations without behavior being dominated by any one.

In normal development, primitive reflexes are inhibited while righting reactions and automatic movements are observed. Protective and equilibrium reactions develop by age 18 months and remain throughout life. Any evaluation and treatment program must also assess normal responses present as well as abnormal primitive reflexes just described (Table 8-3). These normal responses, in addition to being necessary for safe, independent, functional mobility, provide the basis for many treatment procedures and can be used for facilitation and/or inhibition. When primitive reflexes dominate motor behavior, there are techniques for reducing their influence and at the same time encouraging increased control by the more normal responses [26].

These techniques start at the patient's developmental level and follow a progressive sequence. This may mean that some primitive reflexes will not be inhibited until adult responses are more easily achieved. The majority of patients are not strongly dominated by primitive reflexes, but they may lack adequate righting reactions, for example, for safe balance. In this case, such basic reactions can be encouraged before the higher functional activity of gait training begins. At the same time, techniques to inhibit abnormal primitive reflexes can be used. Used in conjunction with

facilitation, these are methods to control and influence primitive reflexes together with tone changes. The patient can be required consciously to go through certain motions that mimic or reinforce normal responses and desired control in an effort to bring these responses to an automatic and functional level. Frequently, this involves putting the patient in a position that offers the least resistance to motion or function, and having the patient think about and perhaps even describe the motion out loud while the therapist guides the activity. For example, equilibrium reactions may not be developed enough to provide safe functional balance in sitting, let alone standing, and primitive tonic neck reflexes may dominate gross motor control. The therapist may want to reduce the influence of head position changes on sitting balance, and at the same time encourage protective extension of the extremities and equilibrium reactions. With the patient sitting on the mat edge and feet flat on the floor, the uninvolved upper extremity is put into a weight-bearing position and held in extension while the patient shifts weight from side to side and looks to left and right. The therapist manually keeps the patient's arm extended, and uses tapping and joint compression to facilitate elbow extension while asking the patient to make a conscious effort to hold the arm straight while turning the head. This task can be incorporated into automatic functions by having the patient perform an activity with the uninvolved hand that also requires head movements, while maintaining a weight-bearing position on the involved arm.

ABNORMAL TONE

Damage to the brain caused by a stroke frequently results in changes in muscle tone and control. Tone changes occur in stages and are used to mark the extent of developing motor control [7, 8, 43]. Initially, there is flaccidity that is followed by spasticity until finally, voluntary motor control develops. These stages are not clear-cut so that throughout recovery, which may reach plateau at any point, there may be spasticity in some muscle groups and weakness in others simultaneously. Complete and careful initial evaluation of tone and its influence on function provides important baseline information against which to measure changes, and help guide treatment.

Many clinical techniques that aim to normalize tone, based on the theories mentioned previously, are available. Although little scientific research has been done to substantiate them [38], clinical observations have provided useful evidence in support of their effectiveness.

Immediately after a stroke there is flaccidity of the involved side [43]. Flaccidity or hypotonia is the total lack of tone and activity in a muscle or muscle group, and absence or decrease of reflex activity. Clinically, flaccidity can be recognized by lack of voluntary active motion, of tone that is ordinarily present in a normal resting muscle, and of normal resistance to passive movement. The longer this condition continues to dominate, the worse the prognosis is for recovery [31]. Seldom does a patient remain in the true flaccid stage; by 48 hours following onset some tone is likely to develop [43].

True flaccidity and severe weakness have clinical consequences and implications for immediate treatment. They can result in edema or swelling of the distal portion of the extremities, and joint integrity can be affected when the protection normally provided by the active muscles is missing. For example, subluxation may occur in the upper extremity. In addition, peripheral nerve and vascular damage may occur because of subluxation, traction, or pressure. The hip may become traumatized with abnormal positioning. The trunk may become misaligned, which contributes to poor body posture and possible damage to internal organs. Sensory loss, cognitive perceptual motor deficits, and apraxia may compound these problems by interrupting the normal feedback mechanism and by interfering with abilities to correct. Flaccidity and severe weakness become more apparent when the patient is tired, anxious, or overworked.

This weakness can persist in the upper extremity even as the lower extremity begins developing tone. One theory suggests that the sensory input provided by weight-bearing on the leg may facilitate an increase of tone [7]. It is not uncommon for a patient to be ambulating with fair lower extremity motor control and retain a persistently flaccid nonfunctional upper extremity.

Evaluation is done by requesting the patient to assist while the therapist moves each joint passively through its full available range of motion, and watches and palpates for changes in muscle tone. The manual muscle testing grading system that records the amount of resistance in a muscle or muscle group is recorded as a letter grade [42]. Generally, in the flaccid or very weak condition, the grades would be zero, trace, or possibly poor. Testing in this way is done only if there is no spasticity or synergy.

Although true flaccidity is seldom seen after the acute phase, continued severe weakness in some muscle groups may persist as tone develops in others. Evaluation is made of the degree and location of weakness, plus indications of developing tone or spasticity. Basic evaluation is supplemented by techniques for assessing the spastic extremity, such as quick stretch and associated reaction, to determine any developing tone, reflex activity, latent spasticity, or beginning synergy. Additional information includes the presence and degree of secondary complications of loss of joint range of motion and integrity, edema, and shoulder subluxation. These problems require prompt attention by all rehabilitation team members.

Loss of passive range of motion can result from weakness if the extremities are not routinely passively ranged from the first day. This range can be evaluated by the standard method of moving each joint as completely as possible and measuring the freedom of motion present [22]. With the hemiplegic patient, joint range may be documented as a fraction of the full normal range [44]. An edematous extremity is puffy and swollen, the skin appears shiny and stretched, and a depression made by pushing down with a finger does not immediately disappear. In the weak hemiplegic extremities, full passive range of motion is maintained or increased by manually ranging the joints. Passive ROM as preventive and active treatment is an integral part of rehabilitation, and is the responsibility of occupational and physical therapy and nursing staffs. It is done carefully, using the traditional methods of passively moving each joint and incorporating normal joint play and biomechanics [31, 42]. Proper positioning and elevation of extremities are important for maintaining range of motion and reducing edema. In addition, edema can be temporarily reduced by elevating the extremity and firmly stroking distally to proximally.

Frequently, paralysis of the extremities is accompanied by facial weakness, which is commonly combined with sensory loss and can be complicated by perceptual impairment and apraxia. The face lacks the usual symmetrical look, with a drooped appearance of the mouth, especially at the corner, cheek, and eye, which becomes more evident when the patient attempts facial expressions. Weakness or impairment may become more apparent when the patient is tired. Facial musculature is tested by requesting the patient to perform specific motions using the mouth, cheeks, and tongue. Control and use are graded as unable, impaired, or normal [44].

Treatment of facial weakness consists of bilateral active resistive exercises and activities done in front of a mirror, and facilitation techniques of tapping, quick stretch, vibration, and ice. Some specific foods and methods for eating can provide stimulation and facilitate normal facial motion, such as drinking a thick milkshake through a straw and sucking on ice. Facial motions are easily and spontaneously incorporated in and reinforced by daily activities.

Shoulder subluxation, the downward dislocation of the humerus, is one of the most common problems for a patient with flaccidity or weakness. In the flaccid extremity, the locking mechanism [3] that ordinarily holds the humerus in place may no longer function adequately. The supraspinatus, part of the rotator cuff muscles, along with all the other scapular and humeral muscles can no longer hold the humerus in place when they are weak or completely paralyzed. The upward position of the glenoid fossa is no longer maintained, as gravity, the weight of the arm, spasticity, or a tendency for the patient to lean toward the hemiplegic side brings the scapula into a downward position (Figure 8-5). The advantage of the locking mechanism is thus lost and the ligaments alone cannot provide the necessary support. Even without complete paralysis, subluxation can occur as the scapular and humeral muscles become fatigued. Prolonged subluxation can cause permanent muscle, vascular, and nerve damage, and can be extremely painful.

Shoulder subluxation is evaluated by gently allowing the arm to hang by the patient's side, and palpating the suprahumeral gap or space between the acromion process and the humeral head. If a gap is present, its size is measured by finger widths. Additionally, if a subluxation is present, the gap should disappear when the humerus is manually approximated into the fossa. This procedure, together with comparison to the sound side, will assist ruling out atrophy and unusual bony prominences.

Prevention or immediate elimination of subluxation is a priority. The most effective pre-

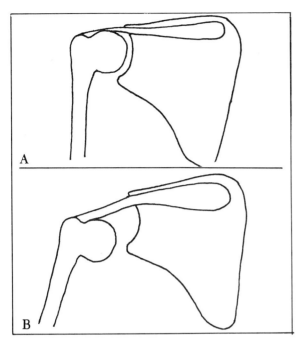

FIGURE 8-5. *Subluxation. A. Position of humerus in the glenoid fossa and the supraspinatus muscle in the locking mechanism. B. Position of the humerus and scapula during subluxation. Note downward rotation of scapula and horizontal motion of humerus.*

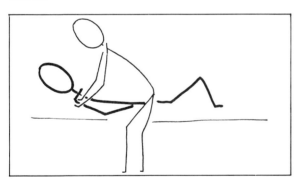

FIGURE 8-6. *Scapular mobilization (see also Fig. 8-7). The therapist manually moves the scapula through range of motion by placing a hand over scapula with fingers on medial border. Humerus is kept approximated in fossa so scapula and humerus work as one unit. Supine. With one hand on scapula and other under axilla, patient's arm relaxed by side, hand on abdomen, and keeping humerus and scapula together, passively: (1) Elevate and upward rotate then depress and rotate scapula downward. (2) Protract and retract scapula by pulling and pushing gently on medial border.*

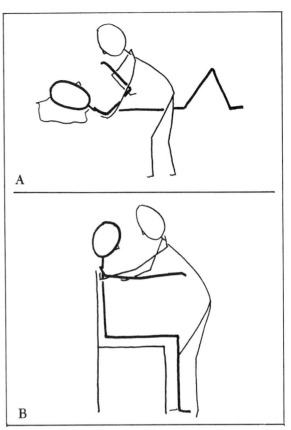

FIGURE 8-7. *A. Supine. B. Sitting. Passively flex humerus between 45° and 90°, staying in pain-free range. Elbow may remain flexed or be extended. Mobilize scapula through following ranges: (1) Protraction and retraction using hand on medial border while passively gently pulling humerus and scapula together foward and back. (2) Upward rotation using hand on medial border and inferior angle of scapula and increasing flexion of humerus gradually (it is important that humerus and scapula work together). (3) With humerus in 45° abduction, passively rotate upward and retract and protract scapula. Increase humeral range as tolerated.*

ventive measure is support of the arm by passively maintaining the humerus in the glenoid fossa. With support, the force of gravity is reduced, articular surfaces are kept together, and pain and potential damage to the surrounding soft tissue can be prevented. In addition, the locking mechanism is in a position to function as tone increases.

An arm sling is one means of support. The type recommended depends on the individual's particular needs and problems, and the therapeutic approach of the rehabilitation team. Any sling should be carefully and routinely evaluated with special attention paid to its effectiveness in eliminating the subluxation and changes in muscle tone, ROM, pain, ease of use, and secondary effects [9]. Slings are most useful when worn during standing, ambulation, and transfer activities, and are not necessary while sitting if a lap board, arm tray, or even pillow is used [7, 9, 42].

Lap trays and arm boards provide good support, and can be adapted for special problems such as edema and contractures, and can allow more freedom of movement and independent ROM. Care should be taken to protect the skin on bony prominences from breakdown.

Support and normal alignment of the humerus and scapula while the patient is in bed are provided with pillows under the scapula and humerus if the patient is immobilized. As the patient gains mobility and is encouraged to move about in bed, techniques for protection and safety are taught. If the patient has the cognitive abilities, responsibility can be given for protecting and positioning the involved arm (Figures 8-2 and 8-3).

A therapy program should be initiated of scapular mobilization and specific exercises to increase pain-free range of motion and tone of the scapular and humeral muscles, especially the scapular upward rotators and supraspinatus portions of the rotator cuff muscles (Scapular Mobilization: Figures 8-6 and 8-7; exercises for subluxation: Figures 8-8 through 8-11). Even as tone increases and the patient

can actively eliminate subluxation, support of the arm may need to continue for some time until muscle endurance allows constant active support. Occasionally, subluxation may be present with spasticity. This happens when the more severely spastic muscle groups pull the scapula into a downward rotated position or pull the humeral head out of the glenoid fossa. In this case, specific techniques and support devices must be consistent with specific program goals.

Treatment of weakness in other body parts, like that for subluxation and facial weakness, consists of applying facilitation methods to increase tone in normal functional patterns, and these exercises can be incorporated into purposeful activities.

After the initial flaccid stage, tone gradually develops and may become exaggerated in the involved side of the body. This hypertonicity is seen clinically as spasticity. It occurs when an upper motor neuron lesion injures the neural components normally responsible for inhibiting or suppressing abnormal reflex activity. This release from higher control allows an unequal excitation of certain muscle groups, usually the antigravity muscles, and reciprocal inhibition of others, usually the antagonists. Spasticity is described as having three components [14]:

1. Increased resistance to passive stretch
2. Hyperactive deep tendon reflexes
3. Clonus, a self-perpetuating, synchronized, exaggerated stretch reflex with such a low threshold that slight passive movement may initiate it

Clinically, it is recognized by an initial free range of movement, then a strong resistance followed by relaxation, frequently called the clasped knife phenomenon.

Spasticity presents many implications for the patient and therapist. It generally is not isolated to a single muscle or even muscle group, but rather exerts its strongest effect on the antigravity muscles that overpower the an-

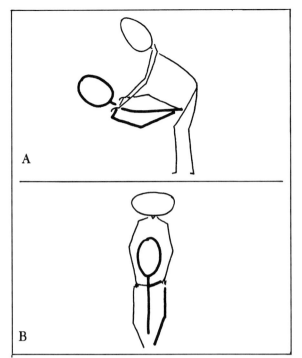

FIGURE 8-8. *Scapula elevation (shrugging). A. Supine. B. Sitting. Active assistance to elevation; tapping on upper trapezius; resistance to active elevation; quick stretch of upper trapezius; associated reactions by resisting sound side; combinations of above.*

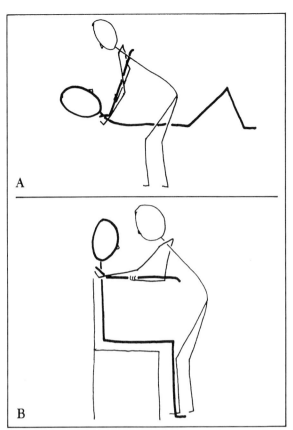

FIGURE 8-9. *Scapula protraction and upward rotation. A. Supine. B. Sitting. With scapula placed in protracted position, patient is asked to "hold," "reach arm forward," or "make arm longer;" quick stretch to scapula protractors then actively assisted through protraction (feel for catching reaction) giving resistance to protraction.*

tagonists to them [14]. This causes muscle imbalance and produces the following classic patterns or synergies, with variations according to theorist [7, 8, 43]:

1. In the upper extremity: A general flexion pattern of scapular downward rotation and retraction; humeral adduction and internal rotation; elbow, wrist, and finger flexion, and forearm pronation
2. In the lower extremity: A general extension pattern of hip adduction and internal rotation; knee and hip extension; and ankle and foot plantar flexion and inversion
3. Trunk and neck muscles: May be shortened resulting in lateral flexion on the involved side

It is also acknowledged that every patient suffering from stroke experiences spasticity to some extent, if even for a brief time, and that it develops through stages [43]. These stages have been described in different ways [7, 8], but it is generally accepted that spasticity usually begins developing in proximal muscle groups after an initial flaccid phase, and increases in severity to a point at which function may be drastically impaired. Its normal course is to resolve slowly as voluntary control increases. This process of development and resolution of spasticity can reach a plateau at any

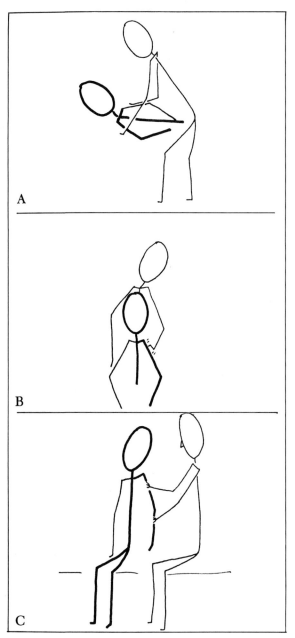

FIGURE 8-10. *Humeral abduction. A. Supine. B. Sitting. Active assistance through 45° of abduction and patient holds; tapping over supraspinatus and deltoid; quick stretch to abductor muscles and ask for active abduction; bilateral resistance to abduction. C. Manually eliminate any gap by positioning humerus in place and asking patient to hold by requesting "reach," "lift arm out to side," or "shrug." Use mirror if helpful.*

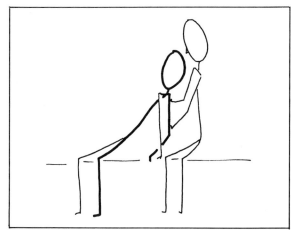

FIGURE 8-11. *Scapular stability. Patient supports some body weight by leaning to side on elbow or hand if possible; repositioning arm further from body and leaning on elbow or hand; leaning on elbow and moving body and scapula up and down.*

time and presents long-range problems of synergy, weakness, muscle imbalance, decreased ROM, and functional limitations. Changes in tone can continue for 12 to 18 months postonset and have been noted to occur as long as three years from onset [31]. It has been noted [30] that recovery of upper and lower extremity function "varies inversely with the degree of spasticity." Many factors influence spasticity and may, in turn, lead to an increase or decrease in function. Medical conditions such as bladder calculi, decubitus ulcers, infection, pain, or constipation, and emotional conditions such as stress, tension, or extreme excitement cause an immediate effect on the degree of spasticity. External sensory stimuli such as a blast of cold air or sudden noise or touch, and internal factors such as excessive effort are also influencing factors. In fact, many therapeutic facilitation and inhibition techniques are based on the premise that particular sensory input can elicit specific motor outputs, and thus when used properly, can promote more normal motor function.

Spasticity, especially when prolonged, and its accompanying muscle imbalance have potentially severe consequences. These include decrease in passive ROM and joint contractures, pain, possible subluxation, abnormal body postures, and even pressure on internal organs. They also affect stability, and thus all functional activities. These consequences can be further complicated when combined with sensory loss and perceptual and cognitive impairment, as the patient has fewer abilities, cues, and body resources on which to rely.

Accurate evaluation of spasticity is a continuous process, with initial assessment providing a baseline on which changes can be measured. Spasticity cannot be evaluated by the traditional methods used to assess strength. Although it is seen as a degree of resistance, it is not under voluntary control and is not indicative of muscle weakness or strength. Rather it is viewed as a muscle imbalance caused by abnormal tone, primitive reflexes, and hyperactive stretch reflex in a muscle group that does not allow reciprocal relaxation of the antagonistic group.

Spasticity is evaluated both as a condition of its own and as it influences posture, motor control, and function. Some therapists [7] assess it in terms of postural tone, balance, reactions, movement patterns, control, and total body motor performance.

Formal evaluation is done mainly by clinical observation and professional judgment during a standard procedure. A quick firm stretch of a muscle group starting in the shortened state, will elicit any abnormal resistance in that group. The amount of resistance encountered and the degree to which it restricts passive ROM can give a reasonable indication of the degree of spasicity. How it is recorded may vary but a common grading system is as follows:

Mild: When slight increased resistance is encountered at the end of the range, but full passive ROM and gross functional coordination may be present
Moderate: When increased resistance is encountered in the middle of the range, with impairment of voluntary function and some possible reduction of passive ROM
Severe: When this increased resistance is encountered in the shortened muscle state, with passive ROM drastically reduced and no voluntary function possible.

As no scientific or completely objective measure has been found, the evaluation tool continues to be the knowledge and skill of the therapist.

Informal methods of assessment provide additional information about spasticity. When it is purposefully elicited, for example, in the elbow flexors by a quick stretch or requested flexion, the time it takes to return from the full flexion position to a normal extended resting angle can give further information about spasticity in that particular muscle group. Reduction of passive ROM of involved joints and actual palpation of the muscle bellies gives information on severity. The amount of voluntary control the patient has available to counteract its influence is also an important indicator of degree and stage of spasticity. This can be seen during functional activities when the patient uses bilateral reciprocal motions or exaggerated effort. The information from these formal and informal methods includes degree, stage of development, and any factors that might directly affect spasticity, and its consequences on performance and safety, some of which might demand priority attention by the therapists.

Treatment generally involves techniques based on the sensorimotor approaches and positioning discussed earlier, to reduce or prevent its effects on motor performance. Figures 8-12 to 8-22 demonstrate possibile ways of increasing normal tone and function of the involved extremities. See Figures 8-23 and 8-24 for rolling and bridging activities to facilitate pelvis and trunk control and bilateral hip and knee control.

Spasticity frequently creates problems that become priorities of treatment. Decreased range of motion or contractures, pain, swallow-

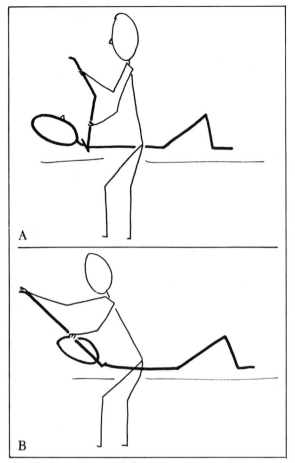

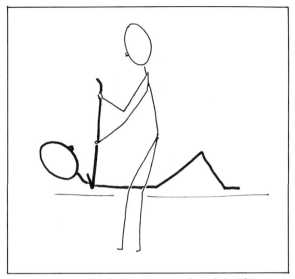

FIGURE 8-13. With spasticity reduced, hold arm at 90° shoulder flexion and elbow in extension as tolerated and use joint compression straight down through arm, then have patient hold position; with minimal support lightly push or tap arm to keep vertical position; place arm slightly off vertical position in various directions and have patient actively bring arm back to upright, add resistance as patient is able. Have patient maintain vertical position while reaching up to include scapula protraction and retraction, flexing and extending elbow, and making and relaxing fist as possible.

FIGURE 8-12. A. If flexion spasticity is present, gradually bring shoulder into flexion, external rotation, and abduction, and elbow, wrist, and hand into extension and forearm into supination using reflex inhibiting positions; slow stretch to spastic muscles; gentle push-pull of humerus; facilitation to elbow extension with tapping, quick stretch, resistance. B. Hold this position (do not go into painful range).

ing difficulties, postural imbalance, and poor trunk alignment jeopardize the patient's safety and demand immediate attention.

To guard against loss of range of motion, a program is provided for hypertonic extremities that includes inhibition techniques of slow stretch, reflex-inhibiting positions, and head positions that promote the desired movements. Passive ROM using these techniques can be done by all members of the team and the fami-

ly. If cognitively and physically capable, the patient can do self-ROM in a group program and individually, using these techniques in addition to bilateral, whole-body mobility and interaction.

Positioning is necessary if the spasticity is so severe that the patient cannot attend to it independently and during sleep. Proper positioning goes on 24 hours a day and requires careful use of sensorimotor techniques. (See Figures 8-1 to 8-4.) Devices and techniques must be used in such a way as not to interfere with the patient's independence and self-esteem.

When spasticity is severe and function and ROM are jeopardized, splinting the upper extremity and bracing the lower extremity may be advisable. The treatment priorities, the patient's level of ability and the philosophy of the rehabilitation facility all help to determine

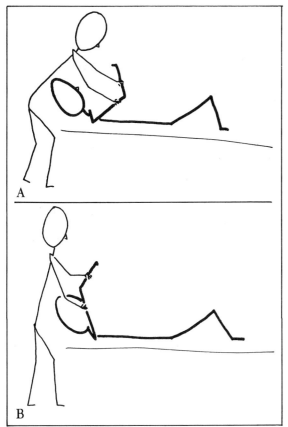

FIGURE 8-14. *Active shoulder and scapula motions. A and B. Use active assistive motion; progressive resistive motions; quick stretch and joint compression combined with first two. Vary previous motions with changes in elbow flexion.*

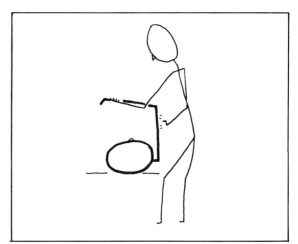

FIGURE 8-15. *Active elbow extension. With 90° shoulder flexion use active assist through full elbow range; quick stretch and tapping to extensors; resistance to extension motion. Combine shoulder and elbow active motions, out of patterns, by having patient hold one joint position and move through other joint motions. For example, hold shoulder in 90° flexion and flex and extend elbow. Facilitate by using tapping, placing, quick stretch.*

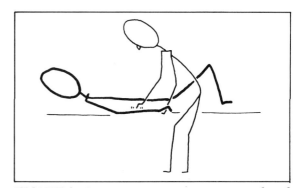

FIGURE 8-16. *Active wrist extension. Arm relaxed with elbow extended over edge of mat, use active assist and resistance to wrist extension; quick stretch with resistance; tapping on extensor surface.*

when either of these is necessary. A variety of wrist and hand splints is used. The basic palmar or resting splint and the dorsal resting splint maintain the wrist, fingers, and thumb in varying degrees of extension, and are available commercially or can be fabricated individually. A basic cone splint can be used in emergency situations to maintain a functional position of the hand, although it does not include the wrist and may be contraindicated in some situations. The sponge, or Bobath splint is a thick piece of foam rubber with five holes cut to accommodate the fingers and thumb [7]. The fingers are positioned in abduction, which also promotes extension, although this splint does not include the wrist. If safe functional transfers and ambulation are priorities and are made possible by bracing, the use of a brace may be a treatment of choice in that particular circumstance. The use of splints and braces, as with any adaptive device, need not be the end result of treatment, but rather means to reach

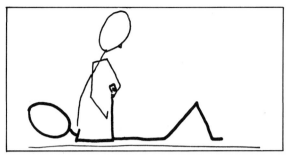

FIGURE 8-17. *Active elbow, forearm, wrist, and hand motions. Patient holding 90° elbow flexion and forearm vertical while supinating and pronating forearm, flexing and extending wrist, and grasping and releasing hand. Vary degree of elbow flexion and extension and return to vertical with and without added weight. Use joint compression, resistance, quick stretch, and tapping with above.*

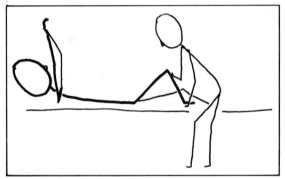

FIGURE 8-18. *Hip control. With hip and knee flexed and foot flat on mat, facilitate hip motions by placing hip in various positions of flexion and having patient hold position with knee upright. Use joint compression and tapping. Place leg in degrees of external rotation and have patient hold then return to neutral. Have patient hold knee upright with hip in neutral while therapist uses resistance. Facilitate ankle dorsiflexion by slow stretch into dorsiflexion; resistance to dorsiflexion; stroking plantar aspect to toes; tapping dorsiflexor surface.*

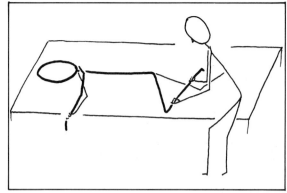

FIGURE 8-19. *Hip and knee control. Lying on sound side facilitate hip and knee control by active assist through range of flexion and extension plus resistance, tapping, joint compression; actively assist 1 joint while others remain stationary, for example, knee flexion and extension while hip remains flexed.*

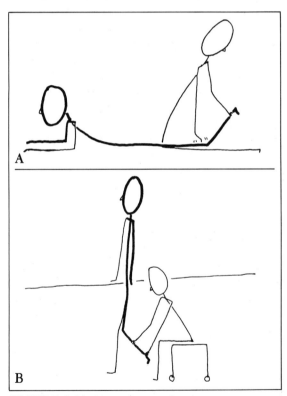

FIGURE 8-20. *Motions out of pattern. A. Prone. B. Standing. Facilitate isolated motions in prone and standing by active flexion of knee with hip remaining in extension, using resistance, tapping, passive range of motion, joint compression.*

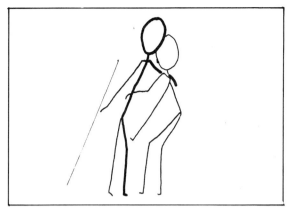

FIGURE 8-21. *Lower extremity control. Facilitate lower extremity control by standing and weight-bearing on extremity and use knee stabilization, tapping.*

eventual increased function and safety without devices.

When spasticity is present in the muscles responsible for swallowing, speech, and facial expressions, techniques to reduce these problems require the skilled approach of the occupational therapist and speech-language pathologist (see Chapter 9).

Pain is a common problem and can severely limit the patient's psychological adjustment and active participation in therapy. It is important for the team and the patient to understand the kinds of pain and possible available treatments (Table 8-4).

### DEVELOPMENT OF VOLUNTARY MOTOR CONTROL

On a progressive continuum of motor return, the patient will begin to exhibit voluntary movement outside of the typical synergistic patterns, permitting increased function. These movements may be incomplete, weak, of low endurance, and awkward, and are probably still influenced by synergy and primitive reflex activity. Their presence indicates clinically that change and resolution of the hemiplegia are continuing, and offers additional alternatives of treatment.

Selective voluntary control in both gross and fine motor activities should be evaluated. Test-

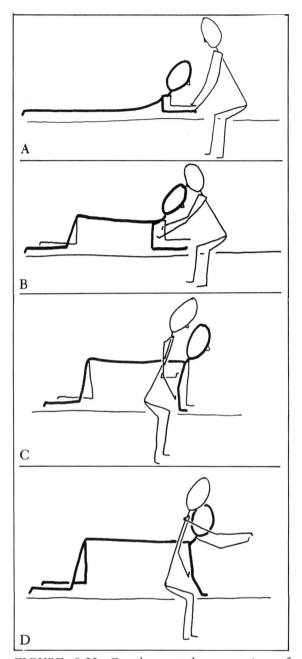

FIGURE 8-22. *Developmental progression of weight-bearing positions as tolerated. Assist patient to assume positions and hold them. Vary positions by leaning to left and right, forward and back, and changing head positions. Facilitate control by tapping, actively assisting, resisting, etc. Have patient use sound arm for activities. Patient might actually crawl with reciprocal motions.*

TABLE 8-4. *Pain*

| Cause and Pathology | Charcteristics | Techniques for Treatment |
|---|---|---|
| Decreased ROM, tightness, and spasticity | Found with spastic conditions and shortening of muscles and tendons<br>Pain increased with passive ROM<br>Common in shoulder, elbow, wrist, hand, hip, ankle, and neck | Prevention<br>ROM to prevent contractures<br>Avoid actual stretching of tight muscles that can lead to more trauma and soft tissue damage<br>Inhibition and relaxation techniques; use of heat, cold, vibration, may have some value |
| Flaccid shoulder results in nonalignment of joint with traction, pressure, and trauma to periarticular structures and brachial plexus injury | Extremity lacks normal tone, is hyptonic<br>Subluxation of shoulder joint; more pain may be present if arm unsupported or with passive ROM past 90 degrees<br>With brachial plexus injury:<br>Atypical return of function<br>Deviation from usual return of function proximal to distal<br>Extensive contractures in fingers<br>Segmental muscle atrophy<br>Sensory changes follow peripheral nerve pattern rather than diffuse sensory loss | Prevention<br>Proper support and positioning of arm at all times with slings, pillows, arm boards, etc.<br>Do not lift or move patient by using involved arm<br>Protection of shoulder and upper extremity until regeneration<br>Careful passive ROM (past 90° only if scapula mobilized)<br>Active ROM<br>Facilitation techniques and scapula mobilization<br>Ultrasound, moist heat with ROM |
| Shoulder-hand syndrome (reflex sympathetic dystrophy) | Shoulder pain referred to hand<br>Wide range of syndromes; any or all of painful vasodilation and vasoconstriction; nonpitting swelling or atrophy of hand and loss of skin lines; changes in skin temperature; frozen shoulder; hand painful in flexion | Passive and active ROM within pain-free range and with no pain after one hour<br>Support shoulder and arm<br>Heat for comfort and preparation for exercises<br>Medications for pain relief<br>Ultrasound followed by passive ROM, scapula mobilization and self-ROM when possible |
| Thalamic pain<br>Part of thalamic syndrome (mild hemiparesis, hemianesthesia, hemiataxia, and pain) | Nonspecific pain in leg and arm<br>Not necessarily associated with tone changes, edema, or other medical conditions<br>Not responsive to medication<br>Severe, persistent, paroxysmal, often intolerable pains of hemiplegic side | No known medical or physical treatment<br>Careful diagnosis necessary to eliminate other possible causes<br>Need to educate patient and family about cause with goal that greater understanding will bring greater tolerance<br>Heat or relaxation exercises may help general level of comfort |

ing includes active range of motion using traditional methods that are possible as spasticity diminishes or disappears; selective movements that require the patient to assume positions out of the synergistic patterns; and reciprocal motions requiring smooth, bilateral coordinated use of hands or feet. Test results can be graded as unable, incomplete, complete with difficulty, or normal. As hand and arm functions increase, standardized tests of hand skills, finger function, and prevocational tasks can be administered [22, 23, 42]. These are particularly useful as they give numerical values to performances that can be objectively compared to past and future scores.

During this stage, the patient may more easily recognize improvements in motor skill and function, which provide rewards and a feeling of success. Increased motor control, especially when accompanied by improved perception, sensation, and cognition, can be an additional motivating incentive and encourage the patient to take more responsibility for continuing to learn through work on home programs. Gait, fine motor, and prevocational tasks call for smooth, coordinated bilateral use of the body, and provide natural ways for the patient to incorporate improvement and treatment techniques used in therapy into daily function.

Some basic principles used in promoting motor control include:

1. Active use of the involved extremities in the normal process of performing all functional activities, e.g., dressing
2. Controlled movements out of the synergistic patterns
3. Moving one joint independently of surrounding joints
4. Motions done slowly with control, incorporating stopping, reversing, slowing down, speeding up, and holding, at all points in the movement
5. Adding weight or resistance and retaining the same control
6. Motions of the upper and lower extremity done in a variety of postures, e.g., sitting, standing, kneeling, with head turned
7. Combinations and variations of these

In addition to the facilitation and inhibition techniques, the use of biofeedback in rehabilitation has increased and is becoming a viable treatment tool for the stroke patient. Preliminary studies by Basmajian have shown that the use of electromyography (EMG) biofeedback combined with therapeutic exercise has produced dramatic effects [4]. Significant increases in strength and ROM of foot dorsiflexion were demonstrated by hemiparetic patients who received both conventional therapy and biofeedback [5]. Reduction of shoulder subluxation and improvement in scapular and humeral mobility were noted in patients receiving muscle reeducation with biofeedback to the shoulder area, specifically for proper scapular position of upward rotation [6]. Relaxation of spastic muscles of the forearm and hand can be modified by this technique to allow increased voluntary use of the hand [4].

FUNCTIONAL PROGRAM
The problems discussed thus far, combined with perceptual and cognitive impairment, contribute to the patient's limitation of function in mobility, balance, transfers, gait, and self-care. A treatment program to deal with them combines facilitation and inhibition techniques with a holistic, functionally directed approach. The program also follows a developmental sequence from simple to complex, primitive to cortical level, gross to fine, patterned motions to isolated control, and proximal control to distal coordination. By providing normal bilateral sensory input and guiding motor performance, increased normal motor output is anticipated. In addition, these techniques, even when broken down into simple steps and repeated, continue to be functionally oriented and purposeful in nature. The procedures suggested are only some of those available. Their use assumes the therapist has a full understanding of the patient's entire condition

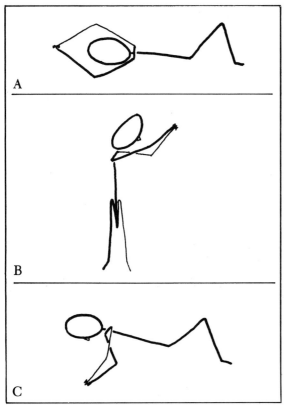

FIGURE 8-23. *Rolling. A. With legs to one side, hold, then roll to other side, upper body relaxed. B. Arms and head to one side, hold, then to other side; lower body relaxed. C. Combine first two motions in opposite directions. Resist or assist patient as needed. Practice separately and together. Combine motions in same direction (one segment at a time) for rolling sequence.*

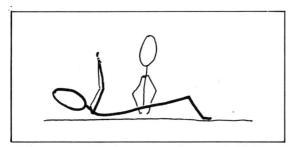

FIGURE 8-24. *Bridging. Raise hips up, hold, lower. Keep knees together and weight evenly distributed. Repeat with knees in more flexion. Use resistance and joint compression. Hold up position and shift weight to left and right keeping knees upright. Hold up position and abduct and adduct knees evenly.*

and needs, and has sufficiently investigated the theories and their rationale.

MOVING AND TRANSFERS
When a patient lacks control of the trunk and proximal joints, difficulty moving in bed is a common problem. The ability to move in bed allows functional tasks to be achieved, such as use of a bedpan, a reach for the call bell, or sitting up. This type of safe and independent movement may be the patient's first experience in regaining body control. Procedures to increase bed mobility, specifically rolling, bridging, and coming to sitting, can start as simple passive activities in the acute phase of illness, and continue in therapy to more sophisticated active fine motor tasks (Figures 8-23, 8-24, 8-25, and 8-26).

A sense of balance depends on a combination of two of three components: vision, proprioception, and labyrinthine function [31]. In addition, to maintain or regain balance depends on muscle strength, control, equilibrium, and adequate mental and perceptual capabilities. Functional balance is a prerequisite for safe transfers, self-care, and ambulation. Balance techniques progress from a broad base with lateral support and low center of gravity, to a narrow base with no support and a higher center of gravity. Activities to promote balance also provide sensory input, require bilateral use of the body, and can assist in increasing confidence. These activities incorporated into early functional mobility and ADL help to develop more normal motor behavior and facilitate carryover of techniques learned in therapy to daily life (Figure 8-27 to 8-40).

Independent, safe transfer from wheelchair to bed, mat, toilet, tub, other chairs, and car is a goal of rehabilitation. In addition, techniques incorporated into transfer training promote increased motor control. To reach a standing position, pulling on the wheelchair or bed rail is strongly discouraged because it is unsafe and may develop into bad habits when gait training begins. Instead, leaning forward to transfer the weight onto the legs and the technique of shift-

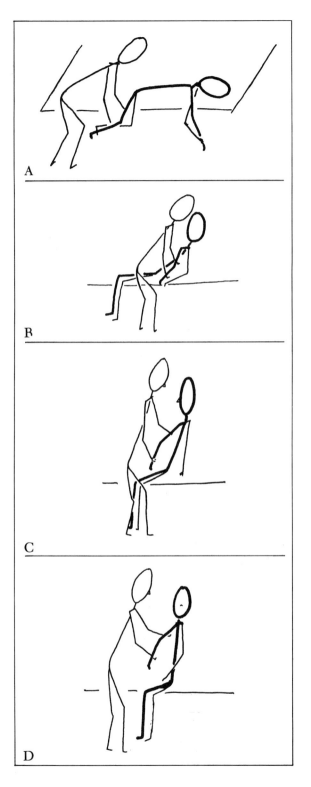

FIGURE 8-25. *To sitting position from sound side. A. Feet over edge, sound foot involved as necessary. Hands clasped together, arms extended. B. Prop up onto sound elbow with head turned toward involved side. Hands are still clasped, if possible, or therapist holds arm extended, and scapula protracted. C. Push up onto sound hand, elbow extended. Hands are still clasped if possible, or therapist holds extended. D. Come to full sitting position, hands in lap, feet flat on floor. Therapist assists balance as needed.*

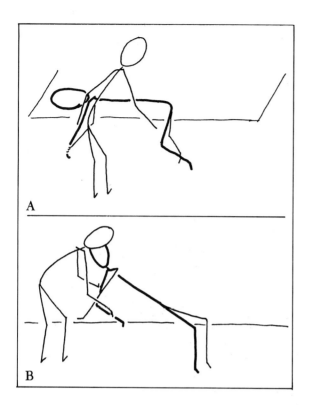

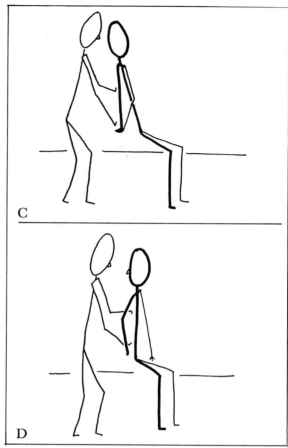

FIGURE 8-26. *To sitting position from involved side. A. Feet over edge, sound foot to help as necessary. B. Prop up onto involved elbow, sound arm help as needed. Therapist helps keep trunk balanced over elbow, feet flat on floor. C. Push up onto involved hand, elbow extended, sound hand helping. Therapist holds some weight if needed, position involved hand flat, and support elbow in extension as needed. D. Come to full sitting with hands clasped in lap.*

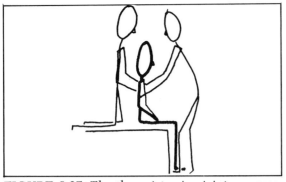

FIGURE 8-27. *The therapists give joint compression straight down through shoulders and trunk. The patient sits on mat or bed edge, feet flat on floor, thighs parellel to floor, weight evenly distributed on both hips, back straight. When maximum support is needed, one therapist kneels behind patient supporting trunk, and the other stands in front.*

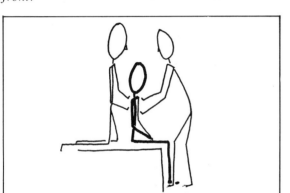

FIGURE 8-28. *Briefly take away support and have patient hold. Do not let patient lose balance; bring back to upright. Use joint compression, verbal and visual cues. Increase time as tolerated.*

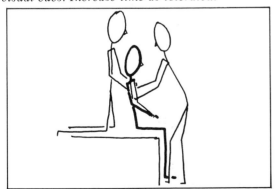

FIGURE 8-29. *Once patient can hold sitting balance for a short time try placing patient slightly off center in various directions and have patient hold position; have patient return to center, with assistance as needed.*

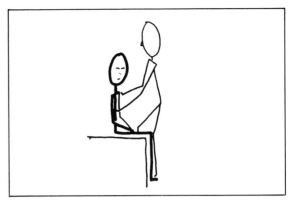

FIGURE 8-30. *When less support is needed. (See Figs. 8-31 to 8-37.) Patient sits unsupported with therapist in front on involved side and slightly forward. Patient keeps balance and takes deep breath and exhales; closes eyes; turns head left, right, up and down.*

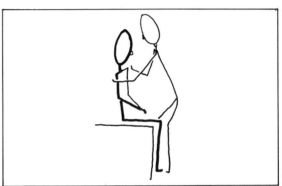

FIGURE 8-31. *Therapist uses following facilitation techniques: (1) Places patient off upright position and has patient hold, then returns to upright, assisting as needed. (2) Gentle, light, quick tapping or pushing in different directions and have patient hold upright. (3) Sustained gentle pushing and patient holds upright. (4) Suddenly take away resistance and patient maintains upright position.*

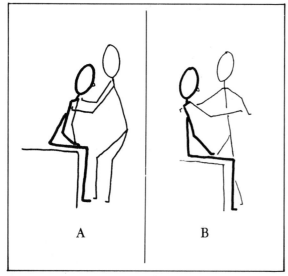

FIGURE 8-32. *Patient performs active motions. A. Lean trunk forward, back, left, right, twist to left, and right to varying degrees. B. Reach sound hand forward, left, right, over head. Combine with trunk leaning. Add weight as tolerated. Try same with involved hand.*

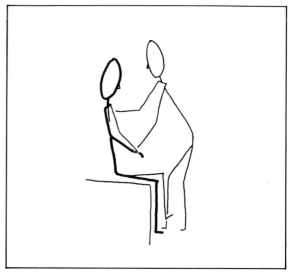

FIGURE 8-34. *Maintain balance and lift up sound knee and foot; lift up involved knee and foot as able; adduct and abduct knees.*

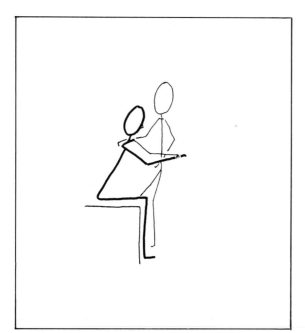

FIGURE 8-33. *Clasp hands together, or with hands under opposite elbows and reach forward, left, right, up, down. Hold positions and combine with trunk leaning.*

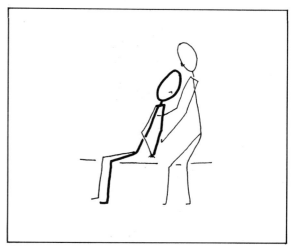

FIGURE 8-35. *Lean to sound side and rest on hand or elbow. Return to upright. Do same on involved side, using sound hand for assist as needed.*

252

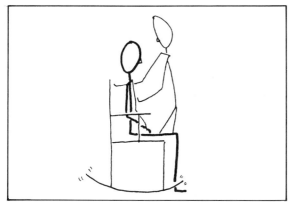

FIGURE 8-36. *Sit in rocking chair, back unsupported. Therapist rocks chair and patient keeps balance.*

ing and sitting is suggested (Figures 8-41 and 8-42).

Generally, it is safer and more independent for the patient to move toward the sound side. Thus it is important to teach this preferred method for transfer, together with sitting and balance activities. It is possible for a patient who has no additional cognitive or balance problems to stand and transfer toward the sound side, using the sound arm and leg for support without additional assistance.

As the therapist cannot guarantee that the patient will only have to transfer toward the sound side, it is suggested that moving toward the involved side be part of training. It also offers the opportunity to apply facilitation and inhibition techniques and to increase use of the involved side in a normal motor pattern. Basic methods are illustrated in Figures 8-43 and 8-44 and are modified for toilet, bathtub or shower, and car transfers. During any motor program and especially during transfer training, it is important to remember good body mechanics. A good back is a precious commodity, and all lifting and moving should be done close to the body, with the knees bent and feet widely spaced for a broad base of support. Heavily or totally dependent patients may require two therapists for transfers and moving.

Although not all patients are alike, there does appear to be a typical gait pattern of hemi-

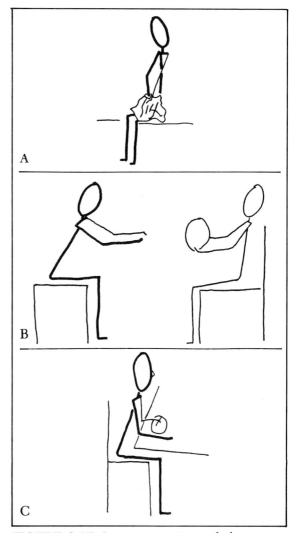

FIGURE 8-37. *Incorporate sitting balance into functional activities as appropriate. A. Dressing. B. Recreational activities. C. At standard table.*

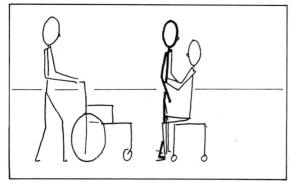

FIGURE 8-38. *Standing balance. Therapist provides support and stability to hips and involved knee, and uses facilitation techniques. (1) Tapping or vibration on knee extensors. (2) Joint compression down on hips. (3) Resistance to hip extension. Have patient keep balance while turning head, lifting sound arm, shifting weight, twisting trunk.*

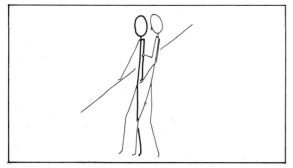

FIGURE 8-39. *The therapist stands on involved side of patient and gives stability to involved knee by placing leg in front. Holding involved elbow in extension, patient leans on hand. Parallel bar or wall is within reach if needed. Vary activity by having patient shift weight to left and right, prevent knee hyperextension; shift weight to sound leg and keep involved leg in place; shift weight to sound leg and reposition involved leg back and forward, assisting with foot as needed.*

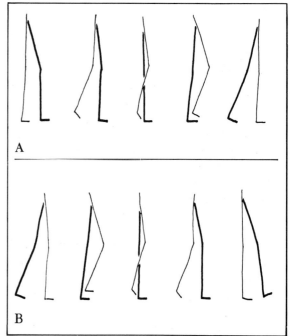

FIGURE 8-40. *Forward-backward stepping sequence with therapist and patient in same position as in Figure 8-39. A. Standing on involved leg, step forward with sound leg and shift weight forward on sound leg. Involved leg stays in place. B. Standing on involved leg, step back with sound leg and shift weight back onto sound leg. Involved leg stays in place. Continue stepping forward and back over involved leg. Vary task by increasing size of step and length of weight-bearing time on involved leg.*

plegia characterized by circumduction of the hip and lack of adequate knee flexion and ankle dorsiflexion during the swing phase. During the initial stance phase the toe makes contact with the floor first because of inadequate ankle and knee flexion. Then, as the body weight is brought over the involved leg, the knee hyperextends, encouraged by the positive support reaction. Actual weight-bearing is avoided as much as possible because of the lack of strength and control to hold the knee in neutral and fear of the leg collapsing. The combined inability to move one joint independent-

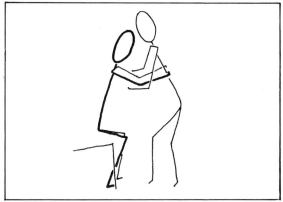

FIGURE 8-41. *Sitting to standing. The therapist's hands are under patient's elbow, patient's hands around therapist's waist or elbows extended, hands clasped together. The patient leans forward so some weight is shifted forward onto legs, increasing amount of leaning and weight-shifting as tolerated. Involved foot is positioned slightly behind sound foot lean and forward so weight is transferred more on involved leg as the patient leans forward.*

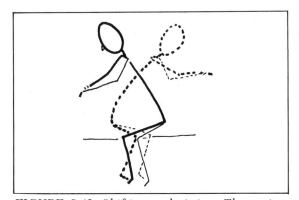

FIGURE 8-42. *Shifting and sitting. The patient transfers all weight to feet as in Figure 8-41, and lifts and moves hips to one side and sits gently on that side. The patient continues moving down one side of mat or bed by this lifting and shifting weight, repositioning feet each time, with assistance as needed. Reverse directions; keeping involved foot behind sound foot, maintain sitting balance and move slowly with control.*

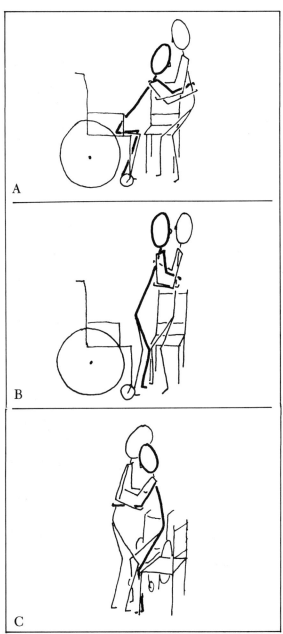

FIGURE 8-43. *Moderate to maximum assistance toward involved side. A. Patient transfers all weight to feet as in Figure 8-41, B. pivots toward involved side, and C. sits by leaning forward. Therapist assists to maintain knee extension and to keep trunk forward, as needed.*

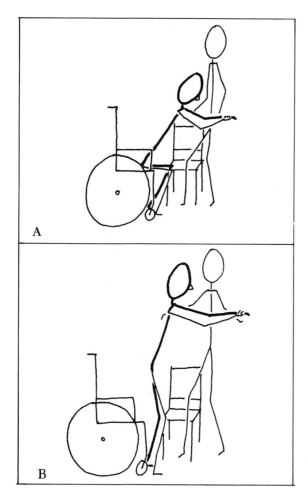

A

B

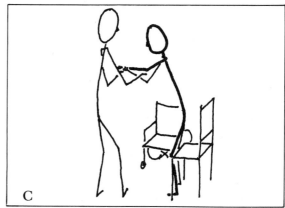

C

FIGURE 8-44. *Minimal assistance or guarding toward involved side. A. With hands clasped together, arms extended, feet positioned under thighs, the patient leans forward to transfer weight to legs and B. come to full standing position; C. pivots toward involved side and returns to sitting by leaning forward. The therapist must watch for knee hyperextension. No flopping down!*

ly of the adjacent joints and adequately bear weight on the weakened extremity creates the quick, unequal awkward gait pattern. This gait is the result of a combination of factors. Weakness or total paralysis may be the primary cause. The presence of spasticity, abnormal reflexes, or contractures can reinforce the pattern and can be further complicated by sensory loss, low endurance, poor balance, perceptual impairment, and apraxia. Evaluation of gait starts with assessment of these factors and their relation to the patient's ability to sit, stand, and move from one position to another. This provides the necessary data for developing a gait program and assessing changes in progress and treatment.

Treatment of gait problems begins before any actual ambulation is initiated. The ability to maintain trunk and head stability, hip and knee control, and sitting and standing balance must be present first, after which gait training or ambulation can begin in earnest. Treatment methods include specific exercise combinations plus guided ambulation practice. The exercises provide opportunities to normalize muscle tone, develop control, and integrate function (see Figures 8-18 through 8-24; and 8-38 through 8-40).

AMBULATION

Once adequate weight-shift and balance are possible, walking can begin. Attention is given to knee stability, equal length of steps, weight-bearing, proper swing through, and body posture. The sound hand uses the parallel bar initially for balance and bearing some of the weight the involved leg is unable to assume, but pulling on the bar for balance is discouraged. In fact, pulling on anything for balance or to assume a standing position is discouraged before it becomes a dangerous habit. Verbal cueing, tactile or proprioceptive stimuli, and gestures by the therapist may assist reeducation. Techniques for dealing with perceptual impairment, apraxia, or cognitive deficits can logically be applied here. (See sections on perception and apraxia.)

The patient may graduate to a cane when safety and function allow, and when it agrees with the therapeutic approach. A broad-based quad-cane may be used initially, and as the patient's stability increases a narrower-based or single-ended cane may be appropriate. Whatever kind is used, the ambulation pattern taught is cane first, then involved leg forward, then sound leg ahead of the cane. When ascending stairs or curbs the sound leg leads to lift the body weight, and the involved leg advances to the same step. When descending, the weak leg is placed first as the sound leg lowers the weight and then steps down with the weak leg.

During ambulation training bracing may be indicated. Like splinting, this may be controversial, but is nonetheless a viable treatment option, and effective for weakness, spasticity, or lack of stability of the lower extremity. With adequate hip extension present, knee stability can be maintained and ankle dorsiflexion controlled with one of several short leg braces. A spring-wire dorsiflexion assist brace can be used for simple footdrop, but cannot provide lateral ankle support or knee stability. A Klenzak dorsiflexion assist or double-action brace assists with dorsiflexion and provides support to the ankle and knee. In addition, it can be adjusted to different degrees of dorsiflexion and can accommodate a prepatellar pad and valgus correction T strap for added support.

## ADL

The term *ADL* (activities of daily living) includes all routine self-care and survival tasks any individual must perform. They usually encompass eating, dressing and undressing, hygiene, and grooming. The primary long-term goal in ADL training is to make it possible for the patient to do these tasks safely and inde-

pendently. Evaluation is accomplished by observing the patient's performance and documenting it with the amount of assistance needed. Self-care assessment forms, such as the Kenny Self-Care Evaluation [31], that designate numerical values for performance are useful for documentation, comparison to reevaluations, and research. Variations of the process, devices, and one-handed methods may allow completion of many self-care tasks that might otherwise be impossible. Greater independence in ADL can provide an increased feeling of success and self-worth [31, 42].

Homemaking skills include meal planning, preparation and cleaning up, laundry, cleaning, shopping, and so forth. Although these skills may not be appropriate for all patients, those who are going home alone or with family will probably have some responsibility or opportunity for some of them. It is important to assess carefully if the patient can do them with complete safety independently, especially using a stove or hot iron, although frequently, a patient will function much better and more safely in the familiar setting. During a home visit some of these tasks can be assessed. Knowing the patient's level of function and anticipated responsibilities will determine the intensity of practice, adaptation of procedures, and the use of devices. Equipment and devices are commercially available for one-handed use, or they can be fabricated for specific needs.

## VISUAL FIELD DEFICITS

Visual impairments that frequently accompany a stroke add to difficulties for the patient and the rehabilitation team. A common visual problem that interferes with the field of vision is *hemianopia* (Figure 8-45). Hemianopia is defined as blindness in one-half of the field of vision of one or both eyes. It results from a lesion to the optic pathways in one side of the brain, which commonly produces a deficit of the opposite visual field, for example, homonymous hemianopia. The patient does not "see"

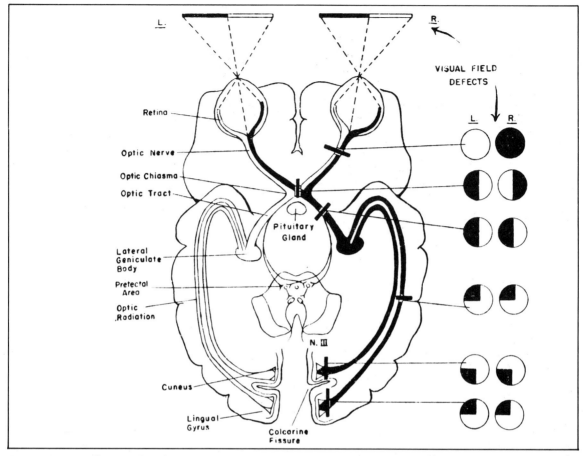

FIGURE 8-45. *The visual pathway. On the right are maps of the visual fields with areas of blindness darkened to show effect of injuries in various locations. (From R. G. Clark.* Manter and Gatz's Essentials of Clinical Neuroanatomy and Neurophysiology *(5th ed.). Philadelphia: Davis, 1975. With permission.)*

stimuli in the involved area and may be unaware of this deficit. It is similar to the fact that we cannot see behind us, and generally are not aware of a lack in our visual field. Any visual information that is not "seen" cannot be acted on, so the patient may not eat the food on one side of the plate, may bump into walls on that side, and so forth. Studies have revealed that the presence of a visual field deficit has an adverse effect on potential overall improvement of the effects of stroke [20]. This condition can be compounded by visual spatial neglect.

Assessment consists of presenting stimuli separately in the left and the right visual fields and simultaneously in both. If the patient is unaware of the stimuli on the involved side during both presentations, homonymous hemianopia is most likely present. Another assessment consists of having the patient bisect each of a collection of lines on a paper put directly in front. If the lines on one side of the paper are missed the presence of a visual field deficit is suspected. During all assessments, the evaluator must carefully observe the patient's performance for compensation that may mask the presence of a deficit. Other limitations and impairments such as communication or cognitive deficits may also influence performance.

Treatment consists of teaching compensation techniques that include arranging the environment and turning toward the involved side so that objects are in the normal visual field. For patients with intact sensation, compensation may occur automatically. These techniques can be incorporated into daily activities and will be most effective if the patient experiences success with a minimum of frustration. The family should also learn them to provide reinforcement and continuity of care.

## COGNITIVE PERCEPTUAL MOTOR FUNCTIONS

A stroke can affect cognitive perceptual motor (CPM) functions including attention, memory, higher intellectual functioning, perception, visual spatial neglect, praxis, and language. Each of these functions is in itself complicated, and their relationships to each other and human behavior are extremely complex. Normal behavior, safe independent functioning, and learning depend on these abilities. The severity of impaired leaning ability, disturbed awareness of self or space, disordered integrative action, and disturbed emotional behavior determines the quality of recovery from stroke [18].

The following section explores each of these deficit areas, with definitions, methods of evaluation, and clinical implications. Treatment techniques and approaches are combined into a total treatment program for cognitive perceptual motor dysfunction. This has been done for several reasons. These deficits frequently manifest themselves in similiar behaviors, but space does not allow attention to the treatment of each one. The section Suggested Reading provides more information of specific conditions. In addition, it is recognized that there is a lack of scientific evidence supporting the value of specific treatments of isolated deficits, making it difficult to justify treatment time for a single purpose. Some techniques and exercises will be discussed, but as functional independence requires CPM abilities, their treatment may be more appropriately incorporated into the rehabilitation program of the total patient.

### ATTENTION

According to one source [40], attention is "the ability to attend to a specific stimulus without being distracted by extraneous environmental stimuli." Before higher cognitive functions of memory, language, and abstract thinking can be evaluated, the patient's ability to sustain attention over time must be determined. A patient who is inattentive or distractible will be unable to process or assimilate information. In addition, anxiety and stress may contribute to distractibility and decrease attention [40]. Inattention may also take the form of denial and neglect. In its severest form, gross denial, the patient will deny paralysis or even illness. (See anosognosia.) Attention is evaluated by asking the patient to count backward from 20 to one, or count to 40 by threes starting at two. Missed or repeated digits, unusually slow response, wrong order, or failure to complete the task may be indications of defective attention. Responses are scored as intact or impaired; aphasia and retardation must be ruled out.

### MEMORY

Memory is a hierarchical process in which information is registered, processed, stored, and recalled. It is a general term for what Straub and Black [40] call a "mental process that allows the individual to store experiences and perceptions for recall at a later time." The process consists of several steps, each of which relies on the normal functioning of the others, and any disruption in the process will result in memory problems. The first step is reception and registration of information through touch, vision, hearing, and so on, and its temporary storage. The next step is the more permanent storage of this information by the active process of repetition and practice. The final step is retrieval or recall of stored information [36]. As different aspects of this memory process are controlled by separate areas of the brain, careful evaluation of the types of memory can help assist in differential diagnosis [40]. In addition, it provides information about the limitations for learning and independent functioning.

The time between presentation of the stimulus and retrieval determines the type of memory. During evaluation and in function, three categories of memory are demonstrated (1) immediate recall or short-term, (2) recent, and (3) remote. The first involves recall of information after a few seconds. Recent memory calls for remembering and retrieving information over hours or days, and in addition, learning new information. Remote memory is the ability to recollect very early experiences and information. Important to memory is the ability of the patient to be oriented to self, place, and time.

Memory is tested in several ways depending on type. For immediate recall the patient remembers verbal and visual lists or collections of shapes, words, or digits. Recent memory is tested by requiring the patient to learn new verbal and visual information and retrieve it after a few minutes, hours, and days. Remote memory is assessed by having the patient recall personal and historical events. Orientation requires the patient to answer questions about identity of self, place, and time. Answers must be verified by the evaluator.

As with any evaluation, care must be taken not to allow other problems such as depresssion or language to influence tests of memory. Impairments in memory will have definite effects on task performance and the ability to learn or relearn. Disruption in any of the steps will limit a patient's ability to learn from therapy and to carry out treatments.

GENERAL INTELLECTUAL FUNCTIONING OR CEREBRATION
General intellectual functioning (GIF), or cerebration, depends on attention, language, and memory. This is the highest level of human functioning that includes the manipulation of the bank of acquired information, and the ability to think abstractly, reason, perform mathematical calculations, solve problems and make judgments [40].

Evaluation of GIF consists of giving the patient a battery of questions and problems consisting of general questions that evaluate the store of knowledge, the ability to solve basic math problems, recognize similarities and differences, sequence patterns and classify groups, solve logical problems, and explain the meanings of proverbs. Performance is scored as intact if answers are correct. Impaired score is given if the response takes a long time, is partially inaccurate, or requires prompting. An absent score is given if the patient attempts to answer but cannot give even a facsimile. In cases where aphasia or language impairment does not allow evaluation, a score of "unable to test" is given, which does not make a determination of GIF status.

Performance in GIF evaluation may be influenced by educational or cultural background and premorbid intellectual capabilities. Impairments may interfere with a patient's ability to function socially and influence safety, and may limit vocational prognosis.

PERCEPTION
Swenson [41] calls perception "the ability to integrate and interpret internal and external sensory information." Generally, the parietal lobes of the brain are responsible for these functions. Impairment in perception is more prevalent in a stroke when the lesion is in the right, usually nondominant, hemisphere. Deficits in motor planning (praxis) and verbal communication are more commonly seen in left hemisphere lesions [34]. (See Chapter 9.) Difficulty with some perceptual and motor planning abilities may be seen with a stroke of either hemisphere.

Studies have shown that lesions of the nondominant parietal lobe resulting in perceptual damage are related to poor prognosis for rehabilitation and functional independence [1, 11, 28]. Perception of stimuli is a prerequisite to learning, and rehabilitation is a learning process, thus it is not surprising that disorders of perception would correspond to limitations in acquiring self-care skills and independence. Components of perception are described below [2, 34, 40].

*Visual spatial neglect*, or unilateral neglect, is a failure to register stimuli and perceptions from one side of the environment and the involved side of the body. The patient is unable to integrate the information and as a result, will ignore the involved half of the body and neglect activity and stimuli in that area of personal space. In contrast to hemianopia, visual spatial neglect is not caused by physical blindness, and the visual fields are intact. This deficit is frequently compounded by a sensory loss, and may be further complicated by a visual field deficit. Testing for this condition involves having the patient draw symmetrical objects from copy or memory, duplicate two- or three-dimensional patterns, complete form boards, select and identify pictures and objects from a list or collection, read and do simple math completion [34]. Missed or incomplete components and lack of detail on one side are indications of visual spatial neglect of that side, and is particularly evident when information is presented on both sides simultaneously. Performance during functional tasks further serves to identify a visual neglect and to demonstrate the extent to which it may interfere with function.

During other evaluations it is important that this not be misinterpreted as apraxia or comprehension, cerebration, or perceptual motor impairment. Adaptation of the testing situation may be necessary to bypass this defect and gather accurate information about other cognitive perceptual areas. As patients with visual spatial neglect may have sensory loss and difficulty learning, they may not be candidates for compensation techniques. More effective may be sensory motor and functional approaches (See Treatment).

*Body image impairment* is the inability mentally and visually to represent and commit to memory the image of one's body, and includes disruption in normal feelings about it.

*Body scheme impairment* or *somatognosia*, is the abnormal perception or awareness of the position of the body and the relationship of its parts. Patients have difficulty not only with differentiating their own body parts and those of others, but also understanding how their body relates to the environment. For both body image and scheme deficits patients may have difficulty following directions that require distinction of body parts, following or copying the therapist's motions, or performing tasks, such as dressing, that rely on an automatic cooperation of body parts and the environment.

*Left-right discrimination deficit* is inability to comprehend and use perception of right and left on the patient's own body, on others, and on objects such as clothes. As with body image impairment, the patient may demonstrate difficulty in tasks such as putting on shoes, and in following directions, for example, "turn left at the stairs."

*Finger agnosia* is difficulty in naming fingers when touched or on command. It is more commonly present in the middle three fingers of both hands, and is frequently seen together with a group of conditions collectively called Gerstmann's syndrome, which includes right-left discrimination impairment, agraphia, and acalculia.

*Agraphia* is inability to write intellegible words, and *acalculia* is impairment in the ability to solve mathmatical problems. (See Chapter 9.)

*Anosognosia* is a severe condition of unconcern for or denial, neglect, and lack of recognition of one's own paralysis. Frequently, a patient may underestimate the extent of disability, may disown the paralyzed limb or feel that it does not belong to his or her body, and thus feel no need to take responsibility for it. The patient may set unrealistic goals and may not appreciate mistakes made in trying to achieve them. Anosognosia can limit ability to learn compensation techniques, follow through on most self-care and self-exercise programs, and benefit significantly from a therapy program. The patient may say things about his or her body like, "I left my arm in the closet," which, although outrageous, is a pretty clear indication of the condition.

*Figure-ground impairment* is difficulty in visually distinguishing a figure from its rival background. Clinically, this may interfere with a patient's ability visually to find objects that are not well defined, leading to frustration, limited attention span, and decreased independent and safe functioning.

*Spatial relations impairment* is inability to perceive the position of an object in relation to oneself and other objects.

*Position in space impairment* is a disturbance in perception or conceptualization of spatial positions such as up, down, in, out, on top, behind, and so forth.

*Form constancy impairment* is inability to perceive or attend to slight differences in shape or form. Items of similiar shape may be confused, for example, a pencil and toothbrush.

*Visual agnosia* is lack of recognition of familiar objects even though the eye and optic tracts are functioning normally. It occurs with a deficit in the area of the cortex that is responsible for interpreting associated visual stimuli with past experience. Various categories include: *simultanognosia*—inability to interpret a whole visual stimulus at a time; *prosopagnosia*—inability to perceive spatial relationships among objects, and between self and objects; and *color agnosia*—inability to recognize different colors.

*Auditory agnosia* is impairment in the ability to recognize or differentiate among sounds.

*Tactile agnosia or astereognosis* is difficulty in recognizing objects when handling them, even though tactile, proprioception, and kinesthetic abilities are intact. As many self-care tasks rely on manipulation of objects without vision, a patient with astereognosis may have difficulties with ADL. If this conditon is combined with neglect or sensory loss, accomplishment of such tasks will be limited. Evaluation for stereognosis is usually part of sensory assessment.

*Impairment of vertical perception* is the inability to determine vertical position of objects or oneself.

It is important to evaluate a patient's perceptual status for several reasons. It gathers the necessary baseline information regarding which perceptual abilities are intact and which are limited. Futhermore, it increases the understanding about how the dysfunctions may influence performance and what capabilities might be intact to allow substitution. Careful assessment will lead to a realistic treatment program and a more cost-effective use of the rehabilitation services.

Perception evaluations may vary. They usually require the patient to copy or draw, arrange items such as puzzle pieces and blocks, verbally identify or discriminate objects and forms, and perform particular motions on visual or verbal command. Responses may be scored as intact if performance is consistently correct, rapid, and conforms to all directions. Impaired scores are given if the final product is inaccurate, if the performance is inconsistent and has significantly diminished qualitative features, and if it is done slowly. Absent score is given if the patient cannot perform any part of the task; however, if inability is caused by communication limitations, apraxia, or lack of cooperation, an unable score is given. Generally, evaluation assesses not only whether or not the patient can perform each task, but how it is done and what particular behaviors influence the results. Some of these behaviors such as trial and error, distractibility, taking excess time, and requiring repeated instruction might account for an imparied score even if the final product or posture is correct. These behaviors or qualitative features should be carefully observed and documented (Table 8-5). Incorrect

TABLE 8-5. *Abnormal Responses That Might Occur in CPM Evaluation*

| Qualitative Features[a] | Critera Adopted |
|---|---|
| Scrawlings | Tendency to limit graphic task to scrawling |
| Increased number of lines | Tendency to overscore lines already drawn |
| Irrelevant graphic material | Tendency to add irrelevant drawings or script (free designs, signature, etc.) |
| Alterations in relative size of the figures[b] | Gross alterations in relative size of figures |
| Piecemeal approach[c] | Tendency to copy designs in fragmentary way, lacking general structure |
| Perseveration | Tendency to reproduce designs in stereotyped way, without reference to the models |
| Excess details | More than usual or necessary amount of details |
| Detail cramped together | Details not in proper relation or proportion to each other |
| Poor planning | Poor ability to devise scheme for doing, making, or arranging (alignment on page, size in relation to page, leaving enough room on page to complete) |
| Poor vertical representation | Appears unaware of what is upright or vertical in environment or in relation to self (alignment of object, symmetricalness in relation to itself, and parts in relation to each other and to page) |
| Unilateral spatial neglect | Neglect (on opposite side to hemispheric locus of lesion) |
| Increased size of the figures | |
| Reduced size of the figures | |
| Difficulty drawing angles | Tendency to reproduce angles as simple curved lines, or to connect the sides of figures by scrawling |
| Oversimplification | Tendency to leave lines or details out |
| Alterations in spatial relations | Gross alteration by displacement, rotation, etc. |
| Increased number of right angles | Tendency to draw right angles when more acute angle indicated |
| Increased number of acute angles | |
| Hesitation | Act of pausing or delaying, stopping momentarily; faltering |
| Frustration | Observed act of bewilderment, confusion with difficulty in completing task; may be verbally expressed or nonverbally seen as refusal to complete |
| Groping | Searching about blindly, hesitantly, or uncertainly |
| Orientation of drawings | Tendency to orientate the drawings diagonally on the paper |
| Limited comprehension interfered with performance | |
| Poor carryover of instructions within category | |
| Distractibility | Attention easily diverted or drawn away |
| Poor error recognition | Cannot identify errors by self or with cues |
| Poor self-correction | If error identified, unable to correct properly |
| Lability interfered with testing | Unsteadiness, quick changes in emotion interfere with testing |
| Fatigue interfered | Fatigue, tiredness interfere with testing |

[a]These qualitative features of abnormal responses might occur during the CPM evaluation. Some relate specifically to graphic material; others are general clinical observations.
[b]Other specific body drawing features: All parts on one side of body missing or specific parts (note which), all parts of both sides drawn on one side, and face not filled in. Profile: (a) Attempt to put all body parts on side body view, (b) which side, and (c) partial profile (not necessarily a negative performance).
[c]Other constructional apraxia characteristics: Incorrect order of numbers on clock, wrong end of matchstick used, inaccurate number of sticks, and inaccurate number of blocks.
Source: From N. Wall. *Hemiplegic Evaluation.* Boston: Massachusetts Rehabilitation Hospital, 1978. With permission.

answers may be the results of problems other than specific perceptual conditions being tested. For example, hemianopia may influence the results of figure-ground tests, yet if the test were administered in the patient's intact visual field, results might be normal.

APRAXIA

Apraxia is the inability to perform purposeful or complex movements despite the presence of intact mobility, sensation, coordination, and comprehension. Although the concept and the purpose of a task are understood, the patient is unable to execute the motion. Harris [21] says that apraxia involves "any movement normally voluntarily initiated, movements of the eyes, face, muscles of articulation, chewing and swallowing, manipulation of objects, gestures with the upper limbs, walking or sitting." The three basic categories of apraxia are discussed: (1) motor, with its subcategories ideomotor and ideational, often the result of a lesion in the dominant hemisphere, (2) constructional, and (3) dressing. The last two are frequently caused by a lesion in the nondominant hemisphere. (See Chapter 9.)

In ideomotor apraxia, the patient is unable to initiate gestures or perform motor tasks on command although the concept is understood. Kinesthetic memory patterns are still intact and the patient is able to describe and carry out automatic activities that rely on habit, but there is a loss of ability to sequence movements, and domination by perseveration of "a continued repetition of movement or work" has been noted [34]. For example, the patient would recognize a drinking glass and explain how one would drink water from it, but when requested, could not pick up the glass and drink. Yet on another occasion, when thirsty, the patient might automatically pick up the glass and drink with no obvious problem. Ideomotor apraxia can be demonstrated in buccofacial, upper limb, lower limb, and whole-body activities. Impairment may be demonstrated in a hierarchy of difficulty. Most difficult is performing a task on

command without the item or clues, for example, asking the patient to demonstrate how to brush teeth. The next most difficult is performing the task by imitating the examiner without the item. The least difficult is having the patient perform the task with the real object on command [40].

Ideational apraxia is the lack of understanding of the overall concept of a task and inability to perform on command or automatically. With this so-called [40] "higher order disturbance" the patient may be able to perform each part of a task, but is unable to integrate an activity consisting of several steps, and cannot describe the process. In addition, there may be failure to recognize how an object is used and also diminished auditory comprehension. This condition is not seen in isolation, but is often combined with other cognitive impairments and is associated with general intellectual deterioration [40]. It will interfere with many routine daily tasks such as preparing a meal or washing up, and can limit a patient's ability to function independently and safely.

Constructional apraxia is impairment in the ability to draw or construct two- or three-dimensional forms or figures from one- and two-dimensional units either on command or spontaneously. A deficit in constructional abilities implies additional faulty visual perception, and what Straub and Black [40] describe as impairment in the ability to "integrate perception into kinesthetic images" and disturbance in translating these images into the necessary "final motor patterns."

Dressing apraxia describes inability to dress, and is not caused by motor performance, but results from deficits of body scheme and spatial relations.

Evaluation of motor apraxia consists of having the patient follow a variety of verbal commands, for example, "show me how you brush your teeth," to imitating the examiner and demonstrating the use of an object. Constructional apraxia includes evaluating the ability to copy two- and three-dimensional forms and drawings and to duplicate three-dimensional designs with matchsticks and colored blocks. Careful observation of the patient during dressing will help to determine if problems are from apraxia. There is a correlation between constructional and dressing apraxia, thus evaluations must consider and accommodate to limitations in other areas. The examiner must be aware of the patient's motor abilities, level of comprehension, primary language, endurance, physical comfort, time of day, emotional state, and hand dominance. For example, it is not uncommon for a patient who has had a stroke resulting in some apraxia to have comprehension difficulties, and all attempts should be made to ensure that a lack of understanding is not called apraxia. Adaptation as necessary and careful administration of the perceptual evaluation along with the entire hemiplegic assessment will allow the evaluator accurately to identify deficit areas and plan a program accordingly. It will also facilitate effective communication of this information to other team members, the patient, and family.*

Clinically, patients with impairment in perception or apraxia or both may behave similarly while performing tasks. Functionally, they may not be able to do simple tasks independently or safely, and be unable to initiate activity even with cueing, or to switch from one task or step to another. There may be difficulties in visually finding or identifying objects that are obvious and necessary for task completion. Some may find it hard to follow even simple directions despite good comprehension, and the same mistakes or new ones may be made in an attempt to correct performance. The patient may perseverate on one motion. During an activity there may be abnormal hesitation, groping, distractibility, and poor planning. These problems can make simple daily tasks seem insurmountable, and demand patience, understanding, and support by team members.

*For a complete evaluation and additional information see the Solet Test for Apraxia; see also reference 4 and 34 at the end of this chapter.

## TREATMENT OF COGNITIVE PERCEPTUAL MOTOR PROBLEMS

In providing a treatment program for the patient with cognitive perceptual motor problems it is essential that the rehabilitation team, the patient, and family work together. Many techniques involve a particular approach during therapy, nursing care, and all functional activities in addition to treatment time specified for working on a problem.

A program can be viewed as having six interrelated components, the priority of which relate to the individual patient and rehabilitation setting. The first is evaluation: treatment cannot be initiated until the specific problems are identified. Time is another, and includes two aspects. One is the time needed for natural recovery to take place, which may be weeks or months. This does not mean waiting for recovery, but rather keeping in mind that although progress may be slow it will be forthcoming. The second aspect is the time it takes for a patient to respond. We all have our own natural rhythm and response rates, and following a stroke, an elderly patient especially may require more time to perform a task. Rushing a patient to respond will only cause frustration for both patient and therapist, and may reduce success. Working with patients whose cognitive impairments limit function and learning requires patience on the part of all involved.

A third component is education—of staff, patient, family, and friends. Only with education, will the rehabilitation team be able to provide continuity of care and unified effort. The patient and family need accurate information about what it is that makes it difficult, impossible, or unsafe for the patient to accomplish some activities and why others must be done in a particular way. Understanding the facts helps reduce misconceptions and allows treatment to be more effective and efficient.

Feedback as a form of education provides accurate information about performance. The patient's own feedback systems may be inaccurate because of CPM or language impairments; from the therapist it must be honest, realistic, and appropriate to the situation and the individual patient, and should provide encouragement. How feedback is provided will depend on the patient's problems and abilities. One with visual perceptual deficits will usually respond better to verbal input, whereas the patient with language impairment may respond best to gestures. Feedback should be consistent and immediate, yet the patient should be given time to perform or correct errors before a response is made. Then timely response can be given to acknowledge accurate performance of successful corrections. It is important not to be patronizing.

The fourth factor concerns the therapeutic relationship. This includes addressing the patient as an adult and showing consideration for cultural orientation, as some treatment approaches may not be received as they were intended. The patient should be part of decision making so that treatment priorities are also the patient's own clearly defined priorities. The therapist should be aware of different individual needs for visual or verbal cues, emotional support, structure, and limits.

The fifth component is the recommended therapeutic program that offers 3 approaches: (1) transfer of training [34], (2) sensorimotor, and (3) functional. Transfer of training is based on the theory [34] that "practice in a particular perceptual task will affect the patient's performance on similar perceptual tasks." In other words, practicing specific perceptual or cognitive exercises will have a positive effect on performance in self-care. Little research has been done, and the results of those studies conducted have been inconsistent [34, 28]. This approach is used in many clinics and does provide an option for treatment. Following is a sample of techniques.

Paper and pencil tasks and exercises such as copying, completing, initiating, and imitating a variety of exercises, for example, mazes, simple pictures, or abstract forms
Use of blocks and cubes, peg boards, matchsticks, puzzles, parquetry board, cards of assorted shapes and colors, and photographs in a variety of ways
Activities and exercises that require the patient to use, identify, and combine body gestures and positions, and identify and accurately manipulate objects in the environment, for example, practicing discriminating left and right body parts, following directions or finding routes on a map

These techniques can be incorporated into the total treatment program in a number of ways:

Maintaining sitting or standing balance while doing the above activities
Weight-bearing on the involved upper extremity; weight-bearing or shifting on the lower extremity while doing above activities
When sitting, actively maintaining the involved arm on the table surface in an extended and protracted position while the other hand does the above tasks
Using the involved arm and hand to perform activities
Modifying the activity to facilitate specific motor performance—weight cuff on wrist, elevated table surface, or blackboard

The sensorimotor approach is based on the theory that perceptual integration and development can be facilitated by providing specific sensory stimulation and controlling desired motor output. The stimulation used and motor responses encouraged follow a developmental sequence and must be carefully integrated. Although little research has been done, activities can be appropriately combined with treatment of motor control and the functional approach mentioned earlier arousing tactile, proprioceptive, and kinesthetic senses through rubbing, tapping, moving, placing, and resisting the body parts. Mat and gross motor programs for functional mobility using weight-bearing, shifting, facilitation, and inhibition techniques are excellent opportunities to employ this approach for perceptual deficits. In addition, verbal and visual cues are used to elicit desired motor responses. For example, the patient with a visual spatial neglect may benefit from weighted, colorful, or ringing bracelets on the involved wrist or ankle, printed signs to "look left," and verbal instructions and feedback from the therapist.

The functional approach is repetitive practice [34] of specific functional tasks that the patient must be able to do to be more independent. This involves treatment of the symptom or particular behavior rather than its cause. The benefits of this approach are several, as it encourages the patient, an adult who is trying to be more independent, to work on activities that are directly relevant to specific age-appropriate needs. It can be efficiently incorporated into the rehabilitation routine by all the team members and family, and does not require additional tools. In these days of skyrocketing health care costs a treatment program that is cost-effective and goal-directed is welcome.

The functional approach involves an effective and alert therapeutic team who have a keen understanding of the patient's problems. It is in part an educational process that involves teaching the patient to compensate by providing information, support, and feedback, and considers the patient's learning style. It also requires that the therapist adapt the environment to facilitate learning and safe function. Some suggestions for this approach are:

1. Use verbal, visual, and tactile cues as helpful and appropriate to aid completion of an activity.
2. Break an activity into manageable parts, for example, during dressing have one garment out at a time.
3. Have the patient practice over and over the task or part of it, such as finding the sleeve of the shirt and putting in the correct arm.
4. Be consistent and systematic in the procedure used for a task.
5. Be concrete, use the real object in a normal way, e.g., real bread and butter or meat, not theraplast, for cutting practice.

6. Provide only enough assistance so the patient can complete a task, and gradually reduce assistance and cues as patient is able to do more.
7. "Use all available channels of learning" [36]; give demonstrations in the intact visual field; sit beside the patient instead of in front to reduce left-right confusion.
8. Have the patient explain the task verbally before starting, and correct any verbal errors before they are put into actions; or have the patient demonstrate the task and correct errors and demonstrate again with corrections before doing the task alone.
9. Establish a routine and associations to draw on and have the patient go through the routine out loud, if possible, before and during a task. This goes along with being consistent in how a task is done, so, for example, when transferring from the wheelchair to the bed have the patient say each step before or while doing it.
10. Educate the patient about existing problems and limitations, and give alternative methods for better performance.
11. Sometimes performance may be better if the patient is allowed to perform the activity spontaneously; for example, position the patient in front of the sink with the necessary shaving supplies, or the one to be used first, and do not give any verbal instructions.
12. Adapt the patient's environment to facilitate performance and allow success; specific adaptations are many, and depend on individual needs. They might include putting markers on clothing or wheelchair brakes, removing clutter and organizing items, color-coding medications.
13. Have the patient wear a watch on the involved arm.
14. Additional suggestions for the apraxic patient might include a functional pattern of movement; kinesthetic and proprioceptive sensory input through use of a particular motion or actively assisting the patient through the motions; initiation of move-

TABLE 8-6. *Differences in Higher Cortical Function with Lesions of the Right and Left Hemispheres.*

| Right Hemisphere | Left Hemisphere |
| --- | --- |
| Impairment of spatial relationships | Finger agnosia |
| Constructional apraxia, left half | Right-left confusion |
| Dressing apraxia | Dyscalculia |
| Visual inattention to left | Agraphia |
| Anosognosia | Aphasia |
| Tactile inattention | Oral apraxia |
| Auditory inattention to left | Decrease in verbal memory |
| | Visual agnosia (dyslexia) |
| | Auditory agnosia |

Source: Adapted from W. Demyer. *Technique of the Neurologic Examination: A Programmed Text* (3rd ed.). New York: McGraw-Hill, 1980.

ment from proximal joints; breakdown of activity and practice of each part; short simple directions; and visual demonstrations that the patient can imitate.

15. Acknowledge successful performance and efforts.

The sixth component is discharge planning, and involves defining the CPM problem areas that continue to interfere with safe independent function, and along with the physical needs, deciding the kind and amount of supervision and assistance that will be required. The continuity of care depends on careful communication among the patient, team members, community, and home service providers. (Table 8-6 provides some general CPM differences between dominant and nondominant lesions.)

EMOTIONAL AND SEXUAL ADJUSTMENT

The person who has suffered a stroke has experienced a catastrophic event and the majority of those seen in rehabilitation will have a lifelong disability. Although the actual physical rehabilitation and treatment may last only weeks or several months, the emotional adjustment can take years or a lifetime.

Approximately 70 percent of individuals with stroke are over 65 years of age [31] and the emotional and psychological changes they might experience must be considered in the adjustment process. (See Chapter 1.) Premorbid personality and cultural and ethnic background are additional factors that must be taken into account.

Emotional lability with uncontrolled swings in mood is not uncommon following stroke. The patient may experience depression and sadness and have good reason to cry; emotional lability, on the other hand, may have no obvious relationship to the immediate circumstances, and crying may stop immediately when the patient's attention is redirected.

Environment can facilitate adjustment to stroke. The patient's room should be arranged to provide social contact and stimulation. This is especially important if the patient has a visual field deficit or spatial neglect, a hearing impairment, sensory loss, or feels frightened or insecure. An atmosphere of respect, support, and encouragement must be maintained. Opportunities should be provided for maximum independence in regular daily tasks. Patients should be dressed in their own clothes and encouraged to socialize and participate in activities.

Educational programs assist emotional adjustment for the patient and family. Daily one-to-one contact with individual health workers provides the most consistent, personal format for this. Individual programs focus on the patient's or family's needs such as medication administration or sexual adjustment, and personalize the material.

Planned group education-discussion programs offer the advantage of patients and families learning with and from their peers. Sharing ideas, fears, and anxieties with someone who is experiencing similar problems eases tension, provides comfort and support, and can facilitate learning. Planned group programs are helpful in dispelling myths, aiding in emotional adjustment, and preparing for discharge. Participation of families in a stroke education program has been shown to decrease anxiety of members, increase understanding of stroke and its implications and of the team approach to rehabilitation, and enhance communication between family and staff [15]. Group programs of range-of-motion exercises and strengthening activities can reinforce individual instruction and provide successful home therapy.

Education can be further reinforced through use of media, such as booklets, films, slides, television, or video tapes. Printed information can be read in privacy and at the reader's own pace, and television and films can have an emotional as well as logical appeal. As with any treatment modality, the material must be carefully selected to meet the needs of all involved, and should be routinely reevaluated.

Sexual activity is an important consideration in the rehabilitation program for both patient and partner. Impotence, anorgasmia, and ejaculatory incompetence are relatively uncommon phenomena for the stroke patient; problems are usually related to the primary physical difficulties of loss of strength, mobility, and motor control, emotional aspects, and the social factors that influence behavior.

Two separate studies [24, 19] found some decrease in libido with differences between left and right hemisphere insult in patients 60 years and younger. With dominant (usually left) hemisphere damage and right-sided paral-

ysis, a decrease in libido may occur; with nondominant hemisphere damage a decrease is unlikely [24]. With dominant hemisphere damage libido is unlikely to increase, whereas with a nondominant lesion an increase is possible. These changes are the same for both sexes. In addition, one study [19] found that "prestroke sexual activity is an excellent predictor of poststroke sexual activity," and that there is a greater likelihood that libido will remain unchanged no matter which hemisphere is damaged except for the direct limitations of the disability and social situation.

The study by Kalliomaki and co-workers [24] found a decrease of 43 percent in the actual frequency of sexual activity or coitus, with 22 percent unchanged (35 percent unusable information). The decrease was significantly more common for men than women. There was no relationship between side of paralysis and frequency of coitus [24]. The fact that there is a greater decrease in sexual activity than there is in interest emphasizes the relationship and conflict between the emotional and psychological factors and the sexual behavior and adjustment.

For those patients over 60 not included in the studies, the process of aging itself may influence sexual functioning. These problems include prestroke illness or limitations, cultural and social pressures, misunderstanding and myths, and lack of a sexual partner. Drugs used to treat hypertension when not carefully monitored and managed can cause impotence or diminished libido [25].

Impairment of communication skills and cognitive perceptual motor abilities may further limit sexual functioning and interest, and influence adjustment. Reduction in sexual activity for aphasic patients may be related to decrease in memory span and emotional concentration [19]. The changes in verbal skills and use of gestures may affect communication and relationship the patient has with the current partner, or attempts at establishing a relationship with a new partner. Visual field deficits and impairments of perception and cognition can further complicate sexual performance and relationships.

A stroke can bring with it a loss of self-esteem, decreased activity, increased financial costs and burdens, depression and frustration, and fear and anxiety for both patient and partner. It is no wonder that sexual activity, along with all other activities, may be impaired. Careful attention to and treatment of these emotional problems can have a positive effect on a patient's sex life. Ford and Orfirer [17] found that for the majority of their patients, the partner's reluctance and concern reduced sexual opportunities. The partner, and even the patient, may assume that onset of a stroke means the end of sex, or that there is actual medical risk associated with resumption of coitus. In fact, the risk is unknown, although it is thought to be highest in patient with stroke caused by intercranial hemorrhage. Kolodny, Masters, and Johnson [25] feel that the risk is actually quite small, and that until more research is done clinicians must use available information, guesswork, and inference.

A program for sexual rehabilitation requires understanding of physical limitations, the patient's social, emotional, and cultural background, the importance of the disability to patient and family, self-perception of the patient, and reaction of the family and staff toward the patient. Goddess and co-workers [19] found that the patients they studied "welcomed open and frank discussions of their sexual needs, desires, practices and futures." This is similar to the permission, limited information, specific suggestions, intensive therapy (PLISSIT) model [10] that suggests a 4-level guide for providing sexual education and counseling. Talking with the patient and partner can relieve some anxiety by acknowledging this topic and providing approval for the interest and concern the patient may have in resuming sexual activity. The subject may be brought up during initial and subsequent evaluations of ADL, household skills, vocational abilities, and home visits. A patient's and partner's misunderstanding of the medical condition and in-

ability to talk about their concerns and needs can be further reduced by providing limited information, in addition to "giving permission." Generally, patients who require more specific information or intensive therapy are referred to a professional trained to deal with a particular problem.

Emotionally and physically, resumption of sexual activity is more difficult for the man [17], probably because of societal stereotypes that are not easily cast off, particularly by older people who may have lived with them for a long time. Physical limitation of strength, control, and mobility may mean he will have to experiment with new positions. He and his partner will have to accept his limitations and make any adjustments with which they are comfortable to continue a rewarding sex life. Women may experience less physical difficulty, but emotionally they must struggle with the same attitudes and reactions as men do.

A therapist dealing with this subject must be aware of her or his own attitudes and feelings about sex, sexual preference, and disability, and refrain from interjecting personal prejudices. At times a patient may seek out a therapist with whom he or she is most comfortable talking about sexual concerns, but more frequently the responsibility for bringing up the subject lies with the health care worker. Sexual activity is one of the most difficult adjustments for a patient and partner to make, and although many deal with this aspect of rehabilitation on their own, support from the rehabilitation staff can make this less painful, contribute to adjustment to the disability, and facilitate optimal resumption of the patient's previous life-style.

VOCATIONAL ADJUSTMENT
When a person has a stroke, the accompanying emotional, functional, and cognitive losses may be further complicated by the loss of material and nonmaterial fulfillment provided through work. Return to work depends on the physical, psychological, and intellectual skills

required, the desire and need to return, and the employer's policies, attitudes, and willingness to adapt the workplace and the specific job. Employment in a new situation will depend on these factors, plus how competitive the job is, and a careful matching of the patient's skills with requirements.

Vocational needs will be limited by the fact that the majority of patients are over the retirement age of 65 years, and only 40 to 60 percent of these achieve complete functional independence [31]. Research has indicated that approximately 30 percent of hemiplegic patients studied were considered employable [31] although the actual number employed was unknown. For those who attempt to return to work, job success after stroke has been related to the involved hemisphere [31]. The patient with a lesion in the dominant hemisphere, even with communication problems, had greater vocational success than the patient with insult to the nondominant hemisphere. The failure of the latter was attributed to difficulty in nonverbal abstract reasoning, and to perceptual distortion that led to poor safety awareness, poor organization and pacing of work, space and time, inefficient use of tools, and decreased attention to quality.

If a new vocation or return to previous employment is a goal, the rehabilitation team must assess the patient's potential employability and make recommendations to the former employer or training program.

Important to returning to work is transportation; accessibility to public conveyance and the patient's ability to drive must be carefully examined. Any number of impairments can limit the patient's ability to drive safely. Some are subtle, such as field deficit, judgment, and attention, and may go undetected by licensing agencies and the patient. Careful evaluation should be performed, however, and necessary restrictions set to ensure the safety of everyone.

## Discharge Planning

Discharge planning is "organized develop-ment of posthospitalization management" [31] that begins on the first day following stroke and is part of the total treatment regimen. In the multidisciplinary rehabilitation program every team member contributes to the discharge process just as they do to evaluation and treatment. The role the member plays in discharge may vary depending on the institution, but the process remains the same.

Functional capabilities such as mobility in the wheelchair or ambulating, self-care, and basic home and communication skills, must all be carefully assessed to determine the patient's level of independence and safety, and amount and kind of assistance that will be needed. Combined with these is the physical set-up in which the patient will be living. A home visit provides valuable information for the entire team to establish the presence of architectural barriers that could limit function and safety such as stairs, curbs, narrow doorways, high sinks, and low bathtubs. The need for equipment and structural modifications will influence function and safety; tub seats, safety bars and rails for tub, toilet, and stairs, and modifications such as ramps, elevators, and lower sinks may be necessary to allow maximum independence. The actual location of the home in regard to shopping, transportation, and social activities is also important.

The community provides many essential links for the patient to aid reintegration to the former life-style. The Visiting Nurse Association (VNA), American Heart Association (AHA), home care agencies, and local city and state services offer indispensable services from daily personal care and medical monitoring to vocational training and recreational activities.

With information about the home environment, a simulated home setting can be provided, reproducing the physical arrangement to anticipate the amount and kind of assistance the patient would have. Some rehabilitation centers may have apartments specifically used for this purpose. The functional living evaluation program (FLEP) [45] was developed to evaluate the patient's ability to manage independently and safely, and to provide an opportunity to practice the skills that will be needed at home. The program goes for 1 week and uses the patient's own room. The criteria for acceptance in the program include imminent home discharge, minimal assistance with self-care and transfers, minimal judgment and safety problems, and willing participation of patient and family. Before beginning, the specific areas evaluated are listed as behavioral objectives, and the skills and functions the patient is expected to do independently are clarified to all team members. At a home visit the family members who are to be involved are taught the techniques they will be required to use. During the program they provide assistance that they anticipate they will eventually give the patient at home. Most patients are expected to get up, bathe at the sink, dress and undress, eat, and get to therapy programs according to their expected level of independence. In addition, they plan and prepare three meals, do laundry, shop, make their beds, and so on, if these activities are expected of them at home. At the end of the week the patient is reevaluated for meeting the defined objectives, and recommendations are made accordingly. The common problems encountered are lack of adequate judgment for personal safety, assistance needed for safe medication administration, and supervision for tub use. Response to this program from the patients and families was overwhelmingly positive. Many patients stated how good it felt to be able to be independent and how it gave them a chance to develop confidence and reduce anxiety.

Assurance of a worthwhile life-style is the ultimate goal of rehabilitation, and discharge planning is the culmination of the skilled efforts and care of the rehabilitation team.

The problems associated with stroke can be complicated and are different for each patient. There are no cookbook answers to any problem, only options, theories, and suggestions. Quality care depends on the therapist being well informed, and inquisitive, as well as sensitive, dependable, and open-minded.

*Acknowledgment is made to Cathy Sangiolo-Gaidis for her review of parts of this chapter.*

# References

1. Adams, F. F, and Hurvitz, L. J. Mental barriers to recovery from strokes. *Lancet* 2:533, 1963.
2. Anderson, C. Parietal lobe syndromes in hemiplegia, a program for treatment. *Am. J. Occup. Ther.* 24:13, 1970.
3. Basmajian, J. V. *Muscles Alive.* Baltimore: Williams & Wilkins, 1974.
4. Basmajian, J. V. Biofeedback in Therapeutic exercise. In J. V. Basmajian (Ed.). *Therapeutic Exercise* (3rd ed.). Baltimore: Williams & Wilkins, 1978.
5. Basmajian, J. V., Kukulka, C. G., and Narayon, M. G. Biofeedback treatment of foot drop after stroke compared with standard rehabilitation technique. Effects on voluntary control and strength. *Arch. Phys. Med. Rehabil.* 56:231, 1975.
6. Basmajian, J. V. ReGenos, E. M. and Baker, M. P. Biofeedback for stroke patients. Presented at the Second Joint Conference on Stroke of the American Heart Association, Miami, 1977.
7. Bobath, B. *Adult Hemiplegia—Evaluation and Treatment* (2nd ed.). London: Heinemann, 1978.
8. Brunstrom, S. *Movement and Therapy in Hemiplegia.* New York: Harper and Row, 1970.
9. Calliet, R. *Shoulder in Hemiplegia.* Philadelphia: Davis, 1980.
10. Chipouras, S., Cornelius, D., Daniels, S. and Makas, E. *Who Cares? A Handbook on Sex Education and Counseling Services for Disabled Persons.* Washington, D.C.: George Washington University, 1979.
11. Cohen, C. A. Perceptual problems in hemiplegia. *South Med. J.* 67:1329, 1974.
12. Critchley, M. *The Parietal Lobes.* New York: Hafner, 1971.
13. Dobie, R. A. Rehabilitation of swallowing disorders. *Am. Fam. Physician* 17(5):84, 1978.
14. Downey, J. A., and Darling, R. C. *Physiological Basis of Rehabilitation Medicine.* Philadelphia: Saunders, 1971.
15. Dzau, R. E., and Boehme, A. R. Stroke rehabilitation: A family team education program. *Arch. Phys. Med. Rehabil.* 59:236, 1978.
16. Fiorentino, M. *Reflex Testing Methods for*

*Evaluating CNS Development* (2nd ed.). Springfield, Ill.: Thomas, 1973.

17. Ford, A. B., and Orfirer, A. P. Sexual behavior and the chronically ill patient. *Med. Asp. Hum. Sexuality* 1(2):51, 1967.
18. Gillingham, F. J., Mawdsley, C., and Williams, A. E. *Stroke.* Edinburgh: Churchill, 1976.
19. Goddess, E., Wagner, N., and Silverman, D. Poststroke sexual activity of CVA patients. *Med. Asp. Hum. Sexuality* 13(3):16, 1979.
20. Hagerer, A. F. Visual field defects and the prognosis of stroke patients. *Stroke* 4:163, 1973.
21. Harris, F. A. Facilitation Techniques in Therapeutic Exercise. In J. V. Basmajian (Ed.). *Therapeutic Exercise* (3rd ed.). Baltimore: Williams & Wilkins, 1978.
22. Hopkins H., and Smith, H. *Willard and Speckman's Occupational Therapy* (5th ed.). Philadelphia: Lippincott, 1978.
23. Jebson, R. H., et al. An objective and standardized test of hand function. *Arch. Phys. Med. Rehabil.* 50:311, 1969.
24. Kalliomaki, S. L., Markkanen, T. K., and Mustonen, V. A. Sexual behavior after cerebral vascular accidents. *Fertil. Steril.* 12:156, 1961.
25. Kolodny, R. C., Masters, W. H., and Johnson, V. E. *Textbook of Sexual Medicine.* Boston: Little, Brown, 1979.
26. Kotte, F. J. Neurophysiologic Therapy for Stroke. In S. Licht (Ed.). *Stroke and Its Rehabilitation.* New Haven: Physical Medicine Library, 1975. P. 347.
27. Krusen, F. H., Kohke, F. J., and Ellwood, P. M. *Handbook of Physical Medicine and Rehabilitation.* Philadelphia: Saunders, 1971.
28. Lorenze, E. J., and Cancro, R. Dysfunction in visual preception with hemiplegia. Its relation to ADL. *Arch. Phys. Med. Rehabil.* 43(10):514, 1962.
29. Mohr, J. P. Cerebral Vascular Diseases. In K. J. Isselbacher, R. A. Adams, E. Braunwald, R. G. Petersdorf, and J. D. Wilson (Eds.) *Harrison's Principles of Internal Medicine* (9th ed.). New York: McGraw-Hill, 1980. P. 1911.
30. Moskowitz, E. Long-term follow-up for the poststroke patient. *Arch. Phys. Med. Rehabil.* 53:167, 1972.
31. Mossmann, P. L. *A Problem Oriented Approach to Stroke Rehabilitation.* Springfield, Ill.: Thomas, 1976.
32. Rusk, H. *Rehabilitation Medicine* (4th ed.). St. Louis: Mosby, 1977. P. 601.
33. Samuels, M. (Ed.). *Manual of Neurologic Therapeutics.* Boston: Little, Brown, 1978. P. 198.
34. Siev, E., and Freishat, B. *Perceptual*

*Dysfunction in the Adult Stroke Patient.* Thorofare, N. J.: Slack, 1976.

35. Silverman, E. J., and Elfant, I. L. Dysphagia: An evaluation and treatment program for the adult. *Am. J. Occup. Ther.* 33(6):382, 1979.
36. Solet, J. *Apraxia: Basic Theory and Treatment.* 1974. Unpublished thesis.
37. Stern, P. et al. Factors influencing stroke rehabilitation. *Stroke* 2:213, 1971.
38. Stern, P., et al. Effects of facilitation exercise techniques in stroke rehabilitation. *Arch. Phys. Med. Rehabil.* 51:526, 1969.
39. Stockmeyer, S. An interpretation of the approach of Rood to the treatment of neuromuscular dysfunction. *Am. J. Phys. Med.* 46(1):900, 1967.
40. Straub, R. J., and Black, F. W. *The Mental Status Examination in Neurology.* Philadelphia: Davis, 1977.
41. Swenson, J. R. Therapeutic Exercise in Hemiplegia. In J. V. Basmajian (Ed.). *Therapeutic Exercise* (3rd ed.). Baltimore: Williams & Wilkins, 1978. P. 325.
42. Trombly, C. A., and Scott, A. D. *Occupational Therapy for Physical Dysfunction.* Baltimore: Williams and Wilkins, 1977.
43. Twitchell, T. Restoration of motor function following hemiplegia in man. *Brain* 74:443, 1951.
44. Wall, N. (Ed.). *Hemiplegic Evaluation.* Boston: Massachusetts Rehabilitation Hospital, 1979.
45. Wall, N., and Neistadt, M. Functional living evaluation program. Unpublished paper, 1979.

## Suggested Reading

Abramson, A. S., and Kutner, B. A bill of rights for the disabled (editorial). *Arch. Phys. Med. Rehabil.* 53:99, March, 1972.

Adams, C. F., and Hurwitz, L. J. Mental barriers to recovery from stroke. *Lancet* 2:533, 1963.

Anderson, T. P., and Cole, T. M. Sexual counseling of the physically disabled. *Postgrad. Med.* 58(1):117, 1975.

Bannister, R. *Brain's Clinical Neurology.* Oxford: Oxford University Press, 1973.

Banus, B. S. *The Developmental Therapist.* Thorofare, N.J.: Slack, 1971.

Bitter, J. *Introduction to Rehabilitation.* St. Louis: Mosby, 1979. P. 112.

Bobath, B. *Abnormal Postural Reflex Activity Caused by Brain Lesions.* London: Heinemann, 1971.

Brennan, J. B. Response to stretch of hypertonic muscle groups in hemiplegia. *Br. Med. J.* 1:1504, 1959.

Domeena, R. Stroke and Sex. In A. Comfort (Ed.).

*Sexual Consequences of Disability*. Philadelphia: Stickley, 1978.

Drachman, D. A. Pain of neurologic interest. *Am. J. Phys. Med.* 45:544, 1967.

Farber, S. D. *Sensorimotor Evaluation and Treatment Procedures*. Bloomington, Ind.: Purdue University at Indianapolis Medical Center, 1974.

Fiebert, I. M., and Brown, E. Vestibular stimulation to improve ambulation after a CVA. *Phys. Ther.* 59:432, 1979.

Fisher, C. M., and Curray, H. B. Pure motor hemiplegia of vascular origin. *Arch. Neurol.* 13:30, 1965.

Fisher, D. W. Adult education theory necessary in health education practice. *J. Am. Heart Assoc.* 19:129, 1975.

Gordon, E. E., et al. Neurophysiological syndromes in stroke as predictors of outcome. *Arch. Phys. Med. Rehabil.* 59:399, 1978.

Green, R. *Human Sexuality*. Baltimore: Williams and Wilkins, 1979.

Health Education Monograph. Definition by Joint Committee on Health Education Terminology. San Francisco: Society for Public Health Education, 1973.

Hurd, M., Farrell, K. L., and Waylonis, G. Shoulder sling for hemiplegia: Friend or foe? *Arch. Phys. Med. Rehabil.* 155:519, 1974.

Jebsen, R. H., et al. Function of "normal" hand in stroke patients. *Arch. Phys. Med. Rehabil.* 52:170, 1971,

Kamenetz, H. L. Occupational Therapy for Stroke Patient. In S. Licht (Ed.). *Stroke and Its Rehabilitation*. New Haven: Physical Medicine Library, 1975.

Kaplan, P. E., et al. Stroke and brachial plexus injury: A difficult problem. *Arch. Phys. Med. Rehabil.* 58:415, 1977.

Knott, M., and Voss, D. *PNF—Patterns and Techniques*. New York: Harper and Row, 1956.

Kukulka, C. G., Brown, D. M., and Basmajian, J. V. Biofeedback training for early finger joint mobilization. *Am. J. Occup. Ther.* 29:469, 1975.

McDaniel, J. W. *Physical Disability and Human Behavior*. New York: Pergamon, 1976.

Moskowitz, E., and Porter, J. Peripheral nerve lesions in the upper extremity in hemiplegic patients. *N. Engl. J. Med.* 269:776, 1963.

Neistadt, M., and Baker, M. A program for sex counseling of the physically disabled. *Am. J. Occup. Ther.* 32:46, 1978.

Newman, M. Recovery after hemiplegia. *Stroke* 3:702, 1972.

Non-paralytic motor dysfunction after stroke. *Br. Med. J.* 1:1165, 1978.

Payton, O. D., Hirt, S., and Newton, R. A. *Scientific Basis for Neurophysiologic Approaches to Therapeutic Exercise*. Philadelphia: Davis, 1977.

Position Paper. *Concept of Planned Hospital-Based Patient Education Programs*. Submitted by Task Force on Patient Education, 1972. Submitted to President's Committee on Health Education, Washington, D.C.

Rood, M. The Use of Sensory Receptors to Activate, Facilitate and Inhibit Motor Responses, Automatic and Somatic, in Developmental Sequence. In C. Sattely (Ed.). *Approaches to the Treatment of Patients with Neuromuscular Dysfunction*. Dubuque, Iowa: Brown, 1962.

Sahs, A. L., et al. *Guidelines for Stroke Care*. U.S. Department of H.E.W., publication No. (HRA) 76–14017. Washington, D.C.: U.S. Government Printing Office, 1976.

Sexual Attitude Reassessment Seminars. Moss Rehabilitation Hospital, Philadelphia, 1977.

Sidman, J. M. Sexual functioning and the physically disabled. *Am. J. Occup. Ther.* 31:81, 1977.

Simon, I. I. Emotional aspects of physical disability. *Am. J. Occup. Ther.* 25:408, 1971.

Solet, J. *Solet Test for Apraxia. Unpublished thesis*, 1975.

Steinbrocker, O. Shoulder-hand syndrome: Present perspective. *Arch. Phys. Med. Rehabil.* 49:388, 1968.

Steinbrocker, O., Spitzer, N., and Friedman, H. Shoulder-hand syndrome in reflex dystrophy of the upper extremity. *Ann. Intern. Med.* 29:22, 1948.

Taylor, M. M. Analysis of dysfunction in left hemiplegia following stroke. *Am. J. Occup. Ther.* 22:512, 1968.

Therapeutic exercise, part 3. *Am. J. Phys. Med.* 46(1):713, 1967.

Trombly, C. A. Effects of selected activities on finger extension of adult hemiplegia patients. *Am. J. Occup. Ther.* 28:233, 1964.

Vinograd, A., Taylor, E. and Grossman, S. Sensory re-training of the hemiplegic hand. *Am. J. Occup. Ther.* 6(5):246, 1962.

Voss, D. Proprioceptive neuromuscular facilitation. *Am. J. Phys. Med.* 46(1):838, 1967.

Weinbroth, S., Esibill, N., and Zuger, R. Factors in the vocational success of hemiplegic patients. *Arch. Phys. Med. Rehabil.* 52:441, 1971.

# 9 STROKE: *Speech-Language Rehabilitation*

*Frances Senner-Hurley and*
*Nancy G. Lefkowitz*

## Speech-Language Problem Areas

The effects of stroke are far-reaching, affecting speech and language, cognition, personality, perception, and motor skills. Symptoms and severity are dependent on site and size of lesion, as well as etiology. Consequently, the speech-language pathologist is faced with a variety of disorders and deficits to diagnose and treat, including aphasia, apraxia, dysarthria, dysphagia, disorientation, confusion, decreased cognition, impaired memory, and attentional deficits.

### APHASIA

Aphasia, the language disturbance that results from stroke, can suddenly disrupt or prevent communication. It is by far the most devastating consequence of a stroke, defined as a symbolic disturbance resulting from cerebrovascular disease. The central language deficits cross receptive functions, that is, auditory and reading comprehension, and expression, that is, verbalizing and writing. There are two major schools of thought regarding aphasia: it is viewed either as a loss of language [80], or interference with available language [72].

Its severity and symptoms are determined largely by the site, size, and etiology of the lesion. Approximately 95 percent of all aphasias result from insult in left hemisphere. It does not only result from stroke, but can also arise from head injury, tumor, surgery, or infec-

tion. In North America, stroke produces an estimated 5000 cases of disabling aphasia per year [25].

### CLASSIFICATION

Since the second half of the nineteenth century, beginning with the work of Broca and Wernicke, a variety of clinical syndromes in the area of aphasia has been described. Over time, several names have been used to describe similar clusters of symptoms. Not only neurologists and speech-language pathologists, but also psycholinguists, neuropsychologists, and neurolinguists have been involved with the study of aphasia and development of nomenclature. The resulting classification systems have a definite bias reflecting the philosophy of their proponents. Once-popular nomenclature, like fashion, may fade away only to reappear at a later point in history. Speech-language pathologists who treat aphasic patients should keep abreast of the changes in terminology, as this facilitates greater understanding of the disorder and allows negotiability among institutions.

In the field of speech-language pathology, the Boston VA Hospital group's neuroanatomical classification system [27] is widely used and accepted. While verbal output, that is, fluency versus nonfluency, is a primary consideration in discriminating among the major aphasic syndromes, other factors contribute to the

**TABLE 9-1.** *Symptoms of Major Aphasic Syndromes*

| Language Behavior | Broca's | Wernicke's | Conduction | Anomic | Global |
|---|---|---|---|---|---|
| Fluency | Nonfluent; awkward articulation, restricted grammar with paucity of grammatical function units | Fluent, relatively normal suprasegmental features; syntax either normal or paragrammatic | Fluent, with frequent pauses for word finding and self-correction of literal paraphasias | Fluent, barring pauses for word finding | Often mute or limited to expletives or stereotypes |
| Auditory comprehension | Superior to all output modalities | Severely impaired | Relatively intact; superior to all output modalities | Range of normal to mild impairment, usually for isolated nouns and verbs | Severely impaired in spite of some evidence of communicative competence |
| Repetition | Reduced, but superior to spontaneous speech production | Severely impaired: often paraphasic or neologistic | Disproportionately impaired as compared to spontaneous speech production | Usually unimpaired | Often absent or limited to single words |
| Paraphasia | Literal and verbal paraphasias | Primary verbal paraphasias; literal paraphasias or neologisms can also occur | Preponderance of literal paraphasias | Infrequent or absent; circumlocutory behavior | May be extended neologistic jargon |
| Naming | Limited, but superior to spontaneous speech production | Usually significantly impaired | Marked by literal paraphasic errors; usually impaired | Various degrees of impairment, often relative to degree of word finding problem | Often absent; at best, severely impaired |
| Writing | Usually impaired; primarily substantives, often with spelling errors | Severely impaired | Impaired; frequent spelling errors | May be normal or agraphic | Absent or limited to copying name |
| Reading | Oral reading limited; comprehension less impaired | Severe impairments in both oral and reading comprehension | Oral reading usually comparable to level of repetition skills; reading comprehension usually unimpaired | May be normal or alexic | Severely impaired; often limited to recognition of own name |

Sources: Adapted from H. Goodglass and E. Kaplan, *The Assessment of Aphasia and Related Disorders*, Philadelphia: Lea and Febiger, 1972; and A. Kertesz, *Aphasia and Associated Disorders: Localization and Recovery*, New York: Grune and Stratton, 1979.

total picture of each one (Table 9-1). The Boston VA group considers Broca's, Wernicke's, conduction, and anomic aphasias as the major clinical varieties.

Yet another syndrome exists that is not included in this description. Global, or total, aphasia is marked by severe to profound deficits in all language areas, and is encountered frequently. At Rusk Institute, four clinical subgroups of global aphasia have been described [30]. The authors find the "varieties" useful, in that they hold implications for treatment planning. Nevertheless, this patient group has the poorest prognosis, as initial severity of deficits has been shown to be the best predictor of eventual outcome [47, 72].

In recent years, clinical varieties of aphasia within the classification system have been discussed in terms of an evolutionary process. Symptomatology is now recognized as dynamic, often following a predictable course over time [47].

In addition to the five major syndromes, there are other less frequently occurring conditions, including transcortical sensory and transcortical motor aphasias [27, 46]. The Boston group has described "pure" aphasias [27], disorders involving a single input or output, such as pure alexia, or pure word-deafness. The concept of a single focus is not universally accepted, in fact, it is in direct conflict with the prevailing definition of aphasia as a multifunction disorder [40, 72].

EVALUATION

The purpose of an initial evaluation is to determine the presence and type of aphasia, to correlate this information with neurological findings to formulate a prognosis, and to identify language strengths and weaknesses that will then serve as a basis for treatment design. Practicing speech-language pathologists make use of a wide range of formal tests (Table 9-2) and informal tasks. Considerations in the selection of testing tools are the patient's deficits, available time, purpose of evaluation, and test availability.

In keeping with the definition of aphasia as a multimodality language disorder, all of the general language ability tests tap auditory comprehension, verbal ability, reading, and writing. The *Boston Diagnostic Aphasia Examination* [27] and the *Western Aphasia Battery* [48] are distinct from the others in that they yield information related to localization. The *Porch Index of Communicative Ability* (PICA) [62] has a multidimensional scoring system that allows for rapid and descriptive recording of observed behaviors; however, its administration mandates successful completion of a 40-hour training program. All three heralded the use of psychometric principles in the evaluation of aphasia [50]. The authors find *Examining for Aphasia* [18] and the *Aphasia Language Performance Scales* [45] useful as screening tools, as they require less time to administer.

The *Neurosensory Center Comprehensive Examination for Aphasia* [79] seems to have gained greater favor among neuropsychologists than speech-language pathologists. Some interesting features of this test are normative data, as well as corrected scores for age and educational level on some subtests.

The *Minnesota Test for Differential Diagnosis of Aphasia* [71] tests a wide variety of tasks within each area. In contrast to the other batteries we have found this one clinically useful with more severely impaired patients, as they are able to respond to the lower-level subtests.

Except for the PICA, which recommends total administration of all 18 subtests in one sitting [62], the other batteries offer greater flexibility during administration. The experienced clinician prudently selects subtests from one or more of the available batteries to obtain a comprehensive profile of each patient's strengths and weaknesses.

The general language batteries are frequently criticized for failing to identify those skills an aphasic patient uses in everyday life [38, 41, 70]. To gain an appreciation of the patient's functional language abilities, Sarno developed

# TABLE 9-2. *Sampling of Formal Tests*

| General Language Batteries | | | Single Modality Tests | | | |
|---|---|---|---|---|---|---|
| Name of Test | Author(s) | Published | Modality | Name of Test | Author(s) | Published |
| Aphasia Language Performance Scales (ALPS) | Keenan and Brassell | 1975 | Auditory comprehension | Auditory Comprehension Test for Sentences (ACTS) | Shewan | 1979 |
| Boston Diagnostic Aphasia Examination (BDAE) | Goodglass and Kaplan | 1972 | | Functional Auditory Comprehension Task (FACT) | LaPointe and Horner | 1978 |
| Examining for Aphasia | Eisenson | 1954 | | Logico-Grammatical Sentence Comprehension Test | Wiig and Semel | 1974 |
| Minnesota Test for Differential Diagnosis of Aphasia (MTDDA) | Schuell | 1965 | | Token Test | DeRenzi and Vignolo | 1962 |
| Neurosensory Center Comprehensive Examination for Aphasia (NCCEA) | Spreen and Benton | 1969 | Reading comprehension | Reading Comprehension Battery for Aphasia (RCBA) | LaPointe and Horner | 1979 |
| Porch Index of Communicative Ability (PICA) | Porch | 1971 | Verbal ability | Boston Naming Test | Kaplan, Goodglass, and Weintraub | 1976 |
| Western Aphasia Battery (WAB) | Kertesz and Poole | 1980 | | Story Completion Test | Goodglass, Gleason, Bernholtz, and Hyde | 1972 |
| | | | | Syllable-Concept Count | Yorkston and Beukelman | 1977 |
| | | | | Word Fluency Measure | Borkowski, Benton, and Spreen | 1967 |

## Functional/Pragmatic Tests

| Name of Test | Author | Published |
|---|---|---|
| Communicative Abilities in Daily Living (CADL) | Holland | 1980 |
| Functional Communicative Profile (FCP) | Sarno | 1969 |

the *Functional Communication Profile* (FCP) [70]. Here, 45 items spanning five areas including movement, speaking, understanding, and miscellaneous, are rated on a nine-point scale, with information obtained through direct observation or an informal interview.

More recently, the *Communicative Abilities in Daily Living* (CADL) [41] became available to tap functional skills using simulated everyday situations. Responses are rated on a three-point scoring system. As the test is designed to measure communicative effectiveness, any mode of response, including nonverbal, is acceptable. Both the FCP and CADL maintain an underlying philosophy that communication is a dynamic interaction, and therefore cannot be assessed by discrete language tasks.

In some instances it is desirable to analyze a specific language skill or modality in greater depth. Several tests are available for assessing auditory comprehension. Of the four noted in Table 9-2, three have certain features in common. The *Auditory Comprehension Test for Sentences* (ACTS) [74], *Functional Auditory Comprehension Tasks* (FACT) [51], and *Token Test* [15] all require nonverbal motor responses. They control for length and syntactic complexity; in addition, ACTS controls for vocabulary level. The ACTS requires a pointing response given an array of four pictures. The FACT uses common objects and objects within the environment as its stimuli, while the *Token Test* makes use of plastic shapes that differ in size, shape, and color; both require pointing or object manipulation in response to verbal commands. The latter is reported to be a sensitive measure of subtle deficits in auditory comprehension, related to infrequency of commands [15]. The *Logico-Grammatical Sentence Comprehension Test* [86], although originally designed for use with learning-disabled children, can provide useful information about a patient's ability to comprehend linguistic concepts in the following areas: comparative, passive, temporal, spatial, and family relationships. In spite of the fact that only the ACTS and the *Token Test* are normed for an adult

aphasic population, all of these can serve as valuable diagnostic tools.

The first test to emerge for assessing reading comprehension was the *Reading Comprehension Battery for Aphasia* [52], designed systematically to evaluate the nature and degree of reading impairment in aphasic adults. Selected stimuli that are relevant to the patient's needs range from single words to paragraphs that require functional reading skills. The information obtained provides guidance as to level, direction, and focus of treatment.

In the area of verbal ability, the *Boston Naming Test* [44] assesses word retrieval in the context of visual confrontation. The pictured items were selected based on frequency of noun occurrence. Although it consists of 85 stimuli, it is rarely administered in its entirety, as there are established criteria for obtaining baseline and ceiling scores. The resultant raw score can be compared to norms for several broad age and educational levels. The test is designed to yield information regarding facilitative techniques for word retrieval, which then has implications for treatment planning.

On the *Word Fluency Measure* [4], the patient is asked to name in one minute as many words as possible that begin with a specific letter. This is clinically useful with a patient who has suspected subtle deficits in word-finding.

The *Story Completion Test* [26, 28] was developed to assess a patient's ability to generate grammatical structures. It consists of a series of incomplete stories that are designed to elicit various syntactic forms based on a hierarchy of complexity.

Yorkston and Beukelman accomplished a *coup de maître* with their *Syllable-Concept Count* [88]. Its development stemmed from their recognition that the verbal subtests in available aphasia batteries failed to differentiate high-level patients from normal speakers, or to demonstrate small changes in performance over time. To rectify this, they created a system to measure verbal efficiency. A description of the "Cookie Theft" picture [27] was analyzed according to the following: (1) number of syllables produced per minute, (2) number of concepts expressed per minute, and (3) number of syllables per concept. Norms for comparison are available on small numbers of normal speakers, fluent aphasics, and non-fluent aphasics. The authors find the *Syllable Concept Count* to be a useful addition in evaluating higher-level aphasic people.

Observation of behavior during testing as well as during informal exchange is important to obtain a total picture of the patient. Sometimes there is a discrepancy between test results and observed behaviors. This occurs most frequently in the area of auditory comprehension, where a patient may be described as having good comprehension in social situations, yet performs poorly on formal tests. This demonstrates the dichotomy between communicative competence versus language function [38, 39, 40]. There are situations in which only informal procedures can be carried out, most often with patients who have profound deficits in auditory comprehension.

No matter what methodologies are employed, evaluation is complete only when all of the data have been interpreted and a treatment plan has been formulated.

## TREATMENT

Maximizing communicative skills is the goal of the two major approaches to aphasia rehabilitation: (1) stimulation-facilitation, and (2) programmed-operant [10, 50].

The former was described by Wepman [83] and Schuell [71]. It is based on the premise that responses can be elicited on an automatic level and then "shifted upward to more intentional use" [2] through choice of facilitators, followed by a gradual fading of cues. This is consistent with the interference theory of language breakdown in aphasia. Several basic principles are inherent to this approach [71]:

1. Sensory input consists of intensive auditory stimulation, with supplementary visual stimulation when appropriate.

2. Each stimulus must be sufficient to elicit a response without forcing.
3. Stimuli may be manipulated by altering length, loudness, and rate of presentation, coupled with repetition.
4. Incorrect responses are not corrected; rather, efforts are directed toward eliciting other correct responses.

In contrast, the programmed-operant approach is based on the tenets of learning theory. It upholds the view that aphasia is a loss of language, and therefore treatment involves re-education. Sarno [10, 80] is credited for first using programmed instruction with aphasics, with recent advocates including Brookshire [5] and Holland [10]. Fundamental steps are [49, 50]:

1. Baseline measures are obtained to allow for periodic measurement of treatment effects. It is essential that both the patient's behavior and the stimulus controls are carefully defined.
2. Behavior is modified through standard conditioning procedures. The programs are constructed either to increase or decrease the frequency of a response, or to establish a new response through successive approximations.
3. Extension of stimulus control, where the process of carryover consists of a systematic shift of a response from the structured clinical situation to more functional spontaneous settings.

It is the authors' belief that in clinical application the division between the two major approaches becomes less distinct. In reality, many treatment programs are hybrids, created from elements of both stimulation-facilitation and programmed-operant approaches [50].

A method used in aphasia treatment that clearly incorporates principles of both is La-Pointe's *Base-10* [49]. This system of measuring patient behaviors requires task specification, establishing criteria, a scoring system, and ten selected stimuli. Baseline measures are obtained, followed by therapeutic intervention using stimulation-facilitation techniques selected to improve performance. Subsequently, changes in performance are measured. This process is repeated over a total of ten sessions, and all of the information is recorded and graphically displayed on a response form. In an age of accountability, *Base-10* allows for documentation of treatment effectiveness.

In 1977, Helm presented a program designed systematically to teach several syntactic structures to Broca's aphasics [34]. Ludlow's work [56] on the recovery of syntax in aphasia provided the foundation for Helm's hierarchical ordering of the following five syntactic structures:

1. Imperative intransitive, e.g., sit down.
2. Imperative transitive, e.g., shut the window.
3. Wh- question, e.g., where is Bill?
4. Declarative transitive, e.g., I eat supper.
5. Declarative intransitive, e.g., he is walking.

Helm recommends that phonology and semantics as well as syntax be controlled and manipulated. Both auditory and visual stimuli are provided in the form of a story completion probe [28] and a picture. Twenty stimuli are presented for each syntactic structure. Other programs appropriate for use with Broca's aphasia are *Melodic Intonation Therapy* [78] and *Amerind* [76], which are described in the apraxia treatment section.

Helm and Benson [36] developed a *Visual Action Therapy* (VAT), which is geared to the globally involved aphasic patient. The ultimate goal of this program is to establish a group of gestural responses that can serve as means of limited output. The VAT consists of a sequence of small increments, beginning with object tracing and picture matching, and proceeding until the patient is able to gesture when the object is removed. The program is based on the premise that limb movements involve less complicated motor sequencing than oral movements, and are therefore more easily acquired.

These programs are aimed at increasing verbal output in the nonfluent aphasic person. A search of the literature failed to reveal a comparable number of programs designed for specific use with fluent patients with auditory comprehension deficits. Other authors [40] have also reported on this inequality of study, conjecturing that comprehension is less studied because it is not an overt behavior.

Following are examples of tasks and programs that are appropriate for use with the auditorily impaired patient. LaPointe [50] described numerous tasks incorporating *Base-10* that are geared toward improving auditory comprehension. Whitney [85] presented comprehension strategies designed specifically for use with the fluent patient. She elaborated on a step-by-step procedure through which the patient is trained to request repeats or to ask that material be presented in written form. For such a program to succeed, the patient must be aware first of deficits and then of the ability to compensate to a degree by using those strategies that yield positive results.

Whitney [85] also described techniques that she termed "stop strategies." These are designed to increase patients' abilities to monitor their own output. They learn to reduce their rates, recognize their own errors, and eventually make their own corrections using word-finding strategies. To facilitate communication with the patient who has auditory comprehension deficits, it is necessary for family, friends, and staff to alter their habitual speaking patterns. For example, shorter phrases with increased pauses allow the aphasic patient more time to receive and process information [5].

Another area that necessitates therapeutic intervention is anomia, a problem pervading all aphasia types. Marshall [57] observed several forms of word retrieval behaviors used by aphasic patients. For example, some are able to retrieve a word after a self-imposed delay.

Others cue themselves through semantic (e.g., I'll have a hot dog ... no, a hamburger) or phonemic association (e.g., I lost my fen, ten, no ... pen). In treatment, it is important to observe which of the tactics the patient uses spontaneously [85]. The patient's awareness of these behaviors can then be heightened, and systematic training ensue's to increase the frequency of use on a volitional level.

Recent attention has been paid to the issue of pragmatics, the ability to convey intent by any means. Holland [38], as a leading proponent of this school of thought, has summarized its implication for treatment as follows:

1. Use a number of contexts other than the nonfunctional diadactic in which therapy presently occurs.
2. Concentrate on relevant communicating and relevant language.
3. Develop a sensitivity to the manner in which aphasics actually communicate by observing, developing, and reinforcing use of other than verbal communicative channels.
4. Help aphasics capitalize on unconventional strategies for negotiating verbal difficulties.

It is beyond the scope of this chapter to enumerate all of the available treatment programs. The diligent clinician is advised to remain current by seeking out new concepts and techniques.

## PROGNOSIS

It is difficult to separate the effects of language treatment from spontaneous recovery. Designing and implementing well-controlled studies that assess the effectiveness of treatment are complicated by the countless variables that influence treatment results. Only two controlled studies [32, 46] that show treatment to be effective can be found in the literature to date. The need for additional data is evident. It is hoped that researchers will continue to produce conclusive evidence supporting language treatment of adult aphasia.

## APRAXIA

Oral apraxia is most often viewed as a sensorimotor disorder of articulation and prosody resulting from brain damage, specifically from involvement of the third frontal convolution, or Broca's area. The possibility of apraxia associated with more posterior, probably parietal lesions, has been raised [84]. It is described as a breakdown in volitional programming of articulatory positioning and sequencing in the absence of severe motor weakness, primary sensory loss, or significant deficit in auditory comprehension [8, 12, 42]. While the majority of speech-language pathologists [8, 12, 65] contend that apraxia is nonlinguistic in origin, Martin [58], who has been a major opponent of this view, describes the condition as a disturbance in linguistic processing. It is not only the basic theory of this disorder that is subject to dispute, but its nomenclature and symptomatology as well [9, 42].

Throughout the literature [8, 9, 42, 65] certain general characteristics of apraxia are identified: visible and audible searching for target phonemes; pronounced difficulty with initiation of speech; fewer errors in automatic, as compared to propositional speech; disruption in normal prosody; inability to self-correct despite recognition of errors; numerous phonemic errors involving voicing transpositions and perseveration; and a highly variable error pattern.

## EVALUATION

The purpose of the initial evaluation is to determine the presence, severity, and type of apraxia, that is, verbal or nonverbal. Through testing, the clinician identifies the patient's capability and explores methods to improve output. These baseline data serve as a starting point for treatment, as well as means for measuring change over time. Regardless of the choice of stimuli, whether it is a formal battery or informal observations, an audiotape or videotape sample should be obtained and kept on file.

Traditionally, speech-language pathologists

evaluated apraxia by analysis of performance on a variety of verbal and nonverbal tasks, many of which were subtests of aphasia batteries. These included automatic speech, such as reciting the alphabet, days of the week, or counting; imitation of words, phrases, and sentences of varying length and phonemic complexity; oral reading of words and sentences; and spontaneous speech. Nonverbal oral motor movements, such as puckering the lips and lateralizing the tongue, were assesssed both individually and repetitively. Performance was scored as correct or incorrect. In 1966, DeRenzi and colleagues [15] reported a test for oral and limb apraxia using a three-point scoring system that offered an improved description of patient behaviors. Darley [12] subsequently published an 11-point graded scoring system that detailed characteristic performances on nonverbal oral motor tasks.

In 1979, Dabul's *Apraxia Battery for Adults* [8] was published. Although it is not yet standardized, normative data are forthcoming. Her battery represents one of the first comprehensive tests designed with an objective scoring system and a systematic set of tasks specifically to evaluate apraxia by six subtests: (1) diadochokinetic rate; (2) repetition of words of increasing length, for example, thick, thicken, thickening; (3) limb and oral apraxia; (4) visual confrontation naming of polysyllabic words, with specific measurement of latency and utterance time; (5) successive repetition of words; (6) inventory of articulatory characteristics using oral reading of the "Grandfather Passage" [82], picture description, and counting to 30.

A checklist of features and a profile sheet appear in the scoring booklet, and are used to verify the presence or absence of apraxia. The number of characteristics exhibited, along with frequency of occurrence, determine severity.

Frequently, neurogenic communicative disorders occur concomitantly. In a review of the files of 100 dyspraxic patients, one-third were found to have accompanying aphasia [37].

Therefore it is necessary to administer selected portions of aphasia/dysarthria/apraxia test protocols to arrive at a differential diagnosis. In spite of a clinician's best efforts to interpret raw data, differential diagnosis is not always clear-cut. When a patient is globally impaired across all language functions it may be impossible to distinguish the motor planning deficits from the central disturbance. During the course of recovery, as symptoms and features change a clearer diagnostic picture should emerge.

TREATMENT

The ultimate goal of treatment is to restore volitional purposive control of articulation and prosody, given the limits imposed by the patient's reduced physiological support for speech [66]. Achieving this objective requires determination and perseverance by the patient and clinician, often over the course of several years.

Rosenbek, one of the more prolific and current authors in the field of apraxia, thoroughly discusses the primary approaches to its treatment and the rationale behind numerous techniques. Based on Luria's work, Rosenbek [64, 65] divided treatment into two main approaches: facilitation and reorganization. Facilitation allows a patient improved access to the phonological system through selected environmental conditions such as imitation or the use of rhythm. Reorganization, which involves relearning, is divided into inter- and intrasystemic forms. Intrasystemic reorganization is the shifting of speech down to a more automatic level, or up to a more volitional, higher cortical level. In this process, speech is an auditory-vocal act. For example, a patient using serialization to arrive at a desired number is reorganizing on an automatic level, whereas the patient who uses learned nonverbal articulatory placement to produce the first sound of a word is reorganizing on a volitional level. Intersystemic reorganization involves the introduction of a system or set of behaviors, such as limb gestures or writing, as part of the speaking act. Most treatment programs make use of both facilitation and reorganization in a systematic manner.

Rosenbek and co-workers [69] published an eight-step task continuum for treatment of apraxic adults that has components of both facilitation and reorganization. The program involves systematic progression beginning with imitation and maximal cueing, and moving to the endpoint of volitional production. Subsequent analysis of this program by its original authors [68] revealed that the eight steps were not a continuum; however, the program, with modifications in sequence order, or omissions of the two steps involving reading, continues to be a viable approach for improving output in some apraxic patients. In a study by Deal and Florance [13] it was found unnecessary to proceed in order through all eight steps of the Rosenbek program. These investigators modified the program further by applying more stringent performance criteria.

Deal and Resler [14] developed a program that shows parallels to that of Rosenbek's group. Prior to initiating this program, a probed spontaneous speech sample is obtained to determine the patient's mean length of utterance. Ten target sentences of controlled length are then constructed, with selection geared toward ultimate incorporation into a dialogue, which the authors refer to as a pseudoconversational paradigm. In teaching volitional control of the ten target sentences, maximal cueing is initially used, followed by systematic fading of cues. Stringent performance criteria are established at each level of the program. Deal and Resler recommend periodic probing to determine if the mean length of utterance has increased; if so, subsequent stimuli are designed to reflect the improved performance. Both programs require painstaking repetitive drill.

In 1974, Sparks, Helm, and Albert [78] developed an ingenious approach to apraxia treatment that stemmed from the assumption that musical, tonal, and rhythmic abilities are housed in the right hemisphere of the brain.

They conjectured that patients with an anterior left hemisphere lesion still had access to the functions carried out by the right hemisphere. This gave birth to *Melodic Intonation Therapy* (MIT), a two-level program of progressive steps in which somewhat exaggerated patterns of rhythm, rate, and stress are paired with the stimuli. This program, like those described previously, relies on simultaneous repetition, followed by fading of cues to reach the eventual goal of volitional production using more normal suprasegmental patterns.

An example of a program that can be used as a facilitator or intersystemic reorganizer is *Amerind* [77]. This is a system of signals based on American Indian sign language, and has been modified and successfully applied with some apraxic patients. The patient acquires a collection of signals that are felt to be universally understood, thus serving as a primary mode of communication. The use of gesture facilitates speech production and may, if paired systematically with speech, reorganize it.

One of the more traditional approaches to treatment, appropriate for use with severely apraxic patients, involves building target sounds from nonspeech gestures, as in placing the teeth together and then adding an exhaled air stream for /s/. Once some consistency in the production of individual sounds is achieved, a program such as the *Moto-Sequential Tactile Therapy Program* [43] can be introduced. This 3-stage program involves auditory, visual, and tactile cues. Stage I consists of diadochokinetic drills of nonsense syllables to teach the topographical cues needed for improved sequencing and accurate self-monitoring. Stage II advances to the production of mono- and polysyllabic words elicited by a variety of stimuli. In stage III, the acquired skills are transferred to structured multiword utterances and ultimately to spontaneous speech.

This list is not exhaustive. Additional programs, techniques, and materials are compiled in several texts [12, 37, 65]. There are similarities running through the previously described treatment programs: repetitive drill is an essential component, and careful selection and ordering of stimuli are necessary gradually to move the patient from dependent to independent speech. Once a program is in operation, periodic review is indicated to determine its appropriateness. Changes are justifiable if they will hasten the patient's progress, and a patient initially treated with one program can progress to another. Determining which is best suited to a patient at different points during recovery requires skillful analysis and flexibility on the part of the clinician.

Severely apraxic patients with concomitant deficits either in language or mental status have a poor prognosis for recovery of functional communication [37, 65], and are unlikely to respond to any program. In spite of this, the authors contend that these patients deserve a trial period of treatment with hopes of effecting positive changes that can improve their quality of life. The trial period also provides a time for the clinician to work with the family, helping them to accept the permanency of residual deficits.

## DYSARTHRIA

In contrast to the aphasias and their language deficits, dysarthrias are a group of related motor speech disorders secondary to central or peripheral neurogenic damage [12, 67]. Historically, dysarthria was viewed as a unitary articulatory disturbance. More recently, the definition has broadened to include coexisting motor disorders in 5 systems: respiration, phonation, articulation, resonance, and prosody [12, 67]. These disorders result from paralysis, paresis, abnormal tone, or incoordination of the speech musculature, with severity dependent on site or extent of lesion. This chapter addresses dysarthria secondary to stroke or head trauma, rather than the progressive conditions secondary to diseases such as amyotrophic lateral sclerosis, multiple sclerosis, Parkinson's disease, and Huntington's chorea. The authors know of no compilation of the incidence of dysarthrias based on individual disease processes.

## CLASSIFICATION

Typically, dysarthrias have been classified by site of lesion or etiology. In 1969, Darley, Aronson, and Brown [11] first reported a classification system based on neurophysiology. They identified clusters of deviant speech characteristics associated with specific neurological disorders from which evolved the following six dysarthric types: flaccid, spastic, hyperkinetic, hypokinetic, ataxic, and mixed. This type of classification system is not merely academic, but provides a theoretical background that relates speech to neurology. For practicing clinicians, the efforts of these investigators served as a landmark that fostered improved differential diagnosis.

## EVALUATION

Evaluation of the dysarthrias, in contrast to the aphasias, consists of nonstandardized batteries. With varying degrees of comprehensiveness, clinicians observe and record behaviors across several areas of measurement during an assessment. The observations are largely perceptual unless the clinician is fortunate enough to have access to sophisticated and often costly equipment, such as spectrographs, biofeedback, electromyographs, or cinefluoroscopes. Without such equipment raw data can be obtained and compared to established norms only for isolated behaviors such as verbal diadochokinetic rates, length of sustained phonation, and number of words produced per minute.

An evaluation typically consists of an oral peripheral examination and analysis of speech production. The structure of individual components of the oral mechanism—lips, tongue, palates, oropharynx, mandible, and dentition—is examined. The larynx is not subject to direct viewing by a speech-language pathologist, as there are few in this field who are trained to perform indirect laryngoscopy. Therefore some structures are only assessed functionally, along any number of the following guidelines: direction and rate of movement, range, force, endurance, and rhythm.

Because language is not limited to isolated oral motor movements or individual syllables, it is necessary to go further and analyze a variety of stimuli. A thorough sampling should include single words and sentences varying in length and complexity, as well as connected speech, and oral reading of a paragraph known in the field such as the "Grandfather Passage" [82] or the "Rainbow Passage" [19]. It is wise to record speech samples on a high-quality audiotape to permit initial analysis and subsequent determination of progress. The speech systems of articulation, phonation, prosody, resonance, and respiration are analyzed by listening to the sample.

An inclusive listing of 38 dimensions described by Darley and colleagues [12] is a valuable resource for identifying individual components and determining the dysarthria type. As there is considerable overlap of symptoms in the various types of dysarthria, the skilled clinician must be able to identify and rank those dimensions that are most deviant to arrive at a differential diagnosis. A severity rating is based on the degree to which intelligibility is compromised. Both the classification system and severity rating are somewhat subjective because of the perceptual nature of the diagnostic process.

TREATMENT

Historically, treatment evolved in direct consequence to the prevailing definition of dysarthria as an articulation problem; that is, the individual articulators were strengthened, followed by traditional articulation drill [83]. The current, more encompassing definition has influenced treatment, which today is based on dual considerations: increasing physiological support for speech, and establishing compensatory strategies making use of residual function [67].

Determining specific treatment objectives is based on interpretation of diagnostic findings. While the dysarthric patient may demonstrate impairments in several systems, the clinician selects those symptoms that when modified will result in the greatest degree of improved intelligibility. Because of the interplay between systems, direct treatment in one area frequently results in improvements in others. The focus of treatment may thus be improvement in one or several of the following areas: respiration, phonation, resonation, articulation, and prosody.

Systematic progressive drill is the rudiment of treatment. For example, rate reduction has long been stressed as a method of increasing intelligibility, in that more precise articulatory contacts can be made. Metronomes, foot tapping, and more recently, a pacing board [35] have been used to facilitate the goal of reduced rate. The clinician must carefully sequence stimuli according to length and propositionality as the patient is moved toward the eventual goal of an internalized slow rate.

Once the patient has achieved effective rate control further gains in intelligibility are possible through direct focus on the prosodic features of speech production, namely, stress and intonation. In teaching the patient to use stress, which may be achieved through a change in pitch or loudness, imitation may be the starting point. The patient needs to be aware that placement of stress alters the meaning of an utterance and is thus a powerful conveyor of intent. For example, GREEN-house differs from green HOUSE (you wouldn't want your Boston ferns in the latter, nor would you want to live in the former!). As the patient progresses, a structured question-answer paradigm can be introduced. For example, to the clinician's question, "Do you like SCROD?" the patient may answer using any of the following contrastive stress patterns [19, 21, 67]:

1. Yes, I like SCROD.
2. No, I DON'T like scrod.
3. No, I like LOBSTER!

It is necessary for the above to take place in less structured activities for carryover to take place.

Further suggestions in treatment planning and direct techniques for modifying problems within each system have been detailed by Rosenbek and LaPointe [67]. Practicing clinicians are urged to refer to their exhaustive work.

Along with direct treatment of symptoms, counseling is an essential part of a program [1]. For most patients and their families, the initial weeks following onset of stroke are difficult ones. The skilled clinician provides information about the nature of the problem and realistic expectations about recovery in an atmosphere of encouragement and hope. Initially, it may be necessary for the clinician to support and stimulate the patient to try as hard as possible. Ultimately, however, the responsibility for change lies not with the clinician alone; the patient must assume an active role and be willing to accept compromised intelligibility for treatment to be successful.

It is not just the patient's motivation and personality that determine the outcome of treatment, as there are some who will remain significantly impaired despite intensive efforts. For these patients, the extent of the neurological deficit is insurmountable for achieving verbal communication. The clinician who continues treatment with the emphasis on verbal skills for a prolonged time period is doing the patient a great disservice, and establishing an alternate mode of communication is indicated. The choice of nonvocal communication is determined by careful assessment of the patient's abilities, limitations, and needs. This may include the joint cooperation of occupational therapy, physical therapy, speech-language pathology, the family, and the patient. The system may be as basic as establishing a yes/no response through a single motor movement such as an eye blink, or as sophisticated as a computerized system costing several thousand dollars. Detailed information regarding alternate modes of communication can be found in *Nonvocal Communication Resource Book* [81], and the quarterly publication, *Commu-*

*nication Outlook* [7], which provides supplementary material and information about current advancements in the field.

MEDICAL INTERVENTION

At various stages during rehabilitation, medical specialties may be consulted regarding specific problems. When there is a significant degree of hypernasality that has not been affected by spontaneous recovery or direct treatment, the patient should be evaluated by an otolaryngologist for surgical intervention, or a prosthodontist for possible fitting of a palatal lift prosthesis. Palatal studies by a radiologist are important in determining the status of the velopharyngeal mechanism and the best type of intervention. Other aberrations in vocal quality such as hoarseness or breathiness also merit the attention of an otolaryngologist or radiologist. Indirect laryngoscopy and electromyographic studies may be performed to assess the functional status of the laryngeal mechanism. When dysphagia is present, the radiologist's findings on a barium swallow or cineradiography will significantly influence the method of treatment. If intelligibility of speech is compromised because of poorly fitting dentures or lack of teeth, referral to dentistry is indicated. As ability auditorily to self-monitor is critical to the success of treatment, if the patient fails audiometric screening, referral to an audiologist is advisable for complete workup and consideration for a hearing aid. Once a supportive device, such as a palatal lift, dentures, or a hearing aid, is obtained, ongoing speech treatment is essential for achieving optimal benefit.

TEAM APPROACH

The dysarthric patient with multiple motor disorders is likely to require the attention of several health professionals. Frequently, the treatment objectives cross disciplines of occupational and physical therapy, respiratory therapy, dietary, and nursing and reinforce one another. For example, the patient with reduced

TABLE 9-3. *The Role of the Right Hemisphere*

| Features and Functions | Behavioral Manifestations of Brain Injury |
|---|---|
| Visual and auditory perception and visual imagery | Disturbed spatial relationships affecting calculations, reading, writing, and comprehension of syntactic structures; Difficulty with dreaming and imagination; Difficulty with facial recognition; Difficulty with feeding and dressing; Difficulty discriminating voices |
| Abstraction | Concrete interpretations; Impaired metaphorical thinking; Personalizing information |
| Emotion and affect | Impaired sense of humor; Difficulty interpreting emotions and moods of others; Marked indifference to own problems; Denial of problems; Flat affect, reduced prosody; Paucity of gestures; Inappropriate jocularity |
| Judgment | Impulsivity; Impaired problem solving and reasoning skills; Misinterpretations; Lack of insight; Embellishments, confabulations, irrelevancies; Inability to formulate a gestalt from the individual parts |
| Organization | Difficulty recognizing relationships among key points of a story; Difficulty relaying a story; Difficulty ordering and sequencing events; Copious output |
| Attention | Distracted by visual and auditory stimuli; Poor eye contact; Internal distractibility |

Data from references 22, 23, 33, 54, 59, 60, 61, 87.

breath support is assisted by deep breathing exercises carried out by a chest physical therapist, a physical therapist, and a speech-language pathologist. The physical and occupational therapists' efforts to improve neck and trunk control affect the patient's airway, while splinting and bracing affect posture and positioning [67]. The result is improved physiological support for speech, which assists the work of the speech-language pathologist. For the dysarthric patient with dysphagia, teamwork of dietary, occupational therapy, physical therapy, speech-language pathology, nursing, and the family are indicated. (See section on dysphagia for further discussion.)

There are instances when simultaneous treatment by two or more professionals is beneficial. For example, there are patients with decreased endurance who can only tolerate a few treatment sessions per day. They may be seen for physical and speech treatment programs while in the supine position, whether in bed or on a mat in the physical therapy suite. As endurance increases, additional treatment sessions are added, enabling each discipline to carry out its own program. Scheduling of the total treatment program requires cooperation of team members. For example, the patient who requires suctioning should be seen by the chest physical therapist, nurse, or respiratory therapist immediately preceding speech treatment in an effort to diminish excessive secretions that interfere with speech production. Ultimately, the aim of this cooperative approach is to maximize the patient's functioning in the shortest amount of time.

TABLE 9-4. *Some Etiological Considerations in Dysphagia*

*Neurogenic Involvement*

> Stroke (cortical and brain stem)
> Head trauma
> Brain tumor
> Multiple sclerosis
> Parkinson's disease
> Amyotrophic lateral sclerosis
> Pseudobulbar palsy
> Polio
> Guillain-Barré syndrome
> Other upper and lower motor neuron diseases
> Senility
> Widespread vascular disease

*Structural Alterations*

> Glossectomy
> Laryngectomy
> Other oral-pharyngeal-esophageal surgical alterations
> Trauma to oral or pharyngeal mucosa (burns, accidents)

*Mechanical Obstruction*

> Head and neck tumors
> Esophageal tumor

*Muscular Dysfunctions*

> Achalasia
> Esophageal reflux
> Dermatomyositis

*Functional and Psychological Causes*

> Depression
> Fear of aspiration (patient with tracheostomy)

Sources: From D. A. W. Edwards, The problem of dysphagia, *Practitioner* 216:631, 1976; K. M. Griffin, Swallowing training for dysphagic patients, *Arch. Phys. Med. Rehabil.* 55:467, 1974; K. M. Griffin, J. Stubbert, and K. Breckenridge, Teaching the dysphagic patient to swallow, *RN* 61: Spring, 1974; and E. H. Silverman and I. L. Elfant, Dysphagia: An evaluation and treatment program for the adult, *Am. J. Occup. Ther.* 33:382, 1979.

RIGHT HEMISPHERE DAMAGE

It has long been known that the left hemisphere of the brain houses language function, while other functions are classically associated with the right hemisphere. A review of the literature [22, 23, 33, 54, 59, 60, 61, 87] yields a sizeable number of functions believed to be mediated by the right hemisphere (Table 9-3).

Unilateral right-sided brain injury may disrupt these functions and produce clusters of deviant behaviors. Gardner and Hamby [23] described patients with lesions of the right hemisphere as having largely intact phonology, syntax, and semantics. In spite of this proficiency with language, they noted frequent disruption of linguistic and paralinguistic features, often displayed as literal-mindedness, inappropriate jocularity, confabulatory output, and nonprosodic or flat delivery.

Others have further described deficiencies in certain aspects of linguistic competence. Myers [59] reported that these patients are often unaware of their environment, and insensitive to both the situation and the effect their message has on the listener. These deficits can be interpreted as a breakdown in pragmatic function [3, 54]. For example, this patient may unintentionally insult someone with a caustic remark without being able to recognize and interpret the receiver's reaction. Thus the patient fails to adhere to traditional boundaries of communication. Myers [60] speculated that the underlying deficit is in processing and interpreting more complex external stimuli, and organizing and channeling internal information.

In recent years, the view of language and communication has broadened thanks to the efforts of linguists and neuropsychologists [3, 22]. This has led to an expanded role for the speech-language pathologist as a communication specialist. Interest was aroused in treating patients who were unable to participate fully in an interactive process. Clearly the patient with right hemisphere involvement falls within this domain and requires the intervention of this professional.

EVALUATION

To delineate the specific behaviors produced by a right hemisphere infarct, which may include communication, perception, and affect, a team approach is recommended. Their diagnostic efforts yield a detailed analysis of the patient's problems, many of which are interrelated. For example, someone with a reading deficit may have a left homonymous hemianopia or left-sided neglect identified by the occupational therapist or neurologist, as well as impairment in interpreting the context of material because of problems with abstraction and judgment.

The speech-language pathologist must draw on a variety of clinical tasks to assess the amount of damage as there is not yet a standardized battery available for use with this population. Several facilities have compiled and presented batteries [23, 54] to identify deviant symptoms. The authors recommend that speech-language pathologists within a given department work together to construct a practical battery. Examples of tasks that yield useful diagnostic information include retelling a story, explaining a joke or a metaphor, and drawing a conclusion and making an inference. Some published tests exist that can be incorporated into the battery. For example, the *Proverbs Test* [29] can provide information about the patient's ability to abstract; *the Logico-Grammatical Sentence Comprehension Test* [86] yields information about the patient's ability to handle five different syntactic structures.

TREATMENT

Treatment is a challenge to the speech-language pathologist, as until recently this condition remained unexplored territory. Although its characteristics have been well described, there is a striking paucity of information regarding therapeutic intervention.

The authors have identified two primary objectives for treatment: (1) to normalize communicative interactions, and (2) to develop compensatory strategies to improve areas of deficit. These objectives may be accomplished pragmatically, cognitively, or through environmental manipulation.

To improve the quality of communicative interactions, it is necessary for the patient to become aware of the rules that govern communication. For example, if a patient lacks focus or organization and rambles as a result, it is the responsibility of the team, which includes the family, to inform the patient of this problem and redirect output by appropriate instructions or questions. This initially involves limiting the patient's output, followed by gradually leading the patient to increase the amount of relevant information conveyed. A model for limiting irrelevant verbal output follows:

| Speech-Language Pathologist | Patient |
|---|---|
| Tell me the name of this. Use only one word to identify it. | Book |
| Good, you gave me just one word. Now, tell me in | Read |

one word what you do with it.

That's right. Now put those words into a short sentence.

I read a book every night, but you know it was cold last night, and . . .

(SLP interrupts): Just a minute. Can you repeat my instructions?

Yes. Use those words in a sentence.

That's right. Why don't you try it again? Use the words *book* and *read* in a sentence.

I read my book at night.

Terrific!

Thus several treatment objectives are met, namely, reduction of rambling and verbosity, and increased concentration and direction to task.

Another major focus of treatment involves training to improve reading and writing performance. Ostreicher [61] and Lehner [54] reported positive response to treatment in these areas. Lehner identified the need for improving visual tracking and scanning skills as a prerequisite for a reading program. Ostreicher [61] described ways to modify and control the environment to compensate for the patient's visual-perceptual deficits. As examples, he advocated placement of the material to the patient's non-involved side, use of bold print as stimuli for reading, and a felt-tip pen as a writing implement. Verbal mediation is another compensatory strategy. For example, the patient who ignores print on the left side of the page needs repeatedly to state at the end of each line how to go about locating the next line of print. The hope is that this volitional action will be integrated into a more automatic pattern over time.

Verbal mediation, or "talking through" a situation may prove to be a useful compensatory strategy for other problem areas as well. In a case study, Myers [59] described a patient who was able to trigger visual memories, visual associations, and facial recognition through verbalizing. Further use of intact linguistic skills was displayed when he purposefully analyzed each element of a situation to recognize the gestalt and draw a conclusion.

Counseling the family is an integral part of the treatment program. As they gain an understanding of the deficits, improved ability to cope with the problems will emerge. In order to ensure the patient's safety, the family must provide supervision in the presence of problems such as impaired judgment, visual-perceptual problems, and impulsiveness.

These very issues of safety will influence decisions regarding the patient's ultimate disposition. It has been the authors' experience that those with right hemisphere damage often require long-term supervision either by a dedicated family member or in residential placement. It is our hope that increased skill in intervention techniques, along with research to document treatment effectiveness, will improve the prognosis for this population.

DYSPHAGIA

Dysphagia, a dysfunction of the swallowing process, requires the skilled intervention of the rehabilitation team. It may result from numerous neurogenic, structural, mechanical, and psychological problems (see Table 9-4). The most immediate physical problems include inadequate nutritional intake and pneumonia.

To treat the patient it is important to have an understanding of normal swallowing, or deglutition. In actuality, swallowing is a single, complex, coordinated physiological process controlled by neural regulation [16]. In practice, however, the act is divided into three stages [16, 30, 53, 75]. During stage one, the buccal-pharyngeal stage, the bolus of masticated food or liquid is passed from the mouth to the pharynx by means of muscular activity. In stage two, the pharyngeal stage, the bolus or liquid reflexively passes through the pharynx to the esophagus. During this stage complex muscular activity brings the vocal cords tightly together while respiration is momentarily inhibited [73], thus preventing the bolus or liquid from entering the airway. The third, or esophageal stage, which is totally reflexive, consists of the material passing from the esophagus into the stomach by peristaltic action [30, 53].

At several of the major Boston hospitals, the responsibility for evaluating and treating the dysphagic patient rests with the speech-language pathologist or the occupational therapist. The following summarizes rehabilitation methods appropriate for use with the patient with neuromuscularly based dysphagia.

EVALUATION

The first step is obtaining a comprehensive history. The major items to be addressed include:

1. Current medical status with primary diagnosis and date of onset.
2. Associated and relevent medical problems, such as diabetes.
3. Nutritional history including food, likes, and dislikes.
4. Present method and status of nutritional intake, e.g., oral, nasogastric tube, gastrostomy.

Once this has been completed, direct evaluation procedures begin with a thorough oral peripheral examination to assess those structures directly involved in stage one of normal deglutition. Lips, palate, jaw, and neck are evaluated with regard to range, symmetry, strength, and coordination of movement. Dentition is also an important consideration, as is laryngeal excursion. During the course of this examination, it is essential to determine the status of the normal adult reflexes. Depending on the site of lesion, normal reflexes, for example, gag and cough, may be absent, diminished, or hyperactive. In addition, the presence of abnormal primitive reflexes such as the rooting and bite reflexes should be determined, as these will influence the treatment objectives.

As sensation plays a role in normal swallowing, it is necessary to determine the integrity of the patient's sensory system. Specific areas that are typically evaluated to find the most sensitive area of the mouth are touch, taste, and temperature. Silverman and Elfant provide detailed instructions as to how to test sensation, together with a recording form with schematic diagrams [75].

The final stage of evaluation is to observe the patient's ability to swallow small amounts of different textures of foods [30, 53, 75]. The food should be placed in the area of the mouth that has been shown to be most sensitive to facilitate a swallow. Griffin [30] advises that this final stage should not be carried out unless the patient has a reflexive swallow, while Silverman and Elfant [75] feel that a spontaneous and voluntary cough is a prerequisite. Several authors [5, 75] strongly advise that suction equipment and trained personnel should be on hand in case of aspiration. All of these procedures, as well as directed treatment, are carried out with the patient appropriately positioned in an upright position with the neck slightly flexed [30, 75] to minimize the risk of aspiration.

The data obtained during evaluation provide the basis for a treatment plan designed to meet the patient's needs. Candidacy must take into account level of alertness, motivation, intellectual functioning, language status, and praxis.

TREATMENT

To carry out effective treatment, the patient should be seated as described, in a nondistracting environment. The authors maintain that treatment should consist of multiple sessions per day. From the inception of the program, the role of each team member should be clearly defined. Often it is the speech-language pathologist and occupational therapist, working singly or jointly, who carry out the early stages of training, with family and nursing staff becoming involved in later stages. The dietitican is involved throughout with selection of foods to maintain nutritional balance. The patient's active participation is dependent on myriad medical and physical factors.

Griffin [31] outlined a five-step training program that consists of the following: (1) exercises to increase strength, coordination and range of movement of the oral peripheral musculature, and assistance for laryngeal excursion; (2) instructions in the basic principles of swallowing; (3) teaching the swallow; (4) the transfer program; and (5) special considerations. Early in the program, together with strengthening exercises, it may be necessary to inhibit any primitive reflexes. Silverman and Elfant [75] and Farber [20] describe specific techniques for this.

In a swallowing program, the level of entry into this program will differ for each patient; some may not need to proceed through all five stages. When training the swallow initially, however, clear instructions and demonstrations are to be prvoided. Training in accomplishing saliva swallowing [30] may precede intake of food substances. The process of initiating a swallow must be brought under volitional control. When the patient is ready to progress to foods, texture and quantity are primary considerations. Often, a consistency such as gelatin is the first to be introduced. Food should be presented in as attractive a manner as possible to stimulate salivation. As soon as the patient is able to tolerate small amounts of a substance, the quantity should be gradually increased, and variety should be introduced in systematic sequence [6, 30, 75]. Clear thin liquids are generally most difficult to tolerate. Some foods such as milk products are contraindicated, as they result in thickened oral secretions.

The transfer program begins when the patient is able to swallow adequately with minimal choking [30]. It is at this time that nursing and family become most involved in carryover to meals. Careful training including observation, however, is mandatory before the clinician relinquishes primary responsibility to other team members.

## Team Approach and Counseling

To achieve a cohesive rehabilitation program, each trained member of the team communicates information related to the patient's treatment to all other involved professionals. Methods of exchange vary from one facility to another, but may include any number of the following: patient care rounds, inservice lectures, written progress notes, direct observation, demonstration, and impromptu discussion. This shared knowledge fosters consistent expectations regarding the patient's level of performance, and reinforces established treatment goals.

Throughout the course of rehabilitation, the team's interactions with the patient and family focus around two major areas: (1) education and counseling, including the nature of the neurological disorder with its many behavioral manifestations, specific strengths and deficits, and understanding of treatment goals and techniques; and (2) facilitation of communication. Counseling may be carried out individually by each caregiver, or as a group in family-team conferences. These are best scheduled at critical points during the patient's hospitalization. Often the first session occurs to summarize the results of the team's diagnostic efforts and to set forth the short- and long-range treatment goals. This is a time for team members to encourage and support the family as they learn to withhold their assistance from the patient to permit realization of greater independence. Over the course of treatment additional conferences are scheduled as needed. A final meeting prior to discharge is desirable to aid and plan for the transition from the hospital to home or to another facility.

It has been said that aphasia is a family illness [55]. This concept holds true for the other neurological disorders as well. Therefore throughout the course of rehabilitation, the family and patient must be assisted as they deal with numerous problems and feelings. It has been estimated that for families of aphasic patients, the adjustment process takes anywhere from three to five years [63], which has direct implications regarding long-term involvement.

The family is not merely a recipient of information and support, but may serve as historians for the patient. The social and occupational history obtained during an interview with members yields valuable information that guides the rehabilitation team as it develops relevant goals. The patient must become an active participant for the program to be successful; with the family acting as an important link in the carryover of treatment goals to a variety of real life situations. In summary, the integrated efforts of the entire team are geared toward one overriding goal—maximal self-sufficiency.

# References

1. American Speech and Hearing Association. *PSB Accreditation Manual: Standards and Procedures for Accreditation of Professional Service Programs in Speech-Language Pathology and Audiology.* Rockville; Md.: American Speech-Language-Hearing Association, 1979.
2. Basso, A., Capitini, E., and Vignolo, L. A. Influence of rehabilitation language skills in aphasic patients: A controlled study. *Arch. Neurol.* 36:190, 1979.
3. Bates, E. Pragmatics and Sociolinguistics in Child Language. In D. Morehead and A. Morehead (Eds.). *Directory in Normal and Deficient Child Language.* University Park; Md.: University Park, 1976.
4. Borkowski, J. G., Benton, A. L., and Spreen, O. Word fluency and brain damage. *Neuropsychologia* 5:135, 1967.
5. Brookshire, R. H. Auditory Comprehension and Aphasia. In D. F. Johns (Ed.). *Clinical Management of Neurogenic Communicative Disorders.* Boston: Little, Brown, 1978.
6. Buckley, J. Dysphagia. Presented to the New England Medical Center's Communication Disorders Seminar's Series, Boston, May, 1979.
7. Chadderdon, L. (Ed.). *Communication Outlook.* East Lansing, Mich.: 1978–80.
8. Dabul, B. *Apraxia Battery for Adults.* Tigard: C.C. Publications, 1979.
9. Darley, F. L. Apraxia of speech: Description, diagnosis, and treatment. Presented to the American Speech and Hearing Association, New York, 1970.
10. Darley, F. L. Treatment of acquired aphasia. In W. J. Friedlander (Ed.). *Advances in Neurology* Vol. 7. New York: Raven, 1975.
11. Darley, F. L., Aronson, A. E., and Brown, J. R. Differential diagnostic patterns of dysarthria. *J. Speech Hear. Res.* 12:246, 1969.
12. Darley, F. L., Aronson, A. E., and Brown, J. R. *Motor Speech Disorders.* Philadelphia: Saunders, 1975.
13. Deal, J. L., and Florance, C. L. Modification of the eight-step continuum for treatment of apraxia of speech in adults. *J. Speech Hear. Disord.* 43:89, 1978.
14. Deal, J. L., and Resler, C. Diagnosis and treatment of apraxia of speech in adults. Presented to the American Speech and Hearing Association, Washington, D.C., 1975.
15. DeRenzi, E., Pieczuro, A., and Vignolo, L. A. Oral apraxia and aphasia. *Cortex* 2:50, 1966.
16. Donner, M. W. Swallowing mechanism and neuromuscular disorders. *Semin. Roentgenol.* 9:273, 1974.
17. Edwards, D. A. W. The problem of dysphagia. *Practitioner* 216:631, 1976.
18. Eisenson, J. *Examining for Aphasia.* New York: Psychological Corp., 1954.
19. Fairbanks, G. *Voice and Articulation Drillbook.* New York: Harper and Row, 1960.
20. Farber, S. *Sensorimotor Evaluation and Treatment Procedures for Allied Health Personnel* (2nd ed.). Indianapolis: Indiana University, 1974.
21. Fisher, H. *Improving Voice and Articulation.* Boston: Houghton Mifflin, 1966.
22. Gardner, H. *The Shattered Mind: The Person After Brain Damage.* New York: Knopf, 1975.
23. Gardner, H., and Hamby, S. The role of the right hemisphere in the organization of linguistic materials. Presented at the International Neuropsychology Symposium, Dubrovnik, Yugoslavia, 1979.
24. Gardner, H., et al. Comprehension and appreciation of humorous material following brain damage. *Brain* 98:399, 1975.
25. Geschwind, N. Foreword. In A. Kertesz. *Aphasia and Associated Disorders: Taxonomy, Localization, and Recovery.* New York: Grune and Stratton, 1979.
26. Gleason, J. B., et al. Retrieval of syntax in Broca's aphasia. *Brain Lang.* 24:451, 1975.
27. Goodglass, H., and Kaplan, E. *The Assessment of Aphasia and Related Disorders.* Philadelphia: Lea and Febiger, 1972.
28. Goodglass, H., et al. Some linguistic structures in the speech of a Broca's aphasia. *Cortex* 8:191, 1972.

29. Gorham, D. R. *Proverbs Test.* Missoula; Mont.: Psychological Test Specialists, 1956.
30. Griffin, K. M. Swallowing training for dysphagic patients. *Arch. Phys. Med. Rehabil.* 55:467, 1974.
31. Griffin, K. M., Stubbert, J., and Breckenridge, K. Teaching the dysphagic patient to swallow. *RN* 61: Sept. 1974.
32. Hagen, C. Communication abilities in hemiplegia: Effect of speech therapy. *Arch. Phys. Med. Rehabil.* 54:454, 1973.
33. Heilman, K. M., Scholes, R., and Watson, R. T. Auditory affective agnosia (disturbed comprehension of affective speech). *J. Neurol. Neurosurg. Psychiatry* 38:62, 1975.
34. Helm, N. Retaining syntax in nonfluent aphasics. Presented to the American Speech and Hearing Association, Boston, 1977.
35. Helm, N. Management of palilalia with a pacing board. *J. Speech Hear. Disord.* 44:350, 1979.
36. Helm, N. and Benson, F. Visual action therapy. Presented to the Boston Area Clinical Aphasiology Group, Boston, 1978.
37. Hill, B. *Verbal Dyspraxia in Clinical Practice.* Carlton, Australia: Pitman, 1978.
38. Holland, A. L. Aphasics as communicators: A model and its implication. Presented to the American Speech and Hearing Association, Washington, D.C., 1975.
39. Holland, A. L. Some Practical Considerations in Aphasia Rehabilitation. In M. Sullivan and M. S. Kommers (Eds.). *Rationale for Adult Aphasia Therapy.* Lincoln, Nebr.: University of Nebraska Medical Center, 1977.
40. Holland, A. L. Some selected aspects of the relationships between comprehension and production of language in adult language. *Allied Health Behav. Sci.* 1:237, 1977.
41. Holland, A. L. *Communicative Abilities in Daily Living.* Baltimore: University Park, 1980.
42. Johns, D. F., and LaPointe, L. L. Neurogenic Disorders of Output Processing: Apraxia of Speech. In H. Whitaker and H. A. Whitaker (Eds.). *Studies in Neurolinguistics: Perspectives in Neurolinguistics and Psycholinguistics,* Vol. 1. New York: Academic, 1976.
43. Jones, F. Moto-sequential tactile therapy: A thesis alternate. Emerson College, Masters degree thesis, 1975.
44. Kaplan, E., Goodglass, H., and Weintraub, S. *Boston Naming Test* (experimental edition). Boston: VA Hospital, 1976.
45. Keenan, J. S., and Brassell, E. G. *Aphasia Language Performance Scales.* Murfreesboro: Pinnacle, 1975.
46. Kertesz, A. *Aphasia and Associated Disorders: Taxonomy, Localization and Recovery.* New York: Grune and Stratton, 1979.
47. Kertesz, A., and McCabe, P. Recovery patterns and prognosis in aphasia. *Brain* 100:1, 1977.
48. Kertesz, A., and Poole, E. The aphasia quotient: The taxonomic approach to measurement of aphasic disability. *Can. J. Neurol. Sci.* 1:7, 1974.
49. LaPointe, L. L. Base-10 programmed stimulation: Task specification scoring and plotting performance in aphasia therapy. *J. Speech Hear. Disord.* 42:90, 1977.
50. LaPointe, L. L. Aphasia Therapy: Some Principles and Strategies for Treatment. In D. F. Johns (Ed.). *Clinical Management of Neurogenic Communicative Disorders.* Boston: Little, Brown, 1978.
51. LaPointe, L. L., and Horner, J. The functional auditory comprehension task. *FLASHA J.* Spring: 27, 1978.
52. LaPointe, L. L., and Horner, J. *Reading Comprehension Battery for Aphasia.* Tigard: C.C. Publications, 1979.
53. Larsen, G. L. Conservative management for incomplete dysphagia paralytics. *Arch. Phys. Med. Rehabil.* 54:180, 1973.
54. Lehner, L. H. Communication deficits associated with right-cerebral brain damage. Presented to the American Speech-Language-Hearing Association, Atlanta, 1979.
55. Linebaugh, C. W., and Young-Charles, H. Y. The Counseling Needs of the Families of Aphasic Patients. In R. H. Brookshire (Ed.), *Clinical Aphasiology Conference Proceedings. 1979.* Minneapolis: BRK, 1979.
56. Ludlow, C. L. The recovery of syntax in aphasia. Presented to the Academy of Aphasia, Albuquerque, New Mexico, 1973.
57. Marshall, R. C. Word retrieval of aphasic adults. *J. Speech Hear. Disord.* 39:53, 1974.
58. Martin, A. D. Some objections to the term "apraxia of speech." *J. Speech Hear. Disord.* 39:53, 1974.
59. Myers, P. S. Profiles of Communication Deficits in Patients with Right Cerebral Hemisphere Damage: Implications for Diagnosis and Treatment. In R. H. Brookshire (Ed.). *Clinical Aphasiology Conference Proceedings 1978.* Minneapolis: BRK, 1978.
60. Myers, P. S. Analysis of Right Hemisphere Communication Deficits: Implications for Speech Pathology. In R. H. Brookshire (Ed.), *Clinical Aphasiology Conference Proceedings 1979.* Minneapolis: BRK, 1979.
61. Ostreicher, H. J. Evaluation and treatment of

right CVA patients. Presented to the American Speech-Language-Hearing Association, Atlanta, 1979.

62. Porch, B. E. *Porch Index of Communicative Abilities*. Palo Alto: Consulting Psychologists, 1967.

63. Riedel, K. Treatment of global aphasia. Presented to Boston Clonical Aphasiology Group, Boston, 1978.

64. Rosenbek, J. C. Treatment of apraxia of speech. Prevention, facilitation, and reorganization. Presented to the American Speech and Hearing Association, Houston, 1976.

65. Rosenbek, J. C. Treating Apraxia of Speech. In D. F. Johns (Ed.), *Clinical Management of Communicative Disorders*. Boston: Little, Brown, 1978.

66. Rosenbek, J. C. Treatment of apraxia of speech. Presented to the Massachusetts Speech and Hearing Association, Hyannis, 1978.

67. Rosenbek, J. C., and LaPointe, L. L. The Dysarthrias: Description, Diagnosis, and Treatment. In D. F. Johns (Ed.). *Clinical Management of Communicative Disorders*. Boston: Little, Brown, 1978.

68. Rosenbek, J. C., et al. Advances in the Treatment of Apraxia of Speech. In R. T. Wertz and M. J. Collins (Eds.), *Clinical Aphasiology: Conference Proceedings*. Minneapolis: BRK, 1973.

69. Rosenbek, J. C., et al. A treatment for apraxia of speech in adults. *J. Speech Hear. Disord.* 38:462, 1973.

70. Sarno, M. T. The functional communication profile. *Rehabilitation Monograph 42, Institute of Rehabilitation Medicine*. New York: New York University Medical Center, 1969.

71. Schuell, H. *The Minnesota Test for Differential Diagnosis of Aphasia*. Minneapolis: University of Minnesota Press, 1965.

72. Schuell, H., Jenkins, J., and Jiménez-Pabón, E. *Aphasia in Adults*. New York: Harper and Row, 1964.

73. Schultz, A., et al. Dysphagia associated with cricopharyngeal dysfunction. *Arch. Phys. Med. Rehabil.* 60:381, 1979.

74. Shewan, C. M. *Auditory Comprehension Test for Sentences*. Tigard: C.C. Publications, 1979.

75. Silverman, E. H., and Elfant, I. L. Dysphagia: An evaluation and treatment program for the adult. *Am. J. Occup. Ther.* 33:382, 1979.

76. Skelly, M., et al. Amerind sign: Gestural communication for the speechless. Presented to the American Speech and Hearing Association, San Francisco, 1972.

77. Skelly, M., et al. American Indian sign (Amerind) as a facilitator of verbalization for the oral verbal apraxic. *J. Speech Hear. Disord.* 39:445, 1974.

78. Sparks, R., Helm, N., and Albert, M. Aphasia rehabilitation resulting from melodic intonation therapy. *Cortex* 10:303, 1974.

79. Spreen, O., and Benton, A. L. *Neurosensory Center Comprehensive Examination for Aphasia*. Victoria, Canada: University of Victoria, 1969.

80. Taylor, M. Language therapy. In H. G. Burr (Ed.). *The Aphasic Adult Evaluation and Rehabilitation: Proceedings of a Short Course*. Charlottesville, N.C.: Wayside, 1964.

81. Vanderheim, G. (Ed.). *Nonvocal Communication Resource Book*. Baltimore: University Park, 1978.

82. Van Riper, C. *Speech Correction: Principles and Methods*. Englewood Cliffs, N.J.: Prentice-Hall, 1963.

83. Wepman, J. H. *Recovery from Aphasia*. New York: Ronald, 1951.

84. Wertz, R. T. Neurologies of Speech and Language: An Introduction to Patient Management. In D. F. Johns (Ed.). *Clinical Management of Communicative Disorders*. Boston: Little, Brown, 1978.

85. Whitney, J. Developing aphasics' use of compensatory strategies. Presented to the American Speech and Hearing Association, Washington, D.C., 1975.

86. Wiig, E. H. and Semel, E. M. Development of comprehension of logico-grammatical sentences by grade school children. *Percept. Mot. Skills*. 38:171, 1974.

87. Winner, E. and Gardner, H. The comprehension of metaphor in brain-damaged patients. *Brain* 100:717, 1977.

88. Yorkston, K. M. and Beukelman, D. R. An analysis of connected speech samples of aphasic and normal speakers. *J. Speech Hear. Disord.* 45:27, 1980.

# 10 BRAIN TRAUMA

*Marilyn Lee Holzer, Denise A. Stiassny,*
*Frances Senner-Hurley, and*
*Nancy G. Lefkowitz*

This chapter offers a multidisciplinary team program for the patient with traumatic brain injury focusing on the cognitive aspects of recovery and rehabilitation. Residual cognitive deficits have been identified as being far more devastating than residual motor problems as the result of head trauma.

Members of the rehabilitation team include a neurologist, social worker, physical therapist, occupational therapist, speech-language pathologist, and nurse. Treatment planning and sharing of information with the family are cooperative efforts. Each member should know the medical, psychological, and social problems of the patient, and the prognosis and aim of rehabilitation.

## Terminology

There are approximately 7½ million people yearly in the United States who incur head injuries [3]. The variable outcome ranges from complete recovery to those who sustain neurological deficits involving both physical and cognitive problems. Traumatic head injury is defined as a blow to the head resulting in damage to the brain. The damage is usually diffuse and widespread, and can be with or without alteration of the individual's consciousness.

More than one-half of all head trauma injuries are caused by highway motor vehicle, especially motorcycle, accidents [3]. Other causes include violent assault, gunshot wounds, drug abuse, and sporting and industrial accidents. Epidemiological studies from the University of Virginia Department of Neurosurgery have provided a sociological profile of populations at high risk for traumatic injuries. These include the adolescent group whose injuries are primarily connected with highway motor accidents, and the geriatric group who sustain most injuries in falls. The man to woman ratio is 3:1, with men suffering not only more frequent but also more serious injuries.

It is not uncommon to find that patients have a history of drug or alcohol abuse, or a past medical history of central nervous system damage. Research has shown that the highest percentage of incidents occur during the months of August and September, and on weekends in the following order of days: Saturday, Sunday, and Friday [32].

Head injuries are caused by acceleration or deceleration or rotation forces acting on the skull that set the brain in motion. In acceleration, the brain moves at a slower rate compared to the object (external to the skull or the skull itself) that strikes the head. The impact site (coup) is the point of highest pressure. However, because of movement of the brain within the skull there is damage to the opposite side of the brain (contrecoup). The skull decelerates when the moving head strikes a solid object. During rotation, the head moves by the combination of hyperextension, hyperflexion, and lateral flexion. On impact, vascular tissues are torn.

As a consequence of these forces the brain is injured through a variety of mechanisms, for example, penetration by foreign matter that causes destruction of tissue along a specific path; compression of tissue by depressed bone fragments; tension that tears the tissues; or shearing. Types of injuries include skull fracture, concussion, contusion, and laceration. Injury caused by an object moving at high velocity can result in a depressed fracture or perforation of the skull. A linear or comminuted fracture that does not disrupt the dura can be produced by an object traveling at low velocity, and is referred to as closed head injury. Concussion can be defined as a transient and reversible loss of consciousness. It results from forces acting on the brain stem causing damage to the reticular activating system. A contusion or laceration signifies visible bruising of the brain to different degrees, plus the presence of blood. Ruptured capillaries and vessels result in hemorrhage, hematoma, and other vascular sequelae. Systemic effects of head trauma can include edema, hypertension, and hypoxia.

## Clinical Aspects

Loss of consciousness, the most common characteristic of severe head injury, generally consists of 5 recovery phases. The depth and duration of each phase varies among individual cases; it cannot be assumed that all patients will progress through each phase.

The first phase, coma, is marked by paralysis of all cerebral functioning. Characteristics include the absence of verbal and motor response and spontaneous eye opening. Also exhibited are reflexive eye movements, hyperactive deep tendon reflexes, and decorticate or decerebrate posturing. Victims may have a lucid period before deteriorating into coma. Recovery is dependent on the severity of trauma.

In the second, semicomatose, phase, the patient begins to withdraw to painful stimuli. In the third phase, the stuporous patient is restless, mute, and responds to simple commands. Responses are disoriented in the fourth, confused, phase. Finally, in the conscious phase, there is recovery of orientation, retention, and insight.

Not all head injuries are severe enough to cause loss of consciousness and long hospitalization. Minor traumas are actually more common than severe ones, and usually require less than 48 hours in hospital. Cerebral injury is mild and generally resolves; however, three-month follow-up studies have shown that some patients with minor head injury become moderately to severely disabled [32]. The patient complains of headaches, vertigo, irritability, insomnia, and concentration or memory problems. There are changes in temperament and emotional disposition that can lead to unemployment and other changes in social status. Patients often fear insanity or an impaired work capacity. This cluster of symptoms has been termed the posttraumatic syndrome, and is more commonly found following minor head injuries than severe ones. It has been difficult to separate the etiology of this syndrome from organic or structural changes, but superimposed psychogenic factors may have to be considered. Studies have shown that this syndrome has significance in patients whose premorbid personality showed behavioral disorders or psychological insufficiency. Early supportive therapy and activation in treatment programs is vital to patients with this disabling condition [19].

PROGNOSTIC FACTORS IN RECOVERY OF FUNCTION

Recovery after severe brain injury may continue over a long period. Generally, the most important stage occurs within the first six months after trauma. Improvements continue throughout the first two years, or longer in younger patients.

It is known that destroyed brain cells cannot regenerate, replace, or repair themselves; thus the potential for successful recovery of func-

TABLE 10-1. *Glasgow Coma Scale*

| Response | Status | Score |
|---|---|---|
| Eye opening (A score) | Spontaneous | 4 |
| | Speech | 3 |
| | Pain | 2 |
| | None | 1 |
| Motor activity (B score) | Obeys | 6 |
| | Localized | 5 |
| | Withdrawal | 4 |
| | Abnormal flexion | 3 |
| | Extension | 2 |
| | None | 1 |
| Verbal activity (C score) | Oriented | 5 |
| | Confused conversation | 4 |
| | Inappropriate | 3 |
| | Incomprehensible | 2 |
| | None | 1 |
| | Responsiveness or coma total 3–15 points | |

Source: From Rehabilitation of the Traumatic Head Injured Adult—Comprehensive Physical Management. Los Angeles: Professional Staff Association of Rancho Los Amigos Hospital, Inc., 1979.

tion and rehabilitation is based on the premise of tissue plasticity, or other parts of the brain taking over the function of the injured parts. Theoretical concepts include substitution of pathways, equipotentiality, regeneration, and collateral sprouting [3]. Brain plasticity is present more in children than adults, whose plasticity has been replaced by increasing functional specialization with age, experience, and language development. Details about such theories do not fall within the scope of this chapter, and readers are referred to neurophysiological and neuropsychological literature.

There are factors in the acute phase that both indicate recovery potential and reflect the severity of brain dysfunction. Clinicians are in agreement about the two most powerful and reliable predictors that change considerably during the first few days after injury. The first is coma, with a direct relationship between its depth and duration and recovery. Generally, the longer the coma, the less satisfactory the recovery. The second is pupil and eye signs. Other signs indicative of a poor prognosis include nonreactive pupils, absence of eye movements and abnormal motor responses. There are four additional factors that are not as significant as these, yet contribute to formulating a prognosis: age, the presence of intracranial hematoma, autonomic central nervous system abnormalities, and extracranial factors such as a prior history of alcohol consumption, or metabolic disorders such as diabetes. The older the individual, the less likely the chance for favorable recovery. Children are known to carry a more promising prognosis than adults. Posttraumatic amnesia has been used as a means to assess the quality of regained cognitive abilities. As it can only be used in retrospect, however, it is not a good early indicator of recovery of function [31].

GLASGOW COMA SCALE
Brian Jennett of the Institute of Neurological Sciences in Glasgow, Scotland, has devised a comprehensive scale that quantifies the severity of central nervous system dysfunction and facilitates arriving at prognosis. The Glasgow Coma Scale (Table 10-1) offers an objective

TABLE 10-2. *Glasgow Outcome Scale*

| Outcome | Characteristics |
|---|---|
| Good recovery | Reintegration into society with ability to pursue previous leisure and occupational goals; may have mild neurological residuals as dysphasia, cranial nerve palsy, slight hemiparesis |
| Moderate disability | Ability to be independent in own care (ADL), and in home and community; vocational goals limited to lower level of responsibility; residual neurological changes may include cognitive changes, dysphasia, dysarthria, hemiplegia, ataxia, or frequent epilepsy |
| Severe disability | Dependent because of cognitive or physical problems; absence of functional language (aphasia or dysarthria) |
| Persistent vegetative state | Without awareness and speech, unresponsive to all external stimuli; may have eye opening, sucking, yawning, or localized responses |

Source: Rehabilitation of the Traumatic Head Injured Adult—Comprehensive Physical Management. Los Angeles: Professional Staff Association of Rancho Los Amigos Hospital, Inc., 1979.

assessment of coma status with results that are consistently reproducible. For these reasons the scale is used by many clinicians (emergency medical technicians, doctors, nurses, and therapists), as it provides an ongoing status report on the patient's condition.

Jennett's scale is based on clinical components that define the coma profile: eye opening, motor response, and verbal response. A numerical value that ranges from no response to normal response is assigned to each. In short, the quality of responsiveness in a patient with head injury can be derived by summing the responses. The final sum ranges from three (least responsive) to 15 (normal). Quantitatively, Jennett defines coma as a score of eight or below. Patients whose profiles fall within a numerical value of less than four usually die. Candidates for rehabilitation have scores within the four to 15 range [32].

The Glasgow Outcome Scale (Table 10-2) indicates that survivors of head trauma can be classified according to their pattern of neurological recovery. Six months postinjury, 90 percent of patients have reached the highest outcome category. Severe disability is the most common outcome at one month postinjury. The best outcome at six months for patients still in the vegetative state at one month, is severe disability. None of these patients improve to the moderate or good neurological recovery category [17].

MEDICAL AND NURSING MANAGEMENT
The initial focus is providing life-sustaining care. Once the patient is medically stable, subsequent treatment is directed toward complications such as seizures, infection, and intracranial hypertension.

Nursing care consists of monitoring vital signs, level of consciousness, and seizure activity, and administering medications. In addition, postsurgical care may also be involved, as is care of the tracheostomy, catheter, feeding tube, cast, and skin [13].

## Cognitive Function and Dysfunction
Cognitive and behavioral changes following traumatic head injury are far more devastating than are residual motor problems. Planning for the individual's social adjustment and reintegration into the community must take into account physical recovery, social-emotional status, and intellectual functioning. The nature and severity of trauma, diffuse or focal, will determine the cognitive functional deficits. There may be severe impairment of some

skills, while others may be spared to varying degrees.

Careful observation provides insight into the patient's approach to task demands and precise areas of limitations. Equipped with this information, the clinician structures therapeutic sessions using tasks that elicit behaviors within the patient's grasp, specifically capitalizing on what the patient can do rather than focusing on deficits. They must bear in mind aspects of the patient's premorbid cognitive status such as level of education, intellectual stability, evidence of learning disability, age, and employment. It would be highly inappropriate to expect the patient to exceed pretrauma levels of intellectual functioning.

The cognitive theory of development proposed by Piaget [28] has been used to interpret behavioral deficits. Its principle is to present the patient with sequential developmental tasks. In this regard, a common assumption is that recovery of cognitive function parallels cognitive ontogeny. Gardner [8] says: "Yet, it is questionable whether the process of development will follow a reversal, in the case of brain damage. Rather, degeneration of behavior is viewed as the transformation of some facets, while others remain resistant to the impact of injury." Whether recovery of function follows the developmental sequence continues to require careful research.

COGNITIVE PROCESSES

Lezak [22] has organized intellectual functioning into 4 classes to describe distinct behavioral characteristics. Class I, receptive functions, involves two interdependent processes: (1) sensation, or the power to appreciate stimuli through the senses and proprioceptively; and (2) perception, the end product of synthesizing sensations into information. These functions form the groundwork for acquiring, processing, classifying, and integrating information.

Expressive functions, Class II, refer to constellations of behaviors such as speaking, writing, drawing, and producing facial and physical gestures. Class III, memory and learning, involves retention and storage of information. Although current research disputes the dual system that represents short- and long-term memory, for clinical purposes three types of memory are tested: immediate, short-, and long-term. Cermak [6] says, "Traditionally, these divisions are based on the amount of time allowed to elapse between the reception of information and the time of its retrieval." Immediate memory is thought to represent information the individual can immediately repeat, for example, saying a series of digits immediately after hearing them. Short-term memory represents the recognition or recall of information several seconds or minutes following presentation, without the benefit of rehearsal [39]. Long-term memory represents a permanent or persistent storage of information over time.

Lezak's Class IV is cognition, or thinking, which she defines as any mental operation that implicitly or explicitly relates two or more bits of information. Under the general heading of cognition she includes the following functions: computations, reasoning, judgment, concept formation, abstracting and generalizing, and organizing and planning.

In addition to the classes of intellectual functions, Lezak describes mental activity variables that contribute to the efficiency of cognitive processes, such as attention (ability to focus on a particular stimulus), concentration (heightened state of focused attention), and conceptual tracking (maintenance of a train of thought).

DYSFUNCTION

Goodglass and Kaplan [12] view patients' cognitive abilities following brain damage as "the complex interaction between the premorbid anatomical organization of cerebral functions and the site(s) of damage to the brain and is reflected by the strategies which the patient brings to bear on the tasks he performs."

The degradation of cognitive processes is seen in the behavior of brain-injured patients in a number of ways. A common characteristic is impaired ability to deal with relationships among objects or concepts and their properties. This deficiency can be seen in a patient who offers literal interpretations of proverbs [11]. Typically, thinking may demonstrate a concrete quality as a result of the loss of higher intellectual functions of abstraction, reasoning, and analysis [22]. Behaviorally, the patient displays decreased responsiveness and attention, and may be extraordinarily slow in orienting to new mental sets or in shifting from one set to another. There is often difficulty producing spontaneous ideas, yet if external structure is given, the patient may respond appropriately. Some may also show signs of perseveration, that is, inability to discontinue a response after it is no longer appropriate to the demands of the task. Recognition of these deficits provides the therapist with insight as to why the patient will have difficulty orienting to activities that demand serial progression. Associated with this is possible difficulty in seeking a new solution when a previous approach has proved inadequate [12]. The patient's approach to novel and even familiar tasks may be fragmented and disorganized.

The phenomenon of stimulus-boundedness is seen when the patient's attention is pulled to a salient feature of a task or situation. Because of this pull the patient fails to grasp the demands of the entire task, and consequently, is unable to plan ahead, initiate activity, or adapt to the demands of changing circumstances [24].

Control of behaviors is a function of the integrative activity of an intact nervous system. Loss of control is manifest in many aspects of behavior. The patient may show poor impulse control, and thus fail to inhibit socially inappropriate activity. Other alterations include tendencies for heightened excitability, aggressiveness, carelessness, and neglect of personal hygiene [22].

Additional change seen as a consequence of brain damage, involves disruption in learning and memory. The ability to learn and remember new information may be deficient as a result of impaired attention, perception, or encoding capacities [12]. Clinically, inability to learn new information and skills subsequent to brain trauma is termed *anterograde amnesia*. *Retrograde amnesia* refers to difficulty remembering events that occurred prior to trauma. During the course of recovery, the clinical phenomenon of *shrinking retrograde amnesia* may be observed. This refers to the individual's capacity for first remembering events most remote in time, and then those closer to the time of injury [12].

LEVELS OF COGNITIVE FUNCTION
The Adult Head Trauma Service at Rancho Los Amigos Hospital has categorized behavior into eight progressive levels of cognitive function that correspond to the classical neurological recovery following coma. Figure 10-1 presents a measure of behavior, which, per level, emphasizes the salient commonly exhibited behavior. It also reflects the rate and quality of recovery and provides the team with a common tool for assessing and documenting a patient's behavior.

SPEECH AND LANGUAGE PROBLEMS
The patient with head injury may exhibit an array of speech, language, and cognitive disorders, depending on the site and extent of damage. Initially, the patient may be mute for time periods ranging from a few days to several months. Following this a number of conditions may arise, some of which may be difficult to distinguish from each other.

One of the more commonly occurring communication problems is *language of confusion*, which has several characteristics: reduced recognition of, understanding of, and responsiveness to the environment; faulty memory; impaired reasoning; unclear thought processes; disorientation in time and space; irrelevant responses; and inappropriate maladaptive behaviors [15, 38]. Most often, confused language is associated with diffuse bilateral lesions of sudden onset. When confusion is present following a unilateral lesion, it tends to be-

RANCHO LOS AMIGOS HOSPITAL
DIVISION OF NEUROLOGICAL SCIENCES
LEVEL OF COGNITIVE FUNCTIONING RECORD

Patient: _____ Date of Birth: _____ RLAH# _____ Unit _____

Date of Onset: _____ Diagnosis: _____

Examiner and Dates Tested

VIII. Purposeful-Appropriate

    a. Alert, oriented; intact recall for past and recent events

    b. Demonstrates carryover for new learning; functions independently within physical capabilities once new tasks are learned

    c. Able to formulate realistic goals for own future; may be candidate for vocational rehabilitation

    d. Able to apply adequate judgment to daily living and community situations relative to premorbid ability level

VII. Automatic-Appropriate

    a. Appropriate and oriented within hospital-home settings

    b. Able to go through daily routine with minimal to absent confusion; depth of recall may be shallow

    c. Demonstrates carryover for new learning although at a decreased rate; requires at least minimal supervision for learning and for purposes of safety

    d. Demonstrates superficial insight into disabilities; decreased judgment and abstract reasoning; lacks realistic planning for own future; prevocational evaluation and counseling may be indicated

VI. Confused-Appropriate

    a. Inconsistently oriented to time and place; recent memory impaired with decreased detail and depth of recall

    b. Follows simple directions consistently; responses are appropriate but may be incorrect if requiring recent memory

    c. Supervised for new learning with little or no carryover, but shows carryover for previously learned skills

    d. Actively participates in therapy programs and demonstrates some purposeful behavior, but remains dependent on external structure

FIGURE 10-1. *Level of cognitive functioning record. Source: Rancho Los Amigos Hospital, Downey, Calif. (With permission.)*

V. Confused-Inappropriate-Nonagitated

    a. Alert, demonstrates gross attention but difficulty maintaining selective attention

    b. Severe impairment of memory functions

    c. Responses fragmented and frequently inappropriate to the situation, reflecting confusion and lack of goal-direction

    d. Agitation in response to external stimuli

    e. Wanders from treatment areas

    f. Absent carryover for purposes of learning; assisted to maximally supervised in activities

IV. Confused-Agitated

    a. Alert and in heightened state of activity but demonstrates severely decreased ability to process environment, responds primarily to own internal agitation

    b. Performs motor activities but behavior essentially nonpurposeful relative to environment

    c. Aggressive or bizarre behaviors

III. Localized Response

    a. Withdrawal or vocalization to painful stimuli

    b. Turns toward or away from auditory stimuli

    c. Blinks when strong light crosses visual field

    d. Follows moving object passed within visual field

    e. Responds to discomfort by pulling tubes or restraints

    f. Responds inconsistently to simple commands

II. Generalized Response

    a. Demonstrates generalized reflex response to painful stimuli

    b. Responds to repeated auditory stimuli with increased or decreased activity

    c. Responds to external stimuli with physiological changes

I. No Response

    a. Complete absence of observable change in behavior when presented visual, auditory, or painful stimuli

FIGURE 10-1. *(Continued).*

TABLE 10-3. *Sampling of Tools for Evaluating Language of Confusion*

| Area | Name of Test | Author(s) and Date |
|------|--------------|--------------------|
| Memory | Wechsler memory scale | Wechsler (1972) |
| Orientation | Orientation and general information items | Wertz (1978) |
| | Orientation subtest from the *Detroit Tests of Learning Aptitude* | Baker and Leland (1967) |
| Reasoning | *Proverbs Test* | Gorham (1956) |
| | Verbal absurdities, likenesses and differences, and social adjustment subtests from the *Detroit Tests of Learning Aptitude* | Baker and Leland (1967) |
| Relevance | Cookie theft analysis | Myers (1979) |
| | Word fluency measure | Borkowski, Benton, and Spreen (1967) |

transient [38]. The majority of language impairments fall within the areas of confused language or cognitive disorganization [14].

As a result of head injury, any of the neurogenic speech-language disorders can occur, either in isolation or in combination. Dysarthria, with or without accompanying dysphagia, may occur as a result of involvement of the upper or lower motor neuron systems, the cerebellum, the extrapyramidal system, or more than one of these areas [38]. Aphasia may be seen if language centers in the dominant, usually left, hemisphere are involved. With closed head trauma, two studies [18, 21] have shown that the most frequent type of aphasia is anomic, followed by Wernicke's [18]. Apraxia of speech, associated with unilateral left hemisphere damage, is an infrequent consequence of traumatic head injury. Damage to the right hemisphere can produce myriad communicative, perceptual, cognitive, and behavioral symptoms. (All of the neurogenic disorders are discussed in greater detail in Chapter 9.)

Often the head-injured patient sustains bilateral frontal damage. When this occurs, affective behavioral disturbances are likely to be present and to interfere with communication. Abulia, a lack of initiative or spontaneity in desired or automatic motor tasks, is one of the possible outcomes of bifrontal injury. Personality alterations may occur; possible manifestations are euphoria or irritability, which do not necessarily represent the patient's mood [16].

EVALUATION

Prior to testing, it is important to obtain neurological data regarding site(s) of lesion to assist in determining which diagnostic tools should be used to evaluate the nature and extent of the patient's communication disturbance(s). If the neurological workup documents brain stem involvement, a dysarthria evaluation is indicated. (See Chapter 9.) If the patient has cortical involvement, differentiation of central language disturbances or cognitive and intellectual deficits is necessary. Therefore testing must include subtests or stimuli from aphasia, memory, orientation, and cognitive areas (Table 10-3). Intelligence testing must be executed by an appropriately trained professional. These diagnostic tools are not applicable only to head-injured patients, but represent a compilation of available materials.

The head-injured patient initially may show fluctuations in performance. As resolution and evolution of symptoms occur, differential diagnosis may not always be clear-cut. Close observation with accurate recording of behaviors, as-

TABLE 10-4. *Overview of Multidisciplinary Approach to Cognitive Rehabilitation of the Traumatic Brain-Injured*

| Approach | Physician | Nursing | Occupational Therapy | Physical Therapy | Speech-Language Pathology | Social Service |
|---|---|---|---|---|---|---|
| Sensory stimulation | Program coordinator; Life sustaining and preventive care; Family consultation | Life-sustaining and preventive care; Reality orientation; Sensory stimulation; Family support | Sensory stimulation; PROM exercises; Reality orientation; Splinting; Normalizing tone; Prefunctional ADL training; Feeding program; Family support | Sensory stimulation; PROM exercises; Reality orientation; LE casts/splints; Chest PT; Standing and mat activities; Feeding program; Family support; | Sensory stimulation; Reality orientation; Feeding program; Family support; | Family consultation; Clarify immediate social situation; Review family resources; |
| Structure | Program coordinator; Special medical services (orthopedist neurologist psychiatrist); Family consultation | Structure unit; Contingency training; Self-care activity; Nutrition; Weekend carryover of weekly gains; Family support | Routine repetition of feeding program, ADL, perceptual and cognitive activity; UE exercises; Gross motor activities; Family support | Mat program: motor control, strength, coordination and endurance exercises; Transfer training; Preambulation and ambulation training; Order ambulatory devices | Memory training; Orientation to time and place; Organizational skills; Cognitive tasks; Reassurance to patient; Family instruction and support | Consultation with other team members; Review family resources; Family group |
| Community discharge planning | Program coordinator; Special medical services; Family Consultation | Instruction in self-medication; Unit ADL responsibilities; Family support | Refine ADL skills; Maximize UE functional status; Home-making and community skill development; Cognitive and perceptual training; Order adaptive equipment; Home visit; Prevocational referral; Family instruction | Maximize ambulation, strength, and coordination; Home visit; Environmental training; Community skill development; Family instruction | Advanced cognitive tasks; Discussion of injury, fears, goals, plans; Use of communicative aids; Family instruction and support | Liaison with community resources; Establish patient groups; Family support group |

Source: Compiled by Marilyn Lee Holzer OTR, Massachusetts Rehabilitation Hospital, Boston.

well as serial testing, is indicated to sort out the major characteristics and arrive at a clear diagnostic picture.

A key to distinguishing language of confusion from aphasia involves comparison of responses on structured versus open-ended language tasks. Because the patient with confused language may exhibit little or no difficulty with syntax, semantics, and phonology, a traditional aphasia battery may fail to detect deficits. In contrast, during open-ended conversation, characteristics of irrelevance and confabulation surface. In addition, test findings show moderate impairments in arithmetic, reading comprehension, and writing to dictation [15], further substantiating a diagnosis of confused language. This patient would also show significant impairments on cognitive and intelligence tests.

To date, a formal battery with norms established for the head-injured population and sensitive to change over time has unfortunately not been published. Several facilities [14, 25] currently use their own diagnostic protocols. The authors urge professionals working with these patients carefully to construct an assessment tool, and use it consistently to document change over time and obtain information on large numbers of patients. Only then will normative, predictive data become reality.

## Rehabilitation

Within recent years, the division of Neurological Sciences at Rancho Los Amigos Hospital has established a model program for effective rehabilitation of patients with brain trauma. Some of the material contained in this section, presented as guidelines for developing treatment programs, is based on information provided by this hospital.

Planning treatment programs for the multifaceted problems that are the results of brain trauma closely relates to the status of a patient's cognitive capacity. Table 10-4 is an overview of a multidisciplinary approach to rehabilitation. Through team conferences the patient's existing level of cognition is deter-

mined. Using this information, team members adopt a unified treatment approach while simultaneously contributing their own professional expertise for that patient's rehabilitation.

Three treatment approaches correspond to specific behavioral characteristics. The patient who demonstrates decreased responsiveness requires sensory stimulation; the agitated, confused patient who behaves inappropriately requires a structured environment; the patient who is ready for reintegration as a productive member of the community requires discharge planning. The clinician must bear in mind that brain damage is not a static phenomenon, and patients demonstrate a wide range of behavior that does not always fall conveniently into an established conceptual framework.

SENSORY STIMULATION

Systematic presentation of external stimuli is provided to prevent sensory deprivation, heighten attention, enhance the patient's comprehension of commands, and elicit appropriate responses that can ultimately be channeled into activities to help prepare the patient for prefunctional adaptive skills. Stimulation techniques are multisensory and include the following:

Auditory: Fast, loud, irregular rhythms such as bells are recommended; a radio is also suitable. Avoid shouting, as it can elicit the startle reflex.

Visual: Bright warm colors promote a facilitative effect. Colored objects such as mobiles, photographs, or paintings should be placed within the patient's field of vision. Television sets may be turned on periodically throughout the day.

Olfactory: Noxious odors such as dilute ammonia, vinegar, and garlic may be used. Similarly, pleasant scents such as coffee, cinnamon, and perfume can be placed close to the patient's nostrils.

Tactile: Bathing provides an excellent opportunity for providing stimulation. The patient can be touched, tapped, or rubbed with assorted textures such as terry cloth, velvet, cotton balls, feathers, and sandpaper. Heat or cold can be applied. If the patient is tactilely defensive, firm application is less offensive than light touch. Body parts should be identified verbally by the therapist as stimulation is applied.

Oral: In combination with oral hygiene, a piece of ice or cotton swab flavored with lemon (sweet or bitter) water can be applied to the lips and tongue.

Kinesthetic: Range-of-motion exercises to the extremities and proper positioning provide kinesthetic input.

Vestibular: A tilt-table, or rocking bed or chair can be used to provide swinging motions. Adjustments can be made for speed, angle, and body position. When applying vestibular stimulation, the patient's blood pressure must be monitored for hypotension.

Therapy is initiated promptly following medical clearance. The stimulation techniques are applied by each team member at intervals scheduled frequently throughout the day. Sessions are brief, lasting approximately 15 minutes. Stimuli are presented one or two at a time, preceded by an explanatory comment. Even though the patient may give the impression of not understanding what is said, it is important to talk to him or her.

The patient should be allowed to respond before repetition of either the same or a novel stimulus. Stimuli should be alternated to prevent an accommodation effect. For example, although a radio and television are facilitative, they should not be run continuously, as the patient will accommodate to its presence. To increase the consistency of response, focus is placed on those stimuli to which the patient is most responsive, followed by those that do not elicit as strong a response.

If the patient fails to demonstrate consistent and appropriate responses after six to eight weeks, the program is usually discontinued. Reevaluations are conducted periodically to note any significant changes that would warrant reinitiating therapy. In special cases a casted extremity might prohibit any external application of stimulation. In the event that serial casting or dropout casts are used, the extremity may be stimulated and ranged as indicated when the temporary device is removed.

REALITY ORIENTATION

In addition to the use of sensory stimulation, the team should engage the patient in a reality orientation program. This provides a repetition of basic personal information that heightens the patient's self-awareness. Information pertaining to the patient's name, location in the hospital, date, year, family member names, home town, and hospital routine is introduced. Again, information must be presented in a brief, succinct, and organized manner.

NORMALIZING TONE

It is not uncommon for the patient who demonstrates decreased responsiveness to have abnormalities of body tone and posture. Treatment requires an understanding of the motor behavior exhibited, including knowledge of normal and abnormal reflex responses.

During normal development primitive spinal and brain stem reflexes gradually diminish so that higher patterns of righting and equilibrium necessary for volitional movement are primary. A consequence of the loss of higher cortical control is that primitive reflexes are released, resulting in abnormal postures that dominate movement [7]. The patient has a variation of abnormal movement, depending on the degree and distribution of tone. Dysfunction can include spasticity; exaggerated co-contraction instead of normal reciprocal innervation, and static (stereotyped) patterns in lieu of normal righting; and equilibrium and other protective reactions [4].

Combinations of patterns are observed in decerebrate and decorticate posturing. In the former, the trunk and all extremities are rigidly extended, internally rotated, and adducted with fingers and wrists flexed. Increased postural righting and vestibular reflexes result in tonic spasms of all antigravity muscles. Decorticate posturing includes flexion of the upper extremities secondary to flexion of the neck; with neck extension the upper extremities extend, and the lower extremities flex [10].

Assessment requires little attention and cooperation, and thus can be carried out with minimally responsive or confused patients. Treatment is directed toward reducing spasticity, inhibiting abnormal reflexes, and facilitating righting and equilibrium reactions. During the process of normalizing tone, serial casting or splinting has been useful. This involves a series of custom-designed splints or casts that gradually decrease deformities and maintain gains from the reduction of spasticity.

PREFEEDING PROGRAM
Bulbar disorders, frequent complications in the head-injured patient, are characterized by impaired swallowing, coughing, chewing, and speaking. The minimally responsive patient often receives complete nutrition and hydration through a nasogastric or gastric tube to compensate for the loss of these functions. When it appears that the patient has adequate cognition, function, and endurance to begin a prefeeding program, the tubes can be gradually removed. Either tube can continue to supplement the diet, especially when complete oral feeding is not feasible.

The prefeeding program should be a coordinated effort of the occupational therapist, speech-language pathologist, nurse, and dietitian. The sessions are conducted in an environment free from distraction and initially are brief, as the patient has fairly low endurance. Proper positioning is important and the choice of food consistency depends on the patient's control of oral musculature.

The program begins with a complete evaluation of the patient to determine problem areas (Figure 10-2). Table 10-5 presents techniques commonly used when evaluating and treating dysphagia. It should be noted that the risk of aspiration must be considered; if the patient gags, coughs, or becomes cyanotic, suctioning is necessary to remove aspirated material.

OCCUPATIONAL THERAPY
A brain trauma evaluation documents the patient's status and also serves as a reference for reevaluating any change in condition. The assessment includes physical status, response to external stimuli, cognition, and self-care skills.

When the patient is able to respond to simple commands, one-step self-care activities are introduced. For example, the therapist provides the patient with a wash cloth for washing the face, eliminating the steps of preparation, such as applying soap. Other activities include eating with a spoon that is already filled with food (if appropriate), and combing the hair. Therapists carefully select activities that will gain the patient's attention and maximize the ability to concentrate. Some examples include identification of differences between two simple or familiar objects, and other tasks that permit manipulation of a minimum number of variables.

Training in bed mobility, including rolling from side to side, sitting up, and balancing are provided. Tossing a large ball is a useful activity to facilitate quick alerting responses. Also, exercises that require gross alternating movements such as swinging the arms in up-down directions with the assistance of overhead pulleys, enable the patient to take a more active role in the program.

The therapist concentrates on maintaining upper extremity joint range of motion through passive exercises. Splints are fabricated as needed to maintain range of motion and prevent deforming effects of abnormal tone. When the patient is able to participate in treatment, progressive exercises are established to facilitate functional use of the upper extremities.

PHYSICAL THERAPY
Some patients develop weakness in the muscles necessary for coughing and breathing. Also, certain conditions warrant tracheostomies

MASSACHUSETTS REHABILITATION HOSPITAL
OCCUPATIONAL THERAPY
PRE-FEEDING EVALUATION

Name:
Diagnosis:
Level of alertness:
Date:            Age:
Onset of Dysphagia:
Present status of food and liquid intake:
      G-tube    IV    puree    semi-solid    solids    liquids    NG tube
Oral intake:    none    assisted    supervised    (self) independent
Communication status:
Praxis:
Present respiratory status:

| O$_2$ | Congestion | | Needs Suctioning | Normal | Trach | |
|---|---|---|---|---|---|---|
| | On Command | Present but not to Command | | Impaired | Absent | Comments |
| **Head Control** | | | | | | |
| Flexion | | | | | | |
| Extension | | | | | | |
| Turn L | | | | | | |
| Lateral Flexion L | | | | | | |
| Lateral Flexion R | | | | | | |
| **Jaw Control** | | | | | | |
| Close | | | | | | |
| Open | | | | | | |
| Lateral Motion | | | | | | |
| **Tongue Control** | | | | | | |
| Protraction | | | | | | |
| Retraction | | | | | | |
| To L | | | | | | |
| To R | | | | | | |
| Elevation | | | | | | |
| Depression | | | | | | |
| **Lip Control** | | | | | | |
| Pursing | | | | | | |
| Retraction | | | | | | |
| Closure | | | | | | |
| Suck | | | | | | |
| Chew | | | | | | |
| Swallow | | | | | | |
| Liquids—cup, straw | | | | | | |
| Semi-solids | | | | | | |
| Solids | | | | | | |
| Cough | | | | | | |

FIGURE 10-2. *Massachusetts Rehabilitation Hospital Occupational Therapy Department, prefeeding evaluation. (Reproduced with permission from the Occupational Therapy Department, Massachusetts Rehabilitation Hospital, Boston, Mass.)*

| Reflexes | Present | Impaired | Absent | Comments |
|---|---|---|---|---|
| Gag | | | | |
| Tongue thrust | | | | |
| Bite | | | | |
| Rooting | | | | |
| Suck-Swallow | | | | |
| TNR | | | | |
| Tonic Labyrinthine | | | | |

Sensory

Present

Impaired

Absent

Right          Left

| Touch | 1 | 2 | 3 | 4 | Comments |
|---|---|---|---|---|---|
| Tongue | | | | | |
| Palate | | | | | |
| Face | | | | | |
| Lips | | | | | |
| Temperature | | | | | |
| Tongue | | | | | |
| Palate | | | | | |
| Face | | | | | |
| Lips | | | | | |

Taste

Present, Absent, Impaired

| | Right | Left |
|---|---|---|
| Bitter | | |
| Sour | | |
| Sweet | | |
| Salt | | |

Additional
Observations

| Food in side of mouth | |
|---|---|
| Drooling | |
| Facial weakness | |

Aspiration

Therapist: _____

M.R.H.
O.T. dept.
1979

TABLE 10-5. *Prefeeding Evaluation and Treatment Techniques*

| Aspect of Feeding | How to Evaluate | Treatment Suggestions |
|---|---|---|
| *Reflexes*<br>Gag<br>Normal reflex: contraction of constrictor muscles of the pharynx. | Touch mucous lining of posterior pharynx, tonsil area, or root of tongue to elicit contraction of pharynx and sometimes a complex movement of retching (tongue humps, evidence of discomfort). Test right and left, avoid carotid arteries. | To facilitate reflex, stretch palatoglossal and palatopharyngeal arches and the uvula. Press firmly on posterior tongue several seconds.<br>To inhibit reflex, walk back on midline of tongue with swizzle stick until just before reflex is elicited. Repeat 5–7 times. |
| Bite<br>Normal 4–7 months. Teeth clamp shut in response to stimulus placed between gums. (Normal biting is not a snapping motion but a sliding of the lower teeth over the upper teeth.) | Place toothbrush handle on crowns of teeth. Reflex present if mouth clamps shut. | To inhibit reflex, patient should be positioned with head upright, chin slightly tucked. If reflex occurs, do not pry mouth open. Wait for spontaneous opening or apply pressure to temporo-mandibular joint thrusting jaw forward to open mouth. Brush lateral borders of teeth and gums with soft toothbrush positioned between teeth and cheeks. Never facilitate masseters if bite reflex exists. |
| Suck-Swallow<br>Normal 0—3–5 months. Suck followed by swallow followed by suck. Each triggers the other reflexively. | Abnormal if the patient is unable to break the suck-swallow pattern voluntarily. | To break the involuntary suck-swallow pattern, place finger in corner of lips to break suction of lips around the straw or nipple. If this is the only means of eliciting a swallow, it may be desirable to maintain the reflex during early stages of treatment. |
| *Involuntary Movements*<br>Tongue thrust<br>Tongue arches, protrudes outside oral cavity and retracts. May be a repetitive motion. | Observe patient's tongue movements. | To facilitate tongue retraction vibrate on either side of the frenulum under tongue inside mouth with finger. Strengthen retraction by resistive sucking of frappes or picking up pieces of paper with end of straw. (1) Place food in corners of mouth or molar region, or (2) apply pressure to tongue as food is deposited on posterior half of tongue. Do not place food in mouth when tongue is protruded. After food is deposited, vibrate forward under chin using either vibrator or fingers. With improvement, place food in more frontal mid-position on tongue. |
| *Voluntary Motor Control*<br>Head<br>Should be able to hold head upright with neck slightly flexed. | Have patient touch chin to chest (flexion), look up at ceiling (extension), | 1. Prone on elbows—hold head up.<br>2. Sitting—have patient turn head side-to-side against resistance.<br>3. Turn eyes, then head. |

TABLE 10-5. *(Continued)*.

| Aspect of Feeding | How to Evaluate | Treatment Suggestions |
|---|---|---|
| | turn to right, turn to left, touch each ear to shoulder on same side (lateral flexion). | 4. Use acrid odors or interesting visual stimuli to elicit spontaneous head turning away from or toward the stimulus. |
| **Jaw**<br>When relaxed, teeth should be slightly apart with jaw directly in midline. Movements of the lower jaw include: elevation, protraction, retraction and lateral motions. | Have patient open mouth, move lower jaw side-to-side, move jaw forward and back. | To stimulate elevation: Vibrate temporalis and masseters. Stretch pressure applied in direction of their muscle fibers.<br>If jaw protracted: Pull quickly out on jaw to quick-stretch digastrics and glenohyoid muscles.<br>If jaw retracted: Do not vibrate posterior fibers of temporalis. Push jaw in for quick stretch of pterygoid and masseter muscles. |
| **Lip**<br>Movements should include pursing, retraction, and closure. | Have patient close lips tightly, pucker lips as to kiss (purse), smile (retract). | 1. Straw with mouthpiece to provide maintained pressure to lips.<br>2. Resistive sucking of frappes or thick liquids.<br>3. Pick up pieces of paper by sucking on straw.<br>4. Vibration and icing of orbicularis oris.<br>5. Quick stretch to orbicularis oris in direction opposite to lip pursing.<br>6. Blowing exercises—bubbles, cotton balls, pinwheel, candle, whistle.<br>7. Practice production of [u],[m], [b], [p],[w] sounds and words.<br>8. Pucker.<br>9. Whistle.<br>10. Tuck lips in.<br>11. Move lips from side to side<br>12. Smiling.<br>13. Alternate pursing and retracting lips. |
| **Tongue**<br>Movements should include retraction, protraction, lateralization, elevation and depression. | Have patient rapidly alternate position of tongue, freely protrude and retract tongue, move tongue around the inside and outside of lips. | 1. To increase lateralization, press swizzle stick intermittently against lateral surface of tongue. Gently push toward other side of mouth. Stimulate both sides several times. Contraindication—tongue thrust.<br>2. To increase elevation:(a) lightly touch swizzle stick or fiber brush to roof of mouth. Hopefully, tongue goes to that spot. (b) Peanut butter on roof of mouth and on upper lip. (c) Practice production of [d],[t], [l],[n],[z],[s] sounds and words. (d) Practice rapid alternating movements of elevating tongue and protruding tongue in sequence.<br>3. For hyper-retracted tongue—push on tongue tip with swizzle stick.<br>4. General exercises: (1) Protrude tongue. Wipe ice cream or jelly off mouth by licking upper lip, lower lip, the corners of the mouth. |

TABLE 10-5. *(Continued)*.

| Aspect of Feeding | How to Evaluate | Treatment Suggestions |
|---|---|---|
| | | (2) Push tongue into cheeks and stick tongue far out. (3) Touch tip of tongue to roof of mouth, touch lower teeth. (4) Clucking tongue. (5) Counting teeth with tongue. (6) Say la, la, ta, ta. (7) Lick lollipop. (8) Lick food off spoon—sticky substances (peanut butter). (9) Place food back on molars. Ask patient to locate it and transfer it to other side of mouth. (10) For strengthening, use tongue depressor to resist movements. |

## Movements Combining Reflex and/or Cortical Control

### Sucking

| | | |
|---|---|---|
| Ability to create pressure changes (suction) in the mouth using the tongue, lips, and buccal movement. | Have patient suck on a lollipop or through a straw while therapist's finger is on opposite end to feel for suction. | Vibration and quick stretch to orbicularis oris by pushing top lip up and bottom lip down. Suck on icepops. Sweetness increases salivation. Suck on cloth soaked in pleasing liquid. Use varied temperature, taste and olfactory stimuli to enhance sensory input. Good lip closure (above) aids sucking. |

### Chewing

| | | |
|---|---|---|
| Food is placed between molars and torn by lateral and rotary jaw movements. Normal chewing is accompanied by tongue lateralization. The tongue moves the food to the chewing surface continually during the process. | Have patient chew canned fruit. Observe up and down or lateral and rotary movement of jaw, lateral movements of tongue. | Before chewing training is initiated, patient should have stable jaw (see jaw control), or therapist may stabilize jaw by placing index finger horizontally below lower lip, the rest of the hand supporting the chin with the thumb anterior to the ear. Facilitate masseters using vibration bilaterally unless bite reflex exists. When pureed foods taken with ease, chewing motion encouraged by passively moving jaw in appropriate rotary manner. Stimulate chewing by massaging masseters, yawning or stretching mouth wide open, closing. Chew gum for 5 minutes. Encourage back and forth and side-to-side motion of jaw. Use different consistencies of food to provide graded resistance to chewing and for strengthening tongue mobility |

### Swallowing

| | | |
|---|---|---|
| Elicited when saliva and food contact the back of the tongue, soft palate, back of pharynx and epiglottis. Normal rate of swallow is 2 per minute (4). | Difficulty swallowing is indicated by drooling, decreased gag reflex, and tongue thrust. Can patient swallow spontaneously or to command? Palpate larynx to feel upward movement | To stimulate swallow: Vibrate laryngopharyngeal musculature. Start under chin and vibrate down either side of larynx to sternal notch. Apply stretch pressure to the pharyngeal constrictor muscles by applying manual traction to the base of the skull in forward and upward direction. Rub back of neck with washcloth. Gentle upward stroking under chin. |

Source: E. H. Silverman and E. L. Elfant, Dysphagia: Evaluation and treatment program for the adult. *Am. J. Occup. Ther.* 33:390, 1979. Used with permission.

to compensate for an obstructed airway, and thus the patient may develop tube irritation, infection, and excessive secretion. Secretions can enter the lungs because of gravitational force, and as a consequence of feeding, food and liquids may do the same. These complications can lead to aspiration pneumonia. When indicated, chest physical therapy is provided to clear the lungs and trachea. Procedures are postural drainage (positioning to assist drainage of secretions by means of gravity) and chest vibration (thumping, percussion, and shaking to dislodge mucus for expectoration). For those patients capable of participating and responding to verbal commands, the therapist will use relaxed and controlled breathing (allows for expansion of lung tissue and mobilization of the rib cage) and coughing (clears excessive secretions from airways) [9].

Patients with brain trauma are susceptible to heterotropic ossification, a condition that causes joint inflammation and stiffness. To minimize the effects of this deforming condition, prevent the development of decubiti, and reduce abnormal tone and postures caused by spasticity it is imperative that the patient be positioned properly at all times. Positioning guidelines for the stroke patient are suitable for the head trauma victim. When necessary, lower extremity splints and abduction rolls may be used. Passive range of motion is provided to maintain joint mobility.

Physical therapists commonly use the tilt-table to provide weight-bearing stimulation. The upright position permits stretching of tight spastic hip, knee, and plantar flexors. Therapy directed toward active control of head and trunk muscles can be initiated, while at the same time, the patient has a better view of the environment from a standing position.

Gross motor movements, both passive and active, are facilitated through a carefully tailored program specific to the patient's motor control profile. Neurodevelopmental techniques are employed. Hydrotherapy can be useful, particularly in providing movement of extremities too weak or painful to move with-out the buoyancy of water. Relaxation for the relief of muscle spasms and pain is an additional benefit of hydrotherapy.

SPEECH-LANGUAGE PATHOLOGY
The speech-language pathologist's role begins when the head-injured patient is functioning at levels II and III [14]. Primary objectives during these stages are to observe behaviors and attempt to increase any responses to sensory stimulation; to determine the presence of any primary receptive or expressive modes; and to carry out a dysphagia program in conjunction with other team members.

STRUCTURED PROGRAM
The focus of the program for the agitated, confused patient with a reduced attention span and inconsistently appropriate response is to create a highly structured environment in which predictable routines are established, distractions are minimized, and excessive demands are not made. Generally, treatment goals emphasize decreasing the patient's agitation, maintaining and increasing selective attention, and improving the patient's ability to process, assimilate, and associate new information with old. With these goals in mind, the quality of purposeful responses will be heightened, and the patient will eventually gain more responsibility in self-care.

Variables within a structured program are adjusted according to the patient's behavior. These include the number (single to multiple), duration (length of treatment), frequency, rate (speed of information presented), and complexity (simple to complex) of stimuli or tasks presented [29]. To foster a relaxed climate in which the patient will experience success and mastery, the variables are controlled in a progressive manner. The patient must never be overwhelmed as a result of adjusting to several tasks or values at once, because these changes will only create frustration and agitation. Similarly, staff must be closely attuned to the patient's tolerance level, and note any signs of fatigue that might result in negative behaviors.

As the patient gains competence, the treatment duration or the rate of task completion may be increased.

The critical issue is not necessarily what task is provided, but rather the reorganizing process it creates. If necessary, maximal assistance is given to allow successful completion, even if this means having the therapist completing it for the patient. The task itself should be familiar, automatic, and repeated daily.

Instructions must be simple, comprehensive, and able to be grasped within the patient's attention span. Using these guidelines, optimal performance can be anticipated and the patient can understand the program's expectations. Directions should be given in a calm and firm tone of voice (but not in a childlike manner) with verbal and physical reassurance. Initially, the patient is treated on a one-to-one basis, and eventually therapeutic sessions are expanded to allow the patient to observe and later join groups.

Staff need to capitalize on those periods in which the patient is least agitated. The therapist should calmly wait out moments of heightened agitation.

Complicating issues of concern of the patient, family members, and staff involve the use of sedating drugs and restraints. These modalities are viewed by both the family and the patient as dehumanizing and as sources of anger. Conversely, staff view them as necessary for patient management to prevent the potential dangers of abusive behavior to self and others, and to reduce the chance of the patient wandering away.

The agitated patient presents a challenging management problem for staff and other patients. Nearly every patient with head trauma will demonstrate some degree of this behavior, varying from thrashing about to physical and verbal abuse. Tragically, there are some who fail to progress through this phase. Staff should not hold the patient responsible for such behavior, as agitation is characteristically seen during the course of recovery. Similarly, staff must work in unison and share the responsibil-

ity of managing and treating the patient. In other words, with these patients it is inappropriate for therapists to defer treatment until they are less agitated.

Two approaches that are not mutually exclusive, and which the staff can use to ensure consistency in structuring the therapeutic environment, include attitude therapy and behavior modification. Attitude therapy can be defined as a process whereby staff and others adopt a particular approach to the patient. Folsom suggests five therapeutic attitudes: kind firmness, active friendliness, passive friendliness, matter-of-factness, and demand [34].

Behavior modification refers to the use of procedures developed to eliminate undesirable behaviors and maximize the probability of productive behaviors [26]. A professional trained in this approach must be consulted before a program is instituted.

OCCUPATIONAL THERAPY
The patient's functional level is determined by assessing sensation, perception, and cognition. In addition, a thorough self-care assessment is made.

A self-care program is provided daily at the appropriate time, and includes hygiene activities at bedside and dressing training using one article of clothing. Training in bed mobility and transfers are initiated as part of the overall program.

Feeding becomes integral to this training. If the patient has swallowing problems, recommedations found in Table 10-5 can be used. Feeding problems secondary to confusion and agitation can be dealt with by minimizing extraneous materials on the food tray, and introducing the meal with a single plate and utensil. Wrappers must be removed. If the patient is unable to use cutlery, it would be appropriate to recommend finger foods. If the patient can hold a fork but is confused about the sequence of eating, the therapist gently guides the patient's hand. Feeding can be accomplished through a graded program, beginning with the patient learning to make correct choices among utensils. Once this is accomplished, a full meal tray may be presented and the patient taught correct sequencing of courses. The therapist may also introduce the importance of neatness and appropriate social behavior so that the patient can eventually eat in the presence of others without reacting to a distracting environment. Conversations should be simple, designed to orient and encourage.

As the patient begins to show interest in the environment, cognitive tasks aimed at stimulating abstract thought are introduced. Concept formation and classification exercises, which begin on a concrete level and progressively move to a more abstract one, are presented. An example might be sorting objects according to two or more dimensions. Therapists can use developmental learning materials (DLM), which offer programs for improving problem solving, sequencing, and memory, as well as time and mathematical concepts. Although these materials have been developed for a younger population, they can be modified for use with adults. Orientation activities that permit the patient's active involvement include keeping a daily log of the therapy schedule. The patient can help create a reality orientation board with information pertaining to the date, weather, name of the hospital, city and state, sports, and hobbies. To help reestablish cultural ties, discussion can follow topics of national foods and music. Eventually, the patient may be able to partake in group activities available for social stimulation.

Perceptual deficits often surface at this level and can be so severe as to preclude effective learning. Their nature depends on the area of the brain that has been damaged. Some common problems include spatial disorientation, object agnosia, distortion of body image, and poor auditory memory [2]. A variety of tools exist for training in specific problem areas including peg boards, parquetry blocks, visual scanning sheets, and puzzles [33, 36]. A mirror can be used to improve body image by encouraging the patient to describe what is seen in the reflection.

Gross motor activities provide a release for excess energy, enhance body awareness through kinesthetic and proprioceptive feedback, and promote motor coordination. A neurodevelopmental treatment approach for the patient's level of motor control is recommended. Automatic activities such as ball-toss and the use of pulleys can be useful. If indicated, a graded strengthening program and fine motor coordination activities should be provided.

PHYSICAL THERAPY
Assessment at this level includes range of motion, muscle strength and tone, sensation, respiratory condition, and ambulation status. The emphasis of therapy is to improve motor performance. Through the application of neurodevelopmental principles, a mat program is designed and such modalities as a balance board, large vestibular ball, and stationary bicycle can be used. Transfer training takes place daily, and includes transfers to a variety of surfaces.

Pre-gait training is provided, and the need for assistive devices is determined and the appropriate equipment made available. Ambulation training usually begins on the parallel bars and progresses to flat surfaces outside them on stairs and rough surfaces as appropriate.

SPEECH-LANGUAGE PATHOLOGY
The considerations in cognitive training for the patient who reaches level IV on the recovery table (see Figure 10-1) must be kept in mind, including session length, frequency of treatment, and stimulus control. Hagen and associates [14] recommend that treatment be carried out anywhere from three to eight times per week. Initially, session length may be only 10 to 15 minutes, but should be increased as soon as the patient tolerates and participates in longer sessions. The amount, complexity, and length of a stimulus, as well as rate of presentation, must be systematically controlled. As the patient improves, one measurement at a time should be increased [24]. At the extreme ends

of the continuum, one might use a photograph of a family member with a patient at level IV, as compared to an article from the New York Times with one at level VIII.

When a patient reaches the confused, agitated state clinical management focuses on reorganization of cognitive abilities. This patient is best treated in a nonthreatening, nondemanding, but highly structured environment with the aim of increasing frequency and consistency of nonagitated responses. Orientation and reassurance are significant aspects of treatment at that time. All tasks are geared toward increasing the patient's attention to environmental stimuli [14, 24].

While at levels V and VI, when the patient is confused and shifting from inappropriate to appropriate, treatment becomes more task-oriented. The patient is expected to participate in a structured, often repetitious program. Facilitation of increased visual and selective attention and visual and auditory retention, and improved orientation and recent memory are primary concerns. Strategies for dealing with impaired memory and orientation include posting a schedule by the patient's bedside and maintaining a calendar of events or daily log. As the patient becomes more capable, considerable emphasis is placed on improving thought organization, which involves sequencing, coding, and categorizing [24].

## COMMUNITY REINTEGRATION

Rehabilitation includes discharge from the hospital and fostering the patient's smooth reentry into the community as a productive member. A patient who progresses to this level is characteristically functional, although residual cognitive and physical deficits require continued therapy to refine skills. Generally, patients within this final phase demonstrate a carryover of new learning so that supervision reaches a minimum or is no longer required. Intellectual capacity for abstract thinking often remains inferior to what it was at the premorbid level.

The team effort is to provide a nonthreaten-ing therapeutic environment in which the patient can learn to function realistically within existing cognitive and physical limitations. At this stage both patient and family take a more active role and work to meet the patient's specific needs. Family members are encouraged to take part in therapy sessions to learn what to expect from the patient.

The discharge program is designed to diminish dependence on the team; thus within the routine of the hospital setting the patient becomes responsible for self-care, care of the personal environment, and completion of the exercise program including arriving on time for appointments. Leaves of absence (LOA) are planned to ease transition from hospital to home. During LOA the patient is able to carry over and test out in the home the skills learned in the hospital, and on return to the hospital, reports any problems encountered so that appropriate therapy can be provided.

Community outings provide opportunities to negotiate doorways, elevators, and curbs, and use public transportation. In addition, they help the patient develop self-esteem and appropriate social behavior. A community outing may begin with a picnic in the park, as this environment is less threatening than a restaurant. Next, a fast-food restaurant could be tried to encourage the patient to interact with the food server, choose from a limited menu, and dine amid some distraction. Finally, a meal in a restaurant encourages the patient to order from a large menu, plan for a tip, and interact with others [29].

### OCCUPATIONAL THERAPY

The focus is on independence in self-care activities, particularly those needed for living at home. When necessary, adaptive equipment and instruction in its use is provided. Tub and toilet transfer training is instituted, and equipment for home use ordered. The strengthening program is continued, as is that designed to improve dexterity, coordination, and manipulation of objects. Tools useful for assessing functional hand use include the Jebson Hand

Function Test and the Minnesota Rate of Manipulation Test.

Functional activities designed to promote concentration, memory, and problem solving are performed at this level. To help the patient retain new learning, mnemonics, or memory cues, can be useful to serve as means of creating associations with material to be learned [39]. Instructions in handling money (using checks, vending machines, making change, balancing a check book, or starting an account) are reinforced. Time concepts (scheduling appointments, planning a daily schedule), use of the telephone (including correct use of the telephone book and contacting the operator), and management of household crises (clogged drains, loss of lights) are also provided as part of the therapy program. Learning can be accomplished through role playing in group or individual sessions.

Levels of skill in basic homemaking and kitchen activities are assessed to identify problem areas. Suggestions are made concerning methods of work simplification and energy conservation, and if needed, adaptive equipment. On a home visit the patient's ability to function in that environment is assessed.

In preparation for return to employment, evaluation of appropriate work skills should take place, such as physical and cognitive requirements, work habits, and production. Assessment of the patient's ability to drive and necessary driver training should also take place.

Brain injury may produce alterations in patterns of sexual behavior. These changes may be considered abnormal because of the situation rather than their intrinsic nature, for example, inappropriate behavior in public places [20]. Kolodny and associates [20] emphasize that most brain-injured patients do not exhibit significant sexual interest.

PHYSICAL THERAPY
Therapy continues to be directed toward maximizing lower extremity strength and coordination. Ambulation training emphasizes safety and increased endurance. The patient learns to negotiate a variety of surfaces, stairs, curbs, escalators, elevators, and the like, and how to get up after a fall.

SPEECH-LANGUAGE PATHOLOGY
When and if the patient recovers to levels VII and VIII, automatic-appropriate and purposeful-appropriate stages respectively, more advanced cognitive training is undertaken. Reasoning, problem solving, judgment, and higher-level organizational and integrative skills receive the greatest attention. Structure is reduced gradually, with addition of independent carryover assignments [24]. It is during this final stage, which may take months or years to reach, that the patient and team members should be addressing life planning, taking into account any long-term residual problems, which are most likely to include deficits in attention, memory, judgment, academics, and abstractions.

Reentry into the community, particularly after lengthy hospitalization, places extraordinary demands on the patient, family, and society. In northern California a program called High Hopes [35] has been developed for the recovering head-injured population to ease their transition from hospital to community. This program can serve as a model for others to develop nationwide. Whenever possible, reentry should be carried out gradually, and with the support of allied health and medical professionals.

## Emotional Issues of the Family
A vital part of rehabilitation that is often overlooked is helping the patient and the family deal with their emotional reactions to tumultuous changes. The catastrophic, sudden onset of head trauma and the realization of the permanence of disability disrupt family cohesion, and members are often unprepared to understand and deal with the physical, psychological, and social dependence of the patient.

The social worker and psychiatrist usually are the team members responsible for counseling the family and assisting in their adjustment. Because of the close working relationship of team, patient, and family, these therapists often provide support and practical management advice, help the family identify needs, and make referrals for appropriate services.

Initially, the family might exhibit shock and a feeling of helplessness on being told of the seriousness of the situation. An empathic and supportive approach must be offered by the team. Subsequent coping mechanisms are often denial and withdrawal. Feelings of retribution may be expressed toward anyone whose possible wrong-doing might be responsible for the patient's condition. It is appropriate for therapists to accept this behavior, while gently interpreting the reality of the situation. At some point the family may exhibit anger, hostility, and resentment toward the staff. By relinquishing any value judgment and guarding against personalizing these reactions, the therapist allows the family to vent their feelings. Using this strategy, the therapist is better able to continue treating the patient [29].

Reactive depression is common as the situation becomes more a reality. This process allows the family to assess the change in family structure and realize its effect on their lifestyle. The team should detect signs of pathological depression and recommend appropriate treatment. Again, the team attitude is empathic, legitimizing the depression by encouraging the family to be aware of and talk about their feelings. By shifting emphasis to the patient's abilities and helping the family to have realistic expectations, the team is able to provide some encouragement, so that with time, the family begins to adapt. The team continues to reinforce the positive rewards of rehabilitation by using tasks that emphasize the patient's functional capacities. Cooperative goal setting also emphasizes the gains of therapy [29].

In perceiving the family's feelings of frustration, disappointment, fatigue, and depression,

Lezak [23] offers six supportive comments she feels the family needs to hear:

1. Feelings of anger, frustration, shame, and sorrow are natural emotional reactions to have toward the brain-injured family member.
2. Providing good care is dependent on the well-being of the care giver, who deserves a respite and occasional self-indulgence.
3. Ultimately, the family must rely on their own conscience despite offers of conflicting, although well-intentioned, advice.
4. A shift in premorbid family relationships can result in intrafamily conflicts; however, it is a natural change that needs to be understood.
5. The lack of improvement in the patient's condition does not reflect the quality of care and concern.
6. It is natural for the primary care giver to have feelings of divided loyalties between caring for the patient and for the rest of the family.

The team is able to assist the family's adjustment through sharing medical information with regard to head trauma. This includes information about brain damage, the prognosis, residual deficits and behaviors, and the roles of team members. This information can be provided in a written booklet, such as *Rehabilitation of the Head Injured Adult—A Family Guide* [30], family instruction, and a support group. Family members and significant others are encouraged to attend and participate in therapy sessions. This helps them decrease feelings of helplessness and isolation, maintain a relationship with the patient, and understand that person's abilities as well as functional deficits. Family involvement enables continuation of the patient's progress after discharge through instruction in procedures, such as stimulation and range-of-motion activities, ambulation, and communication techniques.

A support group provides a forum for families to discuss their feelings, complaints, and questions, as well as gain support from the team and each other. Different facilities offer a variety of groups that range from open, ongoing, drop-in sessions, to a scheduled series of meetings with a speaker representing each discipline. The atmosphere in each case should be comforting, with the rule of confidentiality emphasized.

Patients also need to learn about the behavior they exhibit, and involvement in a peer group can be most useful in this regard. Such a group fosters the development of coping behaviors in an atmosphere that generates the opportunity for feedback, sharing fears, discussing changes in life-style, and preparing for discharge. The group can continue after discharge, giving new and former patients an opportunity for peer support as well as information about community resources.

## Conclusion

Brain trauma is a relatively new area of specialization within rehabilitation. Research is needed in areas such as recovery of function, treatment rationale, and development and standardization of evaluations. Epidemiological studies, such as those conducted at the University of Virginia, are investigating measures for implementing preventive legislation, for example, mandatory helmets for cyclists, and community education on such issues as risks of alcohol consumption. Other issues under investigation are hospital staffing patterns and emergency medical care strategies to decrease mortality [29].

Treatment of head trauma has at times met with disappointment. Unsatisfactory recovery is often viewed as a "failure-oriented" phenomenon, resulting from delayed intervention and fragmented treatment of the unresponsive and difficult-to-manage patient. To achieve maximum success, the team must strive for early intervention that focuses on the primary causes of the patient's symptoms [32].

Sharing mutual goals is essential for enhancement of the program. Team members must adopt a holistic, multidisciplined approach, providing the patient with their individual, professional expertise, while working toward the common goals of improved adaptive learning and a productive life-style.

*Acknowledgment is made to Rancho Los Amigos Hospital in Downey, California for the conceptual framework of the brain trauma patient's cognitive rehabilitation.*

## References

1. Baker, H. J., and Leland, B. *Detroit Tests of Learning Aptitude: A New Instrument of Mental Diagnosis.* Indianapolis: Bobbs-Merrill, 1967.
2. Benton, A. Visuoperceptive, Visuospatial, and Visuoconstructive Disorders. In K. M. Heilman and E. Valenstein (Eds.), *Clinical Neuropsychology.* New York: Oxford University Press, 1979.
3. Berrol, S. Approaches to rehabilitation care of head injured patients. Presented at the 3rd Annual Conference, Head Trauma Rehabilitation—Coma to Community, San Jose, Calif., 1980.
4. Bobath, B. *Adult Hemiplegia: Evaluation and Treatment*(2nd ed.). London: Heinemann, 1978.
5. Borkowski, J. G., Benton, A. L., and Spreen, O. Word fluency and brain damage. *Neuropsychologia* 5:135, 1967.
6. Cermak, L. S. *Psychology and Learning.* New York: Ronald, 1965.
7. Fiorentino, M. R. *Reflex Testing Methods for Evaluating CNS Development* (2nd ed.). Springfield; Ill.: Thomas, 1976.
8. Gardner, H. *The Shattered Mind—The Person After Brain Damage.* New York: Knopf, 1975.
9. Gaskell, D. V., and Webber, B. A. (compilers). *The Brompton Hospital Guide—Chest Physical Therapy* (2nd ed.). London: Blackwell, 1973.
10. Gilroy, J., and Meyer, J. S. *Medical Neurology* (2nd ed.). New York: Macmillan, 1975.
11. Gorham, D. R. *Proverbs Test.* Missoula; Mont.: Psychological Test Specialists, 1956.
12. Goodglass, H., and Kaplan, E. Assessment of Cognitive Deficits in the Brain Injured Patient. In M. S. Gazzaniga (Ed.), *Handbook of Behavioral Neurobiology*, Vol. 2. New York: Plenum, 1979.
13. Guentz, S. Rehabilitation Nursing Techniques. In *Rehabilitation of the Head Injured Adult—Comprehensive Physical Management.* Los An-

geles: Professional Staff Association of Rancho Los Amigos Hospital, 1979.

14. Hagen, C., Malkmus, D., and Burditt, B. Intervention strategies for language disorders secondary to head trauma. Presented to the American Speech-Language-Hearing Association, Atlanta, 1979.

15. Halpern, H., Darley, F. L., and Brown, J. R. Differential language and neurologic characteristics in cerebral involvement. *J. Speech Hear. Disord.* 38:162, 1973.

16. Hecaen, H., and Albert, M. L. Disorders of Mental Functioning Related to Frontal Lobe Pathology. In D. F. Benson and D. Blumer (Eds.), *Psychiatric Aspects of Neurologic Disease.* New York: Grune and Stratton, 1975.

17. Heiden, J. S. Factors Influencing Management and Outcome—Neurological Considerations. In *Rehabilitation of the Head Injured Adult—Comprehensive Physical Management.* Los Angeles: Professional Staff Association of Rancho Los Amigos Hospital, 1979.

18. Heilman, K. M., Safran, A., and Geschwind, N. Closed head trauma and aphasia. *J. Neurol. Neurosurg. Psychiatry* 34:265, 1971.

19. Hook, O. Rehabilitation. In P. J. Vinken and G. W. Bruyn (Eds.), *Handbook of Clinical Neurology.* New York: American Elsevier, 1975.

20. Kolodny, R. C., Masters, W. H., and Johnson, V. E. *Textbook of Sexual Medicine.* Boston: Little, Brown, 1979.

21. Levin, H. S., Grossman, R. G., and Kelly, P. J. Aphasic disorder in patients with closed head injury. *J. Neurol. Neurosurg. Psychiatry* 39:1062, 1976.

22. Lezak, M. D. *Neuropsychological Assessment.* New York: Oxford University Press, 1970.

23. Lezak, M. D. Living with the characteristically altered brain injured patient. *J. Clin. Psychiatry* 39:592, 1978.

24. Malkmus, D. Rehabilitation of traumatic head-injured patients. Course presented at Kent State University, Kent, Ohio, 1978.

25. Michael, L. E., Sinatra, K. S., and Kimbarow, M. L. Language assessment battery for evaluation of closed head-trauma patients. Presented to the American Speech-Language-Hearing Association, Atlanta, 1979.

26. Mussen, P., and Rosenzweig, M. R. *Psychology: An Introduction.* Lexington; Mass.: Heath, 1973.

27. Myers, P. S. Analysis of Right Hemisphere Communication Deficits: Implications for Speech Pathology. In R. H. Brookshire (Ed.), *Clinical Aphasiology Conference Proceedings 1979.* Minneapolis: BRK, 1979.

28. Piaget, J. *The Origins of Intelligence in Children.* New York: Norton, 1952.

29. Rehabilitation of traumatic head-injured patients. Course presented by the Rancho Los Amigos Hospital, Head Trauma Service, Kent State University, Kent, Ohio, 1978.

30. *Rehabilitation of the Head Injured Adult—A Family Guide.* Los Angeles: Professional Staff Association of Rancho Los Amigos Hospital, 1979.

31. Rhoades, M. E., and Garland, D. E. Orthopedic Prognosis of Brain Injured Adults. In *Clinical Orthopedics and Related Research.* Philadelphia: Lippincott, 1978.

32. Rimel, R. Epidemiology and recovery patterns in adult head trauma. Presented at 3rd Annual Conference, Head Trauma Rehabilitation—Coma to Community, San Jose, Calif., 1980.

33. Siev, E., and Freishat, B. *Perceptual Dysfunction in the Adult Stroke Patient.* Thorofare, N. J.: Slack, 1976,

34. Stephens, L. P. (Compiler). *Reality Orientation—A Technique to Rehabilitate Elderly and Brain-Damaged Patients with a Moderate to Severe Degree of Disorientation.* Washington D.C.: APA Hospital and Community Psychiatry Service.

35. Tobias, J. After discharge and community living for the brain-injured adult. Presented at the 3rd Annual Postgraduate Course of the Rehabilitation of the Traumatic Brain-Injured Adult, Williamsburg, Va. 1979.

36. Van Witsen, B., and Connor, F. P. (Eds.). *Perceptual Training Activities Handbook.* New York: Teachers College, 1973.

37. Wechsler, D. *Wechsler Memory Scale Form I.* New York: Psychological Corp., 1972.

38. Wertz, R. T. Neuropathologies of Speech and Language: An Introduction to Patient Management. In D. F. Johns (Ed.), *Clinical Management of Communicative Disorders.* Boston: Little, Brown, 1978.

39. Wingfield, A. *Human Learning and Memory—An Introduction.* New York: Harper and Row, 1979.

## Suggested Reading

Ayres, A. J. *Sensory Integration and Learning Disorders.* Los Angeles: Western Psychological Services, 1975.

Banus, B. S. *Developmental Therapist.* Thorofare, N.J.: Slack, 1971.

Buro, L. K. (Ed.), *The Seventh Mental Measurement Yearbook.* Highland Park, N.J.: Gryphon, 1972.

Dahler, M. A., and Bulich, B. A. (Eds.), *Physical Therapy Manual for Physicans.* Available from

Iowa State Department of Health, Robert Lucas State Office Building, Des Moines, Iowa, 50319, 1968.

Diller, L. A model for cognitive training in rehabilitation. *Clin. Psychologist* 29(2): 1976.

Farber, S. *Sensorimotor Evaluation and Treatment Procedures for Allied Health Personnel.* Indianapolis: Indiana University Foundation, 1974.

Groher, M. Language and memory disorders following closed head trauma. *J. Speech Hear. Res.* 20:212, 1977.

Jamieson, K. G. *A First Notebook of Head Injury* (2nd ed.). London: Butterworths, 1978.

Jebson, R. An objective and standardized test of hand function. *Arch. Phys. Med. Rehabil.* 50:311, 1969.

Jennett, B. et al. Prognosis of patients with severe head injury. *Neurosurgery* 4:283, 1979.

Klatsky, R. *Human Memory—Structure and Process.* San Francisco: Freeman, 1975.

Luria, A. R. *Human Brain and Psychological Processes.* New York: Harper and Row, 1966.

Maier, H. W. *Three Theories of Child Development.* New York: Harper and Row, 1969.

Marmo, N. A. A new look at the brain damaged adult. *Am. J. Occup. Ther.* 28:199, 1974.

Matsutsuya, J. The interest checklist. *Am. J. Occup. Ther.* 23:323 July-August, 1969.

Neistadt, M., and Baker, M. F. *Choices.* Boston: Massachusetts Rehabilitation Hospital, 1978.

Neistadt, M., and Baker, M. F. A program for sex counseling the physically disabled adult. *Am. J. Occup. Ther.* 32:646, 1978.

Silverman, E. L., and Elfant, I. L. Dysphagia: An evaluation and treatment program for the adult. *Am. J. Occup. Ther.* 33:382, 1979.

Singler, J. R. Group work with hospitalized stroke patients. *Social Casework* 56:348, 1975.

Taylor, M. *Adaptive Learning Among Adults with Aquired Cerebral Dysfunction: Problems and Treatment.* Presented at Minnesota Occupational Therapy Association Retreat Workshop, Minneapolis, February, 1971.

Trombly, C. A., and Scott, A. D. *Occupational Therapy for Physical Dysfunction.* Baltimore: Williams and Wilkins, 1977.

Verjaal, A., and Hooft, V. T. Cerebral Concussion. In P. J. Vinken and G. W. Bruyn (Eds.). *Handbook of Clinical Neurology.* New York: American Elsevier, 1975.

Walsh, K. W. *Neuropsychology, A Clinical Approach.* Edinburgh: Churchill Livingstone, 1978.

Williams, M. Traumatic retrograde amnesia and normal forgetting. In G. A. Talland (Ed.). *Pathology of Memory.* New York: Academic, 1969.

# SPINAL CORD INJURY
*Alice Crow Seidel*

## History

The history of spinal cord injury is closely tied to that of neurosurgery and orthopedics. There also is a connection with the industrialization of America, which introduced the use of power engines to drive motors of cars, snowmobiles, and motorcycles. These machines are aligned with speed, and as the power of motors has expanded so has speed increased, together with accidents that often result in spinal cord injury.

Treatment of these injuries reflects the advancements made in neurosurgical and orthopedic procedures. Prior to the discovery of anesthetic and antisepsis, such an injury was likely to be fatal. Paralysis was considered during the Egyptian, Hypocratic, and medieval periods to be hopeless, thus treatment was minimal if even present. During the Renaissance, Ambrose Paré advocated the treatment of spinal dislocations with traction.

Discovery of anesthesia and antisepsis made surgery a relatively less risky procedure. Removal of spinal tumors was considered to be an appropriate option. In 1905, Cushing described contraindications and indications for surgery in the treatment of spinal injury, conditions that continue to be followed today. Present-day research addresses the feasibility of suturing the damaged cord together, and whether regeneration can subsequently occur. Most of this research is being done on animal studies. Additional inquiry has been conducted into methods of minimizing cord damage that may occur during emergency transporta-

tion. Such things as cooling the spinal area to reduce swelling, and positioning the patient during transportation have proved successful in reducing further damage. These techniques are now being used by emergency medical personnel in their management of injured people.

When addressing the history of the treatment of spinal cord injury one must also look at the history of rehabilitation. World Wars I and II signaled an increase in the number of servicemen who survived spinal cord injuries. Following World War II there was a national movement within medicine to address the needs of those with chronic disease and disability, with increased recognition that the spinal cord-injured person could benefit from programs to relearn self-care skills and be vocationally successful. During the 1960s, centers that specialized in treatment and rehabilitation of spinal cord-injured patients were opened. These centers are geographically located to provide a regional network of facilities and personnel equipped to work exclusively with this population. Several of these centers are now engaged in research projects.

## Causes

The causes of spinal cord injury fall into three general categories: (1) traumatic, resulting from car or diving accidents; (2) congenital, such as spina bifida; and (3) degenerative, as in amyotrophic lateral sclerosis. There are processes such as tumors of the spinal cord and spondylitic osteoarthritis in which compression of the spinal cord occurs. In these cases, symptoms resemble those present when spinal cord injury is a primary diagnosis.

Approximately 25 percent of all cases of spinal cord injury are the result of automobile accidents, while only four percent of all cases are caused by disease and tumors [1]. Trauma may be by direct assault as seen in a gunshot or stab wound. In these cases the spinal column is not damaged, but the injury is directly to the cord itself. Indirect trauma in which the spinal column sustains a fracture or fracture dislocation causes spinous bodies to be dislocated and impinge or sever the spinal cord being protected by the column. Such trauma may occur in motor vehicle accidents when the individual is thrown from the car, motorcycle, or snowmobile. Indirect trauma to the cervical cord may be the result of diving into shallow water or other sports-related activity. In addition to the damage caused by dislocation of spinous processes, injury may also result from hemorrhaging within the cord area.

Trauma can cause a complete or incomplete lesion, determined by a thorough neurological evaluation. After a 24-hour period, a complete spinal cord injury is defined as having no "sacral sparing" as evidenced by perineal sensation. In such a case there is complete severance of the cord, with resulting symmetrical loss of motor and sensory function below the lesion site. An incomplete lesion is characterized by the presence of sacral sparing (perineal sensation) and progressive recovery. The cord is thought to be intact at some point, although the exact degree of completeness may not be ascertained until after the swelling and bruising diminish. Often these types of injuries are the results of accidents that do not involve velocity or speed, such as athletic injuries.

Although relatively rare, a patient may sustain a hemisection, or unilateral injury, to the spinal cord causing Brown-Séquard syndrome. This involves spastic paralysis, exaggerated tendon reflexes, and hyperesthesia on the side of and below the lesion. The opposite side of the body demonstrates loss of touch, pain, and temperature below the lesion site.

## Signs and Symptoms

Spinal cord injuries, whether traumatic, congenital, or disease-based, have typical symptomatology. There is symmetrical motor and sensory loss below the site of the lesion, loss of bowel and bladder function, and alteration of sexual function in men. Depending on the level of the lesion, actual motor and sensory loss will vary somewhat from patient to patient. An injury at the cervical levels renders a person quadriplegic, with paralysis of all four extremities as well as in the trunk and abdominal musculature. A paraplegic injury, paralysis of the lower extremity muscles and lower portion of the abdominal and trunk muscles, results from lesions to the thoracic, lumbar, and sacral areas of the spinal cord.

Whether the injury is complete or incomplete will influence the symmetry, as well as the stability, of signs and symptoms. In a traumatic injury the onset of symptoms is sudden, while in a disease process onset is often slow and progressive. All of these variables are considered in the medical workup.

The individual who has sustained a trauma to the spinal cord enters a period of spinal shock immediately following the injury [4]. During this period of two to three weeks there is flaccidity of motor responses and decreased deep tendon reflexes below the site of lesion. In addition, there is decreased blood pressure caused by pooling of blood in the extremities, and atonic bowel and bladder function. During this period, treatment involves bowel and bladder management and correct positioning to prevent further damage to the spinal cord.

Functions necessary for homeostasis, such as digestion, metabolism, circulation, and excretion continue at the spinal level because of autonomic reflex function. In complete lesions above the first thoracic spinal nerve, all control above that level is carried out by the autonomic nervous system. Below $T_2$ the sympathetic system is intact, but function is impaired. Therefore the patient may demonstrate symptoms reflective of control of these functions.

Temperature regulation is difficult during the early posttraumatic period. Symptoms of shivering without drop in body temperature or difficulty adapting to outside temperatures, especially extremes of hot and cold, are seen. Stimulation of the sympathetic nervous system, as when there is distention of the bowel and bladder, produces profuse sweating.

Autonomic hyperreflexia is a phenomenon seen most commonly following damage to the cervical cord. Caused by visceral stimulation or bladder distention, it produces profuse sweating, sudden elevation in blood pressure, flushing, shivering, and nausea. Relief can be achieved by unplugging the catheter if it is stopped up, or by pressing on the abdomen to empty the bladder. Immediate attention to reversing symptoms should be given to avoid elevation of the blood pressure beyond a safe range. It is best to have the physician check the patient after one of these episodes.

Spasticity, the increased stretch reflex, occurs in the muscles below the site of the injury. Spasms can be activated by such things as cold air, light touch, or clothing. They are increased by urinary tract infections, decubitus ulcers, overwork, poorly fitting clothing and equipment, or even by emotional upsets. For most spinal cord-injured patients spasticity is a hindrance rather than a help. Medication such as diazepam can be helpful in controlling its severity and allowing the patient to be more functional. Surgical procedures to cut particular nerves may be necessary in cases of greatest damage.

One of the more debilitating aspects of a spinal cord injury is the interference with bowel and bladder functioning. Lesions above $S_2$ result in a reflexic, automatic, spastic voiding. Below $S_2$, bladder function is described as atonic with an increased capacity, and emptying is dependent on external pressure to the area. Bladder management is an important aspect of the rehabilitation program.

After the period of spinal shock, bowel functioning returns to normal peristaltic activity. When the abdominal muscles are paralyzed the ability to strain is lost, consequently, manual stool removal or use of suppositories is necessary to aid bowel evacuation.

Sexual functioning is tied closely to bladder functioning. Men with complete lesions above $S_2$ level and reflex neurogenic bladders are able to have reflexogenic erections without ejaculation. Patients with atonic bladders and complete lesions below $S_2$ are unable to have erections; men with these injuries are not able to sire children. An incomplete lesion may produce psychogenic erections with ejaculation; these men may be able to sire children. It is important to note, however, that exceptions to these generalities can be found in any group of spinal cord-injured men. Therefore it is important to delay determining sexual potential until after the period of spinal shock and later in the rehabilitation program.

Women with spinal cord injury have minimal, if any, interruption of the menstrual cycle. They are capable of bearing children if provided with the appropriate obstetrical care.

There are some symptoms that are not experienced by all patients with spinal cord injuries, but that are present with particular ones. Respiratory function is important in lesions of the cervical and high thoracic cord areas. Quadriplegics may experience respiratory embarrassment, which necessitates a tracheostomy or respiratory support system. These patients experience a marked decrease in vital capacity, resulting in low general endurance and high susceptibility to upper respiratory infections.

The high-level paraplegic with paralysis to the intercostal and abdominal muscles also experiences a decrease in vital capacity. Difficulty in producing a functional cough and susceptibility to upper respiratory infections are experienced. Vital capacity can be increased through time, and teaching methods for coughing and substitute patterns for breathing and expanding the lungs.

Postural hypotension may be a problem for

the patient who is making the transition from lying flat to upright position. Decreased blood pressure results from the pooling of blood in abdominal and lower extremity areas where the muscles are unable to pump it back to the heart. The patient complains of dizziness, and often blacks out. By tilting the wheelchair backward, and application of a corset and Jobst stockings to aid in returning blood back to the heart, the symptoms are reversed. It is important for the patient and therapist to realize that postural hypotension is a normal response to acclimation to an upright position, and that as the body accommodates to this change the symptoms will diminish.

All patients with spinal cord injury experience sensory deficits and abnormalities. Their types and extent depend on the site of the lesion, and the amount of cord damaged. When there is an incomplete lesion, the patient may retain sensory ability to discern pain, touch, temperature, and position, although other impairment may be present. Two types of pain are distinguishable: one occurs at the injury site and is caused by irritation of spinal roots; the other is more diffuse and involves the portion of the body below the level of injury. It is described as burning, tingling, stinging, aching, pins and needles, and shooting.

Initial diagnostic procedures include a physical examination with special attention to sensory and motor function. Radiological evaluation ascertains the type and extent of bony injury. A lumbar puncture may be performed to assess the extent of damage to the cord. A urological evaluation may determine bladder function. This is important for all types of spinal cord injuries so that appropriate training can be initiated.

## Acute Care

Initial or emergency medical care of the traumatically injured patient is most important in preventing further damage to the cord. The patient should be moved as little as possible. When moving is necessary, the neck and spine should be supported carefully to avoid flexion and rotation. Transportation should be on a stretcher or board, with sandbags or towels around the head and neck and blankets used to maintain body temperature. Bony prominences must be padded to prevent pressure sores that can develop in less than two hours. Immediate care of the paralyzed bladder can be delayed until catheterization can be carried out in strict asepsis of an emergency room. Drugs such as morphine that suppress respiratory function should only be given if there is severe pain, as patients with cervical or dorsal lesions may suffer irreversible respiratory depression if given morphine at this time. Good emergency care may prevent many complications that can set in soon after injury. Because of the specialization and complexity of medical care required, the patient should be transported to a regional spinal cord center for treatment and rehabilitation.

Treatment following energency care focuses on decompressing the spinal cord by reducing compression and stabilizing the vertebral fracture or dislocation through neurosurgical and orthopedic intervention. Urological management is needed to prevent bladder distention and urinary infection. Other areas of concern at this time are proper nutrition to maintain health, medication to control pain, and strict adherence to skin procedures that will prevent decubitus ulcers (pressure sores) from developing. With the high-level quadriplegic, it will be necessary to establish a system for ventilation such as a tracheostomy, or mechanical equipment to assist breathing.

During this time managing spine stability and promoting healing of the fracture site are most important. Immobilization on a Stryker frame or Foster frame is required for a period of six to eight weeks to maintain the spine in a straight position. There is no weight-bearing at any time. The patient may be moved from supine to prone to supine once every two hours so that pressure is distributed on the vertical and dorsal aspects of the body. This change is achieved by strapping the patient onto the frame and manually flipping the frame. Cervical lesions also require traction to the spine to realign the vertebral bodies. This is done by surgically inserting Crutchfield tongs into the skull with five to ten pounds of weight added. Other lesions usually do not require surgical procedures to reduce dislocations and fractures. Fracture reduction in the thoracic and lumbar areas is accomplished by gradual extension of the spine, accompanied by immobilization.

Because of the increased mobility of the area, cervical spine fractures often require internal fusion of the vertebral bodies involved. This is done by grafting a piece of bone, commonly taken from the iliac crest, over the fracture site.

Care of bladder function is carefully addressed. Through the use of an indwelling urethral catheter, bladder distention is avoided. The prevention of infection through using the techniques best suited to the patient is important. Bladder function is of concern even early in the treatment program; intake of adequate and appropriate fluids to minimize formation of calculi is stressed promptly.

Skin care is assumed by the nursing staff with methodical attention to prevent later complications. The patient should be repositioned at least once every two hours, with special attention paid to the buttocks, hips, and heels for any signs of redness or undue pressure. Care must be taken to keep the patient's perineal area dry and clean, especially if there is bladder and bowel incontinence. If there are any areas that show reddened spots that do not disappear 20 to 30 minutes after pressure has been relieved, the area should be padded, and the patient positioned to minimize pressure on these areas. Because the patient will eventually assume responsibility for skin care, education on the procedures the nursing staff follows and their importance is begun early.

Together with healing the fracture site and maintaining healthy skin, proper nutrition is essential. During this period, a diet of high protein and high caloric content is appropriate.

Often, because of a marked decrease in physical activity and psychological depression, the patient does not have an appetite, and intake is reduced. There is a significant loss of weight during the first year following the accident, and often this is not regained. Studies have shown that in lesions involving the cervical and high dorsal areas there are metabolic disturbances in the breakdown of carbohydrates. This abnormality, with decreased physical activity and anorexia, provides partial explanation of weight loss [3]. It is important during this treatment stage to obtain a complete diet history from the patient. Emphasis should be on providing a well-balanced diet, as well as preparing food in favorite ways to facilitate the intake of proper amounts of calories and food groups.

The treatment of pain is a complicated aspect of management. Pain that occurs at the level of the injury as a result of irritation of the spinal roots can be treated by reduction of the fracture dislocation, or decompression of the nerve roots. Immobilization, or in the severest of cases, a rhizotomy, have proved successful in relieving this type of pain.

Pain that is more diffuse and occurs in the paralyzed portion of the body is not as easily treated, probably because it is less localized than pain at the lesion site. It may begin immediately after injury, or years after the initial trauma. It often is most severe in injuries of the cauda equina, although patients with damage at other sites have described it. Treatment is usually not successful, and what relief is achieved is greatly influenced by the patient's activity level and ability to participate in life's activities. Narcotics are not a solution for this pain. The use of an alcohol block has been marginally successful, with relief being for only three to 12 months. Cutting pain pathways in the spinal cord through a spinothalamic cordotomy has provided temporary relief in malignant disease. Surgical procedures for pain are rarely performed on patients with cord injuries, as they carry a high risk factor. The treatment of choice appears to be teaching coping methods and involving the patient in productive activity to occupy mind and body.

## Complications

The three main complications that persons with spinal cord injuries must constantly be aware of are (1) urinary calculi, (2) decubitus ulcers, and (3) muscle spasms. All these, if left untreated, can cause physical discomfort, a marked decreased in physical activity, delay in progress within a rehabilitation program, and in the case of the first two, death. One of the major objectives of treatment programming is education as to methods that when applied will prevent or minimize these complications.

Urinary calculi occur because of hypercalciuria secondary to inactivity and the lack of mobilization of skeletal calcium. The presence of calculi can be prevented through high intake of oral fluid, as much as four liters per day. Also, having the patient change position frequently, either actively or passively, will facilitate the absorption of calcium by the bones. It is for this reason that the more active the patient is the better kidney and bladder function will be. Ambulation, or even standing for a period each day, plus fluid intake in large quantities will serve to keep the incidence of calculi low or nonexistent.

In spite of patient education, decubitus ulcers are frequently seen. They present a major threat to life if left untreated. Even when treated, they usually set a rehabilitation program back many weeks. They can be prevented if the patient and those involved in care are diligent in following some simple procedures.

Pressure sores result from prolonged compression of soft tissue over a bony prominence. They commonly occur over the sacrum, the illiac crest, the trochanters, the heels, or the elbows—all areas that have prolonged pressure over a bone while sitting, lying, or resting one's arms. The continued pressure eventually renders the tissue bloodless, and necrosis develops. When the dead tissue sloughs off, an ulcer remains. If left untreated, secondary in-

fection sets in, and eventually a serious systemic infection can result. Contributing factors in the development of severe pressure sores are malnutrition, maceration of the skin, moistness of the skin because of bladder incontinence or profuse sweating, alcoholism, drug addiction, and a desire for self-destruction. As a result of all of these factors treatment often involves more than removal of pressure from the area, keeping the area dry and clean, or surgical closure. Issues of nutrition, drug addiction, and so forth must be addressed if treatment is to reverse the process.

One means of prevention is patient education as to their causes. Frequent changes of body position, actively or passively; keeping one's body clean and dry; and maintaining proper nutrition are important. Patients must be taught to inspect their skin for the early signs of a pressure sore, and to manage treatment of the early stage to avoid the evolution into more advance stages. Unfortunately, many patients go through the treatment process for a pressure sore before they make a personal commitment to avoid more episodes.

Muscle spasms and their severity vary among individuals. Those with severe spasms often find themselves hindered in reaching their maximal level of self-care independence, and are also susceptible to pressure sores. The presence of severe spasms without a program of passive range-of-motion exercises, predestines the patient to develop contractures in those joints affected. Spasticity is increased in severity when a systemic infection, such as in the urinary tract, is present.

Complications are contractures, a decreased level of independence in self-care, and likelihood of decubitus ulcers because of increased and prolonged pressure on soft tissues caused by the spastic movements. These complications are reversible by modifying the severity of spasms through the use of a muscle relaxant such as diazepam, by surgical intervention, and by a program to provide passive range-of-motion exercises twice daily to the joints. Surgical intervention is the least favored method, because many procedures are destructive to other parts of the nervous system other than those involved in producing spasms. Therefore the decision to use surgical intervention is one of last resort, and is only reached after careful and thorough assessment by the physician of the pros and cons of the procedure for that particular patient.

## Rehabilitation

Rehabilitation requires close cooperation among members of the professional team. Included are representatives of the following medical and health professions: neurosurgery, orthopedics, urology, physical medicine, nursing, physical therapy, occupational therapy, social work, vocational counseling, recreational therapy, and psychology. Each member brings expertise as well as their concern for addressing the patient's needs in a holistic manner. Often, the success of rehabilitation is determined by the team's ability to work collaboratively, in addition to the patient's ability to adapt to the physical and emotional stress of the experience.

An important role for the members of the team is to assist the patient in setting realistic goals. These are goals that are accomplished by completing a series of steps reflective of the patient's maximizing remaining musculature, as well as the social, emotional, and environmental abilities. It is important for therapists to understand that goals are reevaluated regularly, and changed as the patient's physical and emotional status change. It is of major importance that the patient be an active participant in goal setting. This provides the opportunity to be in control of the program and to have some input into its outcome.

One method is the formulation of a contract between the patient and rehabilitation team members to identify (1) goals to be reached, (2) time frame for their completion, (3) activities or steps necessary to be completed, (4) equipment or techniques to be used, and (5) rewards or incentives to be received on completion of

stated goals. Feedback from the contract to the patient and therapist can alleviate misunderstandings about lack of progress or plateaus, and provide a vehicle by which the patient can monitor the outcome. It is suggested that the contract method is similar to an athletic training schedule—a structured step-by-step outline of achieving fitness or a particular goal. In light of the large percentage of patients who were involved in athletics prior to injury, it is understandable why this can be an effective rehabilitation tool.

### PHYSICAL ISSUES

Unlike some other physically disabling conditions in which symptoms are diffuse and fluctuating, a spinal cord injury renders its victim with an exacting motor and sensory loss that corresponds to the level of injury. For example, damage at the seventh cervical level will produce symptomatology that corresponds to the loss of motor and sensory abilities innervated at the seventh cervical spinal nerve and all nerves inferior to that level. To determine the motor and sensory abilities of such an injury, one evaluates the innervation of the remaining (sixth cervical nerves and superior) musculature. Correlation of the motor and sensory systems to the spinal nerves enables the clinician to anticipate remaining function.

The motor and sensory symptoms are best illustrated with a chart (Figure 11-1). It is important to understand that as one moves from cervical to thoracic to lumbar lesions, the potential for function improves. Moving inferiorly down the spinal cord, there are more innervated muscles and sensations that can be used for functional capabilities.

Not all spinal injuries are complete transections of the cord. There may be an incomplete transection that causes motor paresis rather than motor paralysis, sensory loss that may not correspond exactly to the affected dermatome areas, and there may be abnormal rather than complete absence of sensory feedback. The patient with an incomplete lesion often has motor

| C4 | C5 | C6 | C7 | C8 | T1 |
|---|---|---|---|---|---|
| TRAP (Sp Acc N) Diaphragm (Phrenic N) | | | | | |
| | Levator scap Supraspin Teres minor Deltoid Subscapularis Infraspinatus Rhomboids Brachialis Brachioradialis Biceps | | | | |
| | | Supinator | | | |
| | | Teres major Pectoralis major - Clav Serratus anterior Ext carpi rad L | | | |
| | | | Ext Carpi rad B Pronator teres | | |
| | | | Pectoralis major - Sternal Latissimus dorsi Triceps Flex carpi rad Palmaris L | | |
| | | | | Abd poll L Ext poll L Ext dig communis Ext carpi ulnaris | |
| | | | | Flex carpi ulnaris Flex dig superficialis Flex dig profundus Flex poll L Abd poll B Add poll | |
| | | | | | Lumbricales Opponens poll Interossei |

FIGURE 11-1. *Cervical segmental innervation. (From D. J. Wilson, M. W. McKenzie, and L. M. Barber.* Spinal Cord Injury: A Treatment Guide for Occupational Therapists. *Thorofare, N.J.: Charles B. Slack, Inc., 1974. P. 9, Table 1. With Permission.)*

| T2-T12 | L1, 2, 3 | L2, 3, 4 | L4-S2 | L4-S3 | S3-S5 |
|---|---|---|---|---|---|
| Intercostals<br>Long. thoracis<br>Spin. thoracis<br>Rect. abdominis<br>Obliques-ext/int<br>Iliocostalis lumb. | | | | | |
| | Quad. lumb.<br>Iliopsoas<br>Sartorius<br>Add. Longus<br>Pectineus | | | | |
| | | Add. gracilis<br>Add. magnus<br>Add. brevis<br>Obturator ext.<br>Quadriceps | | | |
| | | | Quad. femoris<br>Glat. max.<br>Glut. minimus<br>Glut. medius<br>Hamstrings<br>Piriformis<br>Obt. int.<br>Tensor F.L. | | |
| | | | | Gastrocnemius<br>Soleus<br>Ext./flex. dig. Long<br>Ext./flex. Hall-Long<br>Tibialis post./aut.<br>Peroneus | |
| | | | | | Penis<br>Perineum<br>Scrotum<br>Bladder<br>Rectum<br>Anus |

and sensory abilities that change markedly during rehabilitation. This mandates reassessment and modification of goals to incorporate physical changes.

## PSYCHOLOGICAL ISSUES

Spinal cord injury precipitates psychological symptoms that can be as incapacitating as the paralysis by virtue of the severe amount of stress it produces. Withdrawal from physical activities and sleeping, refusal to eat or speak to visitors, or more severe behavior such as hallucinations and delusions may be seen during the early stages of medical care. It should be noted that such behavior may be enhanced by some of the treatment modalities used to stabilize the spine or avoid infection. Use of the Stryker or Foster frame places the patient in either a prone or supine position, thus limiting visual stimulation to the ceiling or floor, or to items placed within that visual field. To avoid infection while on the Stryker frame, many times these patients are put in a single room under strict isolation precautions. Both of these situations are necessary medical practice, however, they serve to reinforce early emotional reactions to physical changes and stress.

Some of the early psychological problems can be minimized through auditory stimulation of a radio or television, and simple structured board activities that require attention and interaction with another person. The patient should not be allowed to avoid interaction by withdrawal behaviors, however, the staff should acknowledge the difficulties of being physically and socially isolated by the prescribed medical treatment.

Psychological problems that may surface during rehabilitation are most commonly situational. Some behaviors frequently seen are depression and lack of motivation during periods of plateau of progress, and aggressive acting out in response to physical dependence and limitations. General reactions to stress include inability to sleep, regression in social and emo-tional development, and inability to make decisions.

An individual's premorbid methods of coping with stress will surface after the initial life-saving stage of treatment. Often, rehabilitation staff sees psychological problems surface because the process itself is a direct confrontation to the patient of the severity of the disability and its impact on lifestyle. Also, a rehabilitation setting is a safe and accepting one, therefore the patient may feel less threatened and thus less inhibited about demonstrating emotional reactions. After all, the staff will not desert the patient, and help can be obtained for dealing with outbursts.

Psychological adjustment to spinal cord injury is often recognized as occurring in stages. The time span and methods of adjustment vary from patient to patient, and are dependent on premorbid ways of coping and adapting. Some variables are the patient's educational level, cultural and value structures, family cohesiveness, and the person's value of physical prowess, independence, sexuality, and physical appearance. In working with the patient it is important to develop a composite picture of all these areas, insights into which provide an understanding of the patient's situational responses. They may also assist the patient in understanding reactions to the injury and changes in body function.

The adjustment is similar to that of someone with a terminal disease. Theorists feel that the paralysis represents the loss of a body part, and the individual mourns that loss of function [3]. In addition, the individual must reestablish a body image based on remaining function.

Similar to Kübler-Ross's [2] stages of adjustment to terminal disease, the spinal cord-injured person goes through five stages of reaction to the injury: (1) shock, (2) expectancy of recovery, (3) mourning, (4) defense, and (5) final adjustment. For purposes of discussion, these stages are clearly defined; however, in reality a patient does not overtly demonstrate such clear distinctions. Most often the patient vacillates between stages, skips one, or appears to stay at a particular level for an extended period. What is important for both patient and clinician to understand is that one does go through a period of adjustment, and that there are stages or different reactions involved during this time. Patients need to be reassured that they are not psychotic or exceptionally neurotic when they experience periods of intense behavior or reactions. The patient who does not demonstrate some emotional reaction to the injury can be as alarming to the clinician as the one who suffers a severe psychotic break.

During the initial stage, shock, the patient just does not believe that the injury has occurred. Given the sudden onset of injury, disbelief is understandable. To wake up in the morning physically normal and then to end the day paralyzed from the neck down would generate a great deal of disbelief in anybody. Enhancing this may be the fact that the patient never lost consciousness, and remembers the events leading up to, during, and immediately after the accident. The patient may express such things as "I'll be up walking next week," or "It's just a bad dream." During shock there is often a greal deal of denial. It is felt that this enables the individual to direct energy toward staying alive and weathering a critical medical period. Denial is felt to be healthy, and a worthy coping mechanism.

The second stage, expectancy of recovery, is seen most often during acute medical treatment. There remains a hope that after the period of time on the Stryker or Foster frame, it will be possible once again to walk and return to the previous life-style. The patient perceives the injury as a temporary condition. During this period, the patient may try bargaining as a means to ensure speedier recovery. Absolute adherance to the medical regimen and spiritual emphasis by an individual who previously was not religious are two instances of this.

Mourning is the third stage, and is seen as the beginning of a period of realization of the seriousness of the physical changes. Often, mourning begins shortly after rehabilitation is initiated, when the patient receives the signal that there is an element of permanence to the paralysis. Behaviors during this stage can include a sudden and massive constriction of the patient's life in which energies are focused on disabilities and losses, a mood of helplessness and worthlessness, a dominance of self-perception by premorbid comparisons—"I used to be . . ."—or a general period of self-pity and depressive behavior. This stage with its self-directed energies is difficult for family members, and it is important that they have an opportunity to express their feelings about their own reactions toward the patient. They should be made aware of the adjustment stages and accompanying behaviors.

Following mourning, there is a time of reconstruction of the self-image. This moves into the fourth stage, defense of the forming self-image, about which the patient is unsure, not having had an opportunity to try it in surroundings other than the rehabilitation unit. During this period the patient may be angry, and aggressively act out or try behaviors to test others' reactions to the new self-image. It is reminiscent of the adolescent struggling with the dependence–independence conflict in that the spinal cord-injured patient who in many instances actually is an adolescent struggles with the new needs of dependence brought on by paralysis of musculature that previously allowed mobility and physical freedom. During this stage, the patient's energies and anger can often be channeled into intensive rehabilitation programming, resulting in highly productive physical and occupational therapy.

Just as it may be a productive period in therapy, it is also a time of realization of physical limitations as a result of the paralysis. This moves the patient into the final stage of adjustment or coping. The patient moves out of self-centered here-and-now behavior into setting goals for the future. There is concern expressed for education, vocation, relationships with spouses and friends, and long-term quality of life. The patient often demonstrates a willingness to solve problems rather looking to therapists for answers. Moving out of the sheltered setting into the community becomes an important step in testing the new self-image and the new skills acquired through rehabilitation.

## REHABILITATION ISSUES

The rehabilitation process for a person with spinal cord injury offers progress, plateaus, and occasionally regression, while psychological adjustments are made to changed self-image and capabilities. The period begins with the individual being totally dependent on others or equipment to meet daily and bodily needs, and moves through stages to completion of rehabilitation with as much independence as is possible within physical and emotional limitations. During this time there is interaction with a variety of therapists who apply their own expertise to helping the patient achieve the goals that have been set. Every program has objectives and general attributes, as well as precautionary concerns. It should be emphasized that what follow are not recipes for treatment, but approaches to consider in evaluating each patient's physical and emotional characteristics.

### RANGE OF MOTION

Prerequisite to achieving maximum independence in functional activities is maintenance of full passive range of motion in all joints and maintenance and increase of strength of remaining musculature and overall endurance.

Motion within the pain-free passive joint range is of prime importance, as agility and flexibility enable the person more easily to carry out dressing, bathing, toileting, and transferring. All of these require twisting the trunk, bringing the legs to the chest, or bending at the hips to reach the knees and feet. For the high-level quadriplegic, adequate passive range of the shoulder, elbow, forearm, and wrist is necessary to use mobile arm supports and splints. The paraplegic will find flexibility of trunk and legs to be an asset in dressing and bathing. As with all stretching exercises, whether they are done by a therapist or by the patient, it is important to increase passive range of motion in a slow, steady, pain-free way. Because proprioceptive and kinesthetic feedback may be impaired, the patient may overstretch and damage joint support structures without being aware of the injury. It is important carefully to instruct the individual in how to perform flexibility exercises using proper biomechanical dynamics.

### STRENGTH

Strengthening the remaining muscles is generally one of the most important rehabilitation goals. These goals are based on the amount of residual musculature present and its potential use in performing functional activities or operating devices. Although a patient with paralysis from the level of $C_4$ has little remaining musculature, it is important to realize that what there is requires attention to strengthening for its use in using equipment; for example, to operate a hand splint the shoulder, arm, and forearm must be no weaker than a fair grade. Fair-plus elbow flexion is necessary for the performance of a swivel bar transfer. Occasionally, an individual with less than adequate muscle strength will accomplish far beyond the functional capabilities for the injury and residual musculature. Such accomplishments are usually a result of the person's level of coordination, lack of body fat, and exceptional premorbid physical conditioning.

The paraplegic will need to strengthen the upper trunk and upper extremities in preparation for wheelchair or crutch ambulation. Such activities require a strenuous program, especially for the woman who has not developed shoulder and upper back strength prior to injury.

### ENDURANCE

As strength increases, so does endurance. Endurance is defined as the amount of physical output—in length of time or number of repetitions—a person can accomplish before fatigue. Muscle strength is only one part of endurance.

Also included is respiratory efficiency, or the ability of the lungs and heart to exchange oxygen and carbon dioxide and to get the oxygen to the muscles. Patients with injury at the $C_4$ to $C_5$ level sustain paralysis to the diaphragm muscles thus causing respiratory embarrassment. These persons will usually require assistance in breathing through the use of a tracheostomy or respiratory equipment. Cervical cord injuries below $C_5$ will paralyze the intercostal and abdominal muscles, leaving only diaphragmatic respiration. Such respiration is shallow, with the individual initially achieving only 20 percent of normal vital capacity. Besides exhibiting easy fatigability and dyspnea exertion, the individual may be unable to produce a functional cough. With initiation of a rehabilitation program, which includes techniques to improve coughing and activities incrementally to increase endurance and vital capacity, the patient is often able to reach and maintain 60 percent of normal vital capacity. It is important for the therapist to understand that the patient's fatigue may be the result of a decrease in vital capacity as well as muscle strength.

BOWEL AND BLADDER

Bowel and bladder dysfunction creates anxiety and personal discomfort. During spinal shock, these areas are flaccid, and treatment is directed toward preventing complications caused by bowel impaction and bladder distention. Subsequently, a training program will begin with the goals of retaining function and educating the patient in methods of management that will prevent complications. The type of program will depend on whether the patient has an upper motor neuron–reflex emptying bowel and bladder or a lower motor neuron–manual emptying bowel and bladder. It is the responsibility of the physician and nursing staff to oversee the training program. Therapists need to know about the program so that appropriate reinforcement and adequate amounts of fluid can be provided during therapy sessions.

In the upper motor neuron bladder program, the patient must be aware of three goals: (1) to empty the bladder regularly and completely; (2) to maintain urine sterility with no stone formation, and (3) to preserve as near normal capacity and musculature as possible. To meet these goals, the program focuses on having the individual drink a minimum of 3000 milliliters of fluid per day, keep as mobile as possible, and learn a method of intermittent self-catheterization or be on a strict voiding schedule. An important precaution that the individual must be aware of is keeping the regularity of the schedule so the bladder does not become distended. For bowel management, suppositories or digital stimulation to activate the reflex can be used. This routine is also done on a schedule, and its effectiveness is closely tied to diet and regularity of physical activity.

The lower motor neuron bowel and bladder program involves placing the individual on a two-hour voiding schedule. Also, fluids are pushed to maintain the minimum of 3000 milliliters per day. Bowel evacaution is the same as for the upper motor neuron bowel program.

In both programs, the length of time necessary for individuals to obtain control will vary. Often the period of training is prolonged, and can be discouraging to the patient who may be experiencing days of bladder control, and other days of accidents. An understanding staff and family can ease the embarrassment and psychological pain.

SEXUALITY

More information is being generated on this topic about which, as recently as 10 years ago, little was known. Sexual counseling with the spinal cord injured-person is now a role that the occupational therapists or social workers may carry out during rehabilitation.

MOBILITY

The ability to move oneself from place to place is of prime concern. Control over one's mobility signifies ability to determine where one will be at a particular time, and the types of activities one can engage in or observe. All too often rehabilitation professionals see mobility only as ambulation with crutches and lower extremity braces, or the use of a wheelchair.

With the quadriplegic, mobility is possible for all levels of injury. The patient with very high paralysis who lacks control over the use of the upper extremities can use head, voice, or even breath to activate a motorized wheelchair. Adaptations of the wheelchair rims will enable the quadriplegic with extension to propel the chair. The ultimate in mobility is the adapted van that permits independent entry by means of a hydraulic lift, and allows the patient to sit in the wheelchair behind the steering wheel and drive the van with adapted controls.

For the paraplegic patient, mobility is facilitated in two ways: wheelchair, and crutches and braces. The choice between them is influenced by many variables including the level of injury; resulting residual muscle function, especially in the stablizing groups of the abdominal, back, and hip muscles; the distance to be navigated; the age and general physical condition (pain, endurance, weight, deformities) of the individual; and the severity of spasticity.

Four categories of functional ambulation have been identified [5]. They are:

1. Community ambulation: The paraplegic is able to leave home, without assistance, and to walk a moderate distance with braces or crutches. For longer distance a wheelchair is used.
2. Household ambulator: With assistance the paraplegic is able to get up from a chair or bed; and with supervision can ambulate within the confined environment of a house or office. They also may be able to ambulate with supervision to the street and enter a car or van.
3. Exercise ambulation: The paraplegic will attain a standing position with assistance, and may take a few steps using a "drag to" crutch gait. This ambulation pattern is designed for exercise and physiological purpose only, and is not functional.

4. Nonambulatory individual: The paraplegic relies totally on the wheelchair for mobility.

For all spinal cord-injured persons there are immense psychological and physiological benefits to be gained by achieving of mobility. Although a quadriplegic is seldom, if ever, placed in an erect standing position, the very fact of being able to use a wheelchair and maintain a sitting position is an improvement over being supine, prone, or side-lying in bed. Physiological benefits that improve bladder drainage and heart-lung pumping action, and a variance of pressure spots are achieved from being able to assume the sitting position. Psychologically, the visual perception of the environment is enhanced by sitting, and interaction with others and the environment takes on a more normal perspective.

The paraplegic should be encouraged to spend some part of each day standing up. This is possible for those with the highest level of thoracic injury by means of a standing belt that works on the principle of the device used by telephone linemen to maintain position on the pole. A "Stand Alone" is a mechanized standing belt that can provide security for the high-level paraplegic with minimal strength of abdominal and back musculature. The benefits of standing include improved bladder function, relief of pressure over sacral and ischial areas, minimized effects of nonweight-bearing on bones, and emotional uplift from viewing the environment from an upright position.

SELF-CARE

As the patient's mobility problems are resolved, there often is an associated renewed interest in self-care independence. Paraplegics often can achieve independence quickly and with minimal problems, thus leaving their energy to be focused on ambulation. The quadriplegic patient's self-care presents a greater challenge. In all cases, resolution of these issues leading to independence is a process of trying techniques and equipment that use the patient's remaining muscles and biomechanics to their fullest. Some of these techniques have been successful for some spinal cord injured patients; however, they may not be successful for every patient at all times. Therefore it is important to involve the patient in problem solving with the therapist and allow the patient to try individual approaches to the tasks. The therapist's role becomes one of giving support and reviewing ideas the patient presents. As a result, therapists can use their expertise to discourage the use of techniques that may be harmful or use poor body mechanics. Such an approach serves as an educational tool to aid the patient in becoming familiar with the variables that must be addressed when confronted with a self-care problem.

Beginning a self-care program is dependent on several factors. One of the most important to consider is the medical stability of the patient. Even while on a Stryker frame (but beyond the early acute phase) simple self-care skills can be initiated; such tasks as feeding, oral hygiene, and shaving will minimize feelings of dependency and helplessness. Most of these tasks are best accomplished from the prone position. Adaptive equipment should be provided to enable a quadriplegic to grasp silverware, toothbrush, or electric razor. The paraplegic, because of normal upper extremity musculature, usually does not need such equipment. In all cases, it is important that objects be placed so as not to force the patient to assume a position other than the one stabilized by the frame.

Once the patient is removed from the frame, usually six to eight weeks following the injury, a stablizing brace is applied. For the quadriplegic it is a neck brace that does not allow flexion or extension, and only limited rotation of the neck. The paraplegic is placed in a back brace that limits rotation, and flexion and extension of the spine. These braces are worn until the injury site is completely healed as indicated by roentgenogram.

Self-care during this period will become more active than during the initial phases, however, it will be limited by decreased mobility created by the brace. During this period a quadriplegic can begin to do limited upper extremity bathing and dressing, as well as continue with previous activities. Although the self-care goals are limited at this time it is important that they be carried out. These activities require use of the remaining upper extremity musculature and therefore encourage movement and become a part of the strengthening exercises that are so important in attaining independence in the more complex areas of self-care.

Limitations that the paraplegic experiences from wearing the back brace are primarily in the area of reaching the feet and objects that are not within arm's length. The majority of these patients can achieve independence in most self-care activities in spite of a brace. Adaptive equipment such as bath brush with an extended handle, or assistance in bathing the back may be necessary. Long-handled reachers or assistance may be required in starting lower extremity clothing up over the feet.

On removal of the brace, the patient is able to participate in an active program to accomplish the final steps toward maximal independence. Figure 11-2 presents suggested goals for particular levels of disability. As with ambulation, the level of independence depends on the patient's remaining musculature, endurance, weight, age, preaccident physical condition, and overall motivation.

HOME CARE

Home management for the person who lives alone or with a partner is an important aspect of independent functioning. Included are those skills necessary for the maintenance of a house or apartment, meal preparation, laundry, cleaning, budgeting, and money management. If appropriate, child care and other tasks performed to contribute to the family are included in the objectives set for the patient's present or anticipated life-style. Variable goals are influenced by the role the patient has within a family, whether the home is to be a house or apartment, the presence of an attendant, and

| Quadriplegics | | | | | Paraplegics | | | |
|---|---|---|---|---|---|---|---|---|
| C$_4$ Neck Upper Trap | C$_5$ Shoulder Biceps | C$_6$ Wrist Extension | C$_{7,8}$ Triceps Weak Hand | X—Most patients<br>•—Some patients<br>Consider age, weight and sex; complete or incomplete lesion | T$_{1-8}$ Chest | T$_{9-12}$ Trunk | L$_{1-12}$ Hip Flexion | L$_{3-5}$ Knee |
| | | | | *Cough* | | | | |
| | X | X | | With glossopharyngeal breathing | | | | |
| | | | X | Manual (self) | | | | |
| | | | | Independent | X | | | |
| | | | | *Relief of Skin Pressure* | | | | |
| | • | | | Assisted | | | | |
| | | • | | Independent with equipment | | | | |
| | | X | X | Independent | X | X | X | X |
| | | | | *Wheelchair Propulsion* | | | | |
| | • | | | Electric | | | | |
| | X | | | With handrim projections | | | | |
| | | X | X | With friction surface handrims | | | | |
| | | | | With standard handrims | X | X | X | X |
| | | | | *Bed Transfer* | | | | |
| | X | | | Assisted with swivel bar | | | | |
| | | • | | Indep. with loops & sliding board | | | | |
| | | X | | Indep. with sliding board | | | | |
| | | | X | Independent | X | X | X | X |
| | | | | *Car Transfer* | | | | |
| | X | | | Assisted with sliding board | | | | |
| | | X | X | Indep. with sliding board | | | | |
| | | | X | Independent | X | X | X | X |
| | | | | *Wheelchair into Car* | | | | |
| | | • | X | Indep. with loop on wheelchair | | | | |
| | | | • | Independent | X | X | X | X |
| | | | | *Driving with Hand Controls* | | | | |
| | | X | X | With swivel cuff | | | | |
| | | | | With swivel knob | X | X | X | X |

FIGURE 11-2. *Functional goals for patients with spinal cord injury. Source: Adapted from information available from: Spinal Injuries Service Rancho Los Amigos Hospital, Downey, California.*

| Quadriplegics | | | | | Paraplegics | | | |
|---|---|---|---|---|---|---|---|---|
| C$_4$ Neck Upper Trap | C$_5$ Shoulder Biceps | C$_6$ Wrist Extension | C$_{7,8}$ Triceps Weak Hand | X—Most patients<br>•—Some patients<br>Consider age, weight and sex;<br>complete or incomplete lesion | T$_{1-8}$ Chest | T$_{9-12}$ Trunk | L$_{1-12}$ Hip Flexion | L$_{3-5}$ Knee |
| | | | | *Toilet Transfer* | | | | |
| | | • | | Assisted | | | | |
| | | • | • | Independent with equipment | | | | |
| | | | • | Independent | X | X | X | X |
| | | | | *Bath Transfer* | | | | |
| | | • | • | Assisted with seat & sliding board | | | | |
| | | • | • | Indep. with seat & sliding board | X | • | | |
| | | | | Independent to tub | • | X | X | X |
| | | | | *Ambulation* | | | | |
| | | | | Physiological with L.L.B. | | • | | |
| | | | | Functional with L.L.B. | | | • | • |
| | | | | Functional with S.L.B. | | | | X |
| | | | | *Dressing* | | | | |
| | | X | | With assistance | | | | |
| | | • | X | Indep. with equipment | X | | | |
| | | • | • | Independent | • | X | X | X |
| | | | | *Feeding* | | | | |
| X | • | | | Assisted | | | | |
| | • | X | | Indep. with equipment | | | | |
| | | X | X | Independent | X | X | X | X |
| | | | | *Bathing and Showering* | | | | |
| | X | X | | Assisted | | | | |
| | | | • | Indep. with equipment | X | | | |
| | | | • | Independent | • | X | X | X |
| | | | | *Bowel and Bladder Care* | | | | |
| | | X | | Assisted | | | | |
| | | • | X | Indep. with equipment | | | | |
| | | • | • | Independent | X | X | X | X |
| | | | | *Home Management* | | | | |
| | | X | X | Assisted | | | | |
| | | | • | Indep. with equipment | X | | | |
| | | | | Independent | | X | X | X |

economic situation. Because the majority of spinal cord-injured patients are between the ages of 18 and 22 years, many have not established a living situation away from the home or college-based setting. Thus many return to the family on discharge from a rehabilitation program, and as they develop more self-confidence and maturity, issues of life-style and the responsibilities of home management surface. At this time, the patient may reestablish contact with rehabilitation personnel for assistance in resolving problems that might arise as a result of these issues. In addition, it might be worthwhile to seek out other spinal cord-injured persons who have lived successfully and independently within the community.

One recently conceived alternative to nursing home life is independent living. The thrust of it is development of accessible housing, whether apartments, single family, or multiple family dwellings, and the provision of support systems within a community, such as personal care attendants, homemaker aids, and transportation. Independent living alternatives enable the severely disabled person to live outside a nursing home, yet receive necessary assistance in self-care and home management. The handicapped individual becomes the employer of the aides, making the arrangement a business one. These units have been most successful in areas with a high population of young adults who are students or employed nearby. This population understandably appears to be the most motivated to avoid the nursing home setting.

VOCATIONAL ISSUES
Vocational decisions are usually part of the later stages of rehabilitation, as in the early stages there are other concerns perceived to be of higher priority. The issue of employment is nevertheless essential to address, as it represents a sense of productivity and worth to the individual, family, and society. For the person with a spinal cord injury who holds a job, questions such as "How will I support my family?" and "Can I return to my job?" surface early.

This person needs to become familiar with possible modifications of an existing job so that, for example, it can be performed from a wheelchair. Employment alternatives may also need to be discussed, and if a change is necessary, retraining that must be completed and where it will take place. Evaluation for and development of adaptive equipment for the quadriplegic patient to carry out job tasks may be required.

For those who are not currently employed, evaluation of vocational interests in terms of capability, and selection of an appropriate educational or training facility are part of the process.

COMMUNITY ISSUES
Employment and education often represent the patient's initial contact with community attitudes toward the physically handicapped. In addition to architectural barriers, there will be attitudinal barriers to face. The latter are more subtle and often demonstrated by social isolation or a general uneasiness in relating to a disabled person. It is in the handicapped person's best interest to be aware of existing civil rights to be able to participate fully as citizens within the community. The person may want to join a local chapter of the National Spinal Cord Injured Foundation, which offers a support and a resource group for community improvement.

FAMILY ISSUES
The family aids the individual in adjusting to the community. Their attitudes help shape the individual's self-perception. The members play a critical part in carrying through rehabilitation concepts and procedures. They should be regularly appraised of the patient's status—new skills gained, new equipment obtained, or reasons for lack of progress. All too often the family is left out of the rehabilitation process, which can cause them to have feelings of alienation. These feelings may lead to lack of follow-through at home of techniques learned in therapy, or members might be totally over-

whelmed by the handicapped person and not know what to expect.

To maximize participation, the family should be included in therapy sessions as appropriate. A group setting may be helpful as it can provide an opportunity for them to discuss their feelings and concerns with others in similar situations. Communication among all members should be encouraged, and developed if it is not already present. Whenever a family member is expected to carry out a specific therapeutic technique, thorough instruction should take place including safety precautions and why the technique is being used. Such instruction is best provided several times, as the initial session may be overwhelming and result in decreased ability to listen, observe, and retain the instructions.

FOLLOW-UP CARE

The time following discharge from the rehabilitation program is critical in the patient's adjustment to disability. The major focus of follow-up care is to prevent situations, medical or otherwise, that may lead to the need for further hospitalization. In additon, it includes referral to resources and agencies within the community.

Two of the most common situations that require attention are urinary tract infections and pressure sores. Both can be prevented if the patient judiciously follows the preventive regimens that are prescribed. Urinary tract infections can be minimized through the intake of large amounts of fluids, yearly evaluation of kidney function, and following the prescribed bladder management program. The patient should be educated with regard to anatomy and function of the urological system, and the consequences of failing to follow the recommended program.

Pressure sores are also preventable. The patient needs to know their causes and consequences. Procedures such as changing body position in the wheelchair and bed, performing skin inspection daily, and keeping skin clean and dry must be taught. Part of the edu-

cational program can be pictured showing the evolution of a pressure sore and the medical treatment required to repair it. Information about nutrition and general health is also appropriate.

Prevention of deformities is part of follow-up. These usually result from a combination of spasticity, inadequate range-of-motion exercise program, and poor body positioning. If the patient is unable to maintain a prescribed program of stretching exercises, then it is necessary to teach the exercises to family members or an attendant. Immediately after discharge from the rehabilitation program, a visit by a physical therapist in the patient's community may be beneficial in initiating home exercises. The more contacts within the community that the patient has, the greater is the possibility to be physically active, and thus diminish the potential of developing joint and body deformities.

Another aspect of deformity prevention is appropriate positioning. Especially critical is the selection of a wheelchair that fits the patient's body, and also meets mobility needs. Modifications of the chair must be made as the patient alters physically and as muscle atrophy occurs, which in turn changes the contours of the body and its position within a wheelchair. The patient must know where to go for wheelchair maintainence and modifications.

Follow-up by the vocational rehabilitation counselor is critical to successful vocational placement. There must be a smooth transition between the rehabilitation counselor and the counselor who is based in the home town. It is recommended that the latter visit the prospective client in the rehabilitation unit just prior to discharge, after which early and consistent contact will make the transition less traumatic for the patient. Very often the rehabilitation counselor is the only person from a community-based agency with whom the patient has long-term contact. The goal of such contact is the placement of the client in employment or a training program for future employment.

One of the most recent developments in follow-up care is peer counseling. This involves coming together of the newly injured person with other spinal cord-injured people who are already functioning in the community. Such a relationship provides a resource for information as well as support. The model has been highly successful because of the sharing of expertise specific to spinal cord injury, and the personal level of emotional support among the participants.

Another area of follow-up that should be addressed concerns securing financial assistance to live independently. This includes social security, state social service monies, and funds from various state agencies such as vocational rehabilitation. Many times a peer counselor can be of assistance in methods of managing the bureaucracy of these agencies.

Rehabilitation of spinal cord-injured patients presents a challenge to professional staff and to patients and their families. As new techniques are developed and refined the length of time needed for rehabilitation becomes shorter and shorter. There is a concerted effort to return the individual to the home as quickly as possible. It is felt by many rehabilitation personnel that rehabilitation in its truest sense occurs when the person returns home, and begins to perform a productive role within the community and home setting.

## References

1. Cull, J. G., and Hardy, R. E. *Physical Medicine and Rehabilitation Approaches in Spinal Cord Injury.* Springfield, Ill.: Thomas, 1977.
2. Kübler-Ross, E. *On Death and Dying.* New York: Macmillan, 1969.
3. Ruge, D. *Spinal Cord Injuries.* Springfield, Ill.: Thomas, 1969.
4. Wilson, D. J., McKenzie, M. W., and Barber, L. M. *Spinal Cord Injury—A Treatment Guide for Occupational Therapists.* Thorofare, N.J.: Slack, 1974.
5. Yashon, D. *Spinal Injury.* New York: Appleton-Century-Crofts, 1978.

## Suggested Reading
### GENERAL INFORMATION

Braakman, R., Orbaan, J. C., and Dishoeck, M. B. Information in the early stages after spinal cord injury. *Paraplegia* 14(1):95, 1976.

Bracken, M. B., et al. Relationship between neurological and functional status after acute spinal cord injury: An epidemiological study. *J. Chron. Dis.* 33(2):114, 1980.

Chawla, J. C., et al. Techniques for improving the strength and fitness of spinal injured patients. *Paraplegia* 17(2):185, 1979.

Eisenberg, M. G., and Falconer, J. A. *Treatment of the Spinal Cord Injured: An Interdisciplinary Perspective.* Springfield, Ill.: Thomas, 1978.

Family practice grand rounds. Rehabilitation of a young quadriplegic: A team approach. *J. Fam. Prac.* 10(3):517, 1980.

Ford, J. R., and Duckworth, B. *Physical Management for the Quadriplegic Patient.* Philadelphia: Davis, 1974.

Garret, J. F., and Levine, E. S. *Rehabilitation Practices with the Physically Disabled.* New York: Columbia University Press, 1973.

Gerhart, K. A. Increasing sensory and motor stimulation for the patient with quadriplegia. *Phys. Ther.* 59(12):1518, 1979.

Hachen, H. J. Spinal cord injury in children and adolescents: Diagnostic pitfalls and therapeutic considerations in the acute stage (proceedings). *Paraplegia* 15(1):55, 1977.

Hall, W. J., Green, B., and Colandonato, J. P. Spinal cord injury: Emergency treatment. *Emerg. Med. Serv.* 5(3):28, 1976.

Hamilton, B. B., et al. A basic evaluation framework for spinal cord injury care systems. *Paraplegia* 14(1):87, 1976.

Jenkins, W. M., et al. (Eds.). *Rehabilitation of the Severely Disabled.* Dubuque, Iowa: Kendall/Hunt, 1976.

Lawson, N. C. Significant events in the rehabilitation process: The spinal cord patient's point of view. *Arch. Phys. Med. Rehabil.* 59(12):573, 1978.

Little, N., et al. *Rehabilitation of the Spinal Cord Injured: Selected Readings.* Fayetteville, Ark.: University of Arkansas Vocational Rehabilitation Research and Training Center, 1974.

McGee, M., and Hertling, D. Equipment and transfer techniques used by C6 quadriplegic patients. *Phys. Ther.* 67(12):1372, 1977.

Pasley, A. Ambulation program for patients with thoracic spinal cord lesions. *Phys. Ther.* 54(5):372, 1975.

Richards, B. An evaluation of home care after spinal cord injury. *Paraplegia* 12(14):263, 1975.

Talbot, H. S. The holistic approach to spinal cord injury. *Paraplegia* 17(1):32, 1979.

Tator, C. H., and Rowed, D. W. Current concepts in the immediate management of acute spinal cord injuries. *Can. Med. Assoc. J.* 121(11):1453, 1979.

Trombley, C. A., and Scott, A.D. *Occupational Therapy for Physical Dysfunction.* Baltimore: Williams and Wilkins, 1978.

Yeo, J. D. First-aid management of spinal cord injuries. *Med. J. Aust.* 2(10):531, 1979.

## NURSING

Hanson, A. M. Towards independence for paraplegics. *Canadian Nurse* 72(12):24, 76.

Henrikson, J. D. Part III: Activities of daily living; specialized care of the spinal cord injured patient. *J. Pract. Nurs.* 26(8):17, 1976.

Henrikson, J. D. Part V: Secondary health problems; specialized care of the spinal cord injured patient. *J. Pract. Nurs.* 26(10):218, 1976.

McKibbin, B. Part I: The clinical team in action—The management of spinal injuries—Medical management. *Nurs. Mirror* 143(22):47, 1976.

Mountjoy, S. The clinical team in action—The management of spinal injuries—Community care. *Nurs. Mirror* 143(22):57, 1976.

Rogers, M. A. *Paraplegia: A Handbook of Practical Care and Advice.* London: Faber and Faber, 1978.

Shipp, M. The clinical team in action—The management of spinal injuries—Social implications. *Nurs. Mirror* 143 (22):55, 1976.

Silva, A. The clinical team in action—The management of spinal injuries—Physiotherapy. *Nurs. Mirror* 143(22):51, 1976.

Stauffer, S. A master plan for teaching the patient with spinal cord injury. *RN* 42(7):55, 1979.

Sutton, F. The clinical team in action—The management of spinal injuries—Occupational therapy. *Nurs. Mirror* 143(22):53, 1976.

Vincent, P. J., Smith, J., and Danglason, E. Treatment of patients with spinal cord injuries. *Can. Nurs.* 71(8):26, 1975.

Walsh, J. J. The spinal cord disabled. *Nurs. Mirror* 142(5):53, 1976.

## SEXUALITY

Anderson, T. P., and Cole, T. M. Sexual counseling of the physically disabled. *Postgrad. Med.* 58(1):117, 1975.

Becker, E. F. *Female Sexuality Following Spinal Cord Injury.* Bloomington, Ill.: Cheever, 1978.

Cole, T. M. and Stevens, M. R. Rehabilitation professionals and sexual counseling for spinal cord injured adults. *Arch. Sex. Behav.* 4(6):631, 1975.

Comarr, A. E., and Vique M., Sexual counseling among male and female patients with spinal cord and/or cauda equina injury. *Am. J. Phys. Med.* 57(3):107, 1978.

Connie, T. A., et al. Physical therapists' knowledge of sexuality of adults with spinal cord injury. *Phys. Ther.* 59(4):395, 1979.

Eisenberg, M. G., and Rustad, L. C. Sex education and counseling program on a spinal cord injury service. *Arch. Phys. Med. Rehabil.* 57(3):135, 1976.

Evans, R. L., et al. Multidisciplinary approach to sex education of spinal cord-injured patients. *Phys. Ther.* 56(5):541, 1976.

Griffith, E. R., and Frieschman, R. S. Sexual function restoration in the physically disabled: Use of a private hospital room. *Arch. Phys. Med. Rehabil.* 58(8):368, 1977.

Mooney, T., Cole, T., and Chilgren, R. *Sexual Options for Paraplegics and Quadriplegics.* Boston: Little, Brown, 1975.

Romano, M. D., and Lassiter, R. E. Sexual counseling with the spinal cord injured. *Arch. Phys. Med. Rehabil.* 12:568, 1972.

## LEISURE ACTIVITIES

Bleasdale, N. Swimming and the paraplegic. *Paraplegia* 13(2):124, 1975.

Geis, G. C. A therapeutic aquatic's program for quadriplegia patients. *Am. Correct. Ther. J.* 29(5):155, 1975.

Rogers, J.C., and Figone, J. J. The avocational pursuits of rehabilitants with traumatic quadriplegia. *Am. J. Occup. Ther.* 32(9):471, 1978.

## BOWEL AND BLADDER

Finkbeiner, A. E., Bissada, N. K., and Redman, J. F. Urologic care of the patient with a spinal cord injury. *J. Arkansas Med. Soc.* 74(8):301, 1978.

Kuhn, H. M., et al. Intermittent catheterization as a rehabilitation nursing service. *Arch. Phys. Med. Rehabil.* 55(10):439, 1974.

Sperling, K. B. Intermittent catheterization to obtain catheter-free bladder function in spinal cord injury. *Arch. Phys. Med. Rehabil.* 59(1):4, 1978.

## PSYCHOLOGICAL ADJUSTMENT

Roessler, R., and Bolton, B. *Psychological Adjustment to Disability.* Baltimore: University Park, 1978.

Santana Carlos, V. M. Importance of communication in counseling the spinal cord injury patient. *Paraplegia* 16(2):175, 1978.

Stewart, T. D. Spinal cord injury: A role for the psychiatrist. *Am. J. Psychiatry* 134(5):538, 1977.

Trieschmann, R. B. The role of the psychologist in

the treatment of spinal cord injury. *Paraplegia* 16(2):212, 1978.

## VOCATIONAL

Alfred, W. G. A longitudinal study of the course of vocational development following spinal cord injury. *Int. J. Rehabil. Res.* 2(4):544, 1979.

El Ghatit, A. Z., and Hanson, R. W. Educational and training levels and employment of the spinal-cord injured patient. *Arch. Phys. Med. Rehabil.* 60(9):405, 1979.

Weiss, M. (Ed.). *Early Therapeutic Social and Vocational Problems in the Rehabilitation of Persons with Spinal Cord Injuries.* New York: Plenum, 1977.

# INDEX

premorbid personality, 145
self-perception, 145
rest and, 128
sexual problems, 145–146
subacute phase, 140–141
surgery and, 147–148
treatment program, 127
Ribs, movement of during inspiration and expiration, 200
ROM. *See* Range-of-motion
Rule of nines, 154

SACH foot, 84, 86, 87, 89
Scarring, hypertrophic, 159–160
Scleroderma, 117–118
Self-care, 124
Senescence, defined, 1
Sensation, 124
defined, 101
Sensibility, defined, 101
Sensory loss, 5
Sexual dysfunction, 64
Sexuality, 32–33
Shoulder
dislocation, 95
frozen, 94
orthopedics, 94–95
rotator cuff tears, 95
Silastic Medical Elastomer, 160
Simultanognosia, 262
Sjögren's syndrome, 114–115, 146
Skin
anatomy and physiology of, 151–152
care of in burns, 162
SLE. *See* Systemic lupus erythematosus
Smoking, and coronary artery disease, 177
Social gerontology, theories of, 30–32
Social security, 4
Somatognosia. *See* Impairment, body scheme
Spasticity, 238–245, 327
Speech language, problem areas, 275
Speech-language rehabilitation, 275–296
team approach and counseling, 293–294
Speech reading, 8
Spinal cord injury, 325–346
acute care, 328–330
causes of, 325–326
complications, 330–331
functional goals for, 340–341
history of, 325
rehabilitation, 331
physical issues, 331, 334
psychological issues, 331, 334–336
rehabilitation factors, 336–344
bowel and bladder, 337
community attitude, 342
endurance, 336–337
family adjustment, 342–343
follow-up care, 343–344
home care, 339, 342
mobility, 337–338
range of motion, 336
self-care, 338–339

sexuality, 337
vocational, 342
signs and symptoms, 326–328
Spinal deformity, severe, and pulmonary dysfunction, 202
Spirometry, 205
Splints, 130–136
ankle, 135
design of, 130–131
dynamic, 161
elbow, 134
feet, 135–136
full-hand resting, 131–132
hand, 131
knee, 134–135
precautions, 131
resting, 94
serial static, 161
shoulder, 134
static, 161
thumb carpometacarpal stabilization, 134
ulnar drift
metacarpal, 133–134
protective, 133
wrist stabilization, 132–133
Spondylitis, ankylosing, 116–117
common deformities, 116–117
symptoms of, 116
therapeutic measures, 117
Spouse, loss of, 24–25
Starling's law, 172–173
Static positions, avoiding prolonged, 137
Stimulation, electrical, 130
*Story Completion Test*, 279
String wrap, 91
Stroke, 225–274, 275–296
acute phase, 226–229
cognitive perceptual motor functions, 259–265
apraxia, 264–265
attention, 259
cerebration, 260
perception, 260–264
emotional and sexual adjustment, 268–270
etiology of, 225–226
rehabilitation, 225–274, 275–296
activity of daily living (ADL), 257
ambulation, 256–257
discharge planning, 271–272
functional program, 247–257
motor control, development of voluntary, 245, 247
reflex behavior, primitive, 232–235
sensation, 229, 232
speech language, 275–296
tone, abnormal, 235–245
visual field deficits, 257–259
vocational adjustment, 270–271
Stroke volume, 173
Subcutaneous tissue, 152
Support groups, 26–27
for families of older people, 26–27
for individual with age-related problems, 26
Swan neck deformities, 102, 113, 114
Swan neck splint, 102

Swanson MP arthroplasty, 148
*Syllable-Concept Count,* 279–280
Synovectomy, 147
Systemic lupus erythematosus (SLE), 115, 118
   signs and symptoms of, 118
   therapeutic measures, 118

Task orientation, 28
Telescopic aid, 16
Teletypewriter terminals (TTY), 9
Tendolysis, 102
Tennis elbow. *See* Epicondylitis
Tennis elbow strap, 96
Tenosynovectomy, 147
Therapy programs, 25–29
Thumb
   gamekeeper's, 98–99
   injuries, 98–99
Tinnitus, 6
Toes
   claw, 113
   cock-up, 113
   hammer, 113
*Token Test,* 279
Total hip replacement (THR), 147–148
Traction, 130
Transfers, 126
Transportation, 126
TTY. *See* Teletypewriter terminals

Ulnar drift, 113, 114
   splints, 133–134
Ulnar or lateral pressures, avoiding, 138
Upper extremity ROM exercises, 141–142

VAT. *See Visual Action Therapy*
Ventilation, 201
Visiting Nurse Association, 271
*Visual Action Therapy* (VAT), 281
Visual acuity, guide based on, 10
Visual acuity and visual field, guide based on, 10
Visual loss, 9–10
   blind techniques, 17
      organization, 17
      sensory information, 17
   communication aids, 17
   devices for, 15–17
   education, 11
   environmental modification techniques, 11, 14
   evaluation, 10–11
   functional changes, 10
   instructional media sources, 12–13
   personal care aids, 17
   rehabilitation, 11
Visual spatial neglect, 261

Weber two-point discrimination test, 101
Weight bearing classifications, 73
*Western Aphasia Battery,* 277
*Word Fluency Measure,* 279
Workplace, 126–127
Wrist,
   tendon laceration, 101–104
Wrist support
   plastic shell, 100
   and resting splint, 100

Z-shaped deformity, 113, 114